Clinically Oriented Regional Anatomy

Qiang Ding • Yongjie Zhang • Chao Qin
Editors

Clinically Oriented Regional Anatomy

Springer

PEOPLE'S MEDICAL PUBLISHING HOUSE

Editors
Qiang Ding
General Surgery
The First Affiliated Hospital of Nanjing
Medical University
Nanjing, China

Yongjie Zhang
Human Anatomy
Basic Medical Sciences School of Nanjing
Medical University
Nanjing, China

Chao Qin
Urology
The First Affiliated Hospital of Nanjing
Medical University
Nanjing, China

ISBN 978-981-95-9887-8 ISBN 978-981-95-9888-5 (eBook)
https://doi.org/10.1007/978-981-95-9888-5

Jointly published with People's Medical Publishing House, PR of China

This Springer imprint is published by the registered company Springer Nature Singapore Pte Ltd.
The registered company address is: 152 Beach Road, #21-01/04 Gateway East, Singapore 189721, Singapore

Foreword

Sophisticated and enigmatic, the human body is the most fascinating artifice crafted by Nature. Despite its evolution over tens of thousands of years, knowledge about the human body remains to be refreshed. It was not until 1543, when Andreas Vesalius, the greatest anatomist and physician during the Renaissance, published his monumental work *The Structure of the Human Body*, that humans caught the first direct look at their own bodies. Due to his pioneering work in human anatomy, Vesalius blazed a path to modern medicine. Born in Brussels, Belgium, in 1514, Vesalius started to study philosophy and art at K. U. Leuven at the age of 15 and then received a master's degree. Spurred by his grandfather, dean of the medical school at K. U. Leuven, he went to study medicine at the University of Paris in France and the University of Padua in Italy in 1533. Interrupted by war, he returned to the University of Leuven in 1536 to continue his fascination with human anatomy. Thereafter, he went to Italy again, where he obtained his doctorate in medicine on 5 December 1537 at the University of Padua after passing an examination and defending his thesis, and on the second day, he was appointed Professor of Surgery, undertaking a dual role as lecturer and anatomist. Thirty kilometers east of Brussels lies a beautiful township, Leuven, home to the University of Leuven, which is nearly 600 years old. Here, I spent five fruitful years from 1995 to 2001 obtaining my Ph.D. Leuven still has many streets, buildings, and institutions named after Vesalius. Walking around Leuven, you suddenly realize how close you are to this star of the Renaissance, and you can even feel the artistic and scholarly aura he exuded 500 years ago. I am honored to have become his alumnus, someone Vesalius would never have expected to meet generations later.

Modern surgery cannot develop without modern anatomy. A specific structure serves as a carrier of a specific function. Each discovery in human anatomy ushers in a new understanding of body functions. Jiang Tongyu, a professor of Nanjing Medical University, has been respected as the father of layered anatomy. Based on his experience and practice, he proposed a concept and a methodology of continuous layered anatomy, which were embodied in the *Continuous Layered Anatomy Atlas*, published in 1954, and the *Human Anatomy Atlas*, published in 1955, two textbooks selected by the Ministry of Health for medical schools across China. Up to now, the two books have been published in more than 247,600 copies. I once attended his class, in which all students were shaped by his wisdom and enthusiasm in human anatomy. He taught us using words that were easily understood but greatly inspiring. If you let me name a textbook that has most powerfully promoted me into my career as a surgeon, it should be *Regional Anatomy*, which is still in my hand. A good surgeon should grow on a foundation of solid knowledge, rich experience, and sharp insight into anatomy. A perfect surgery depends on a surgeon's decision-making based on his or her understanding of anatomical structures at different layers. On an optimal plane, a surgeon can predict the positions of critical structures, such as vessels, nerves, ureters, and the bile duct, thus making the surgery safe and fluent. No surgeon can stand out without a good mastery of anatomy. Clinicians should keep studying, experiencing, and practicing. Surgery-related adverse events often arise from misjudgment, especially in cases of anatomical variations, and may be followed by devastating results. I feel fortunate to have been instructed by my teachers who devoted their knowledge, experience and skills, morality, and talents, all of which have kept polishing surgery into a more beautiful discipline and myself into a more qualified surgeon.

Zhong Shizhen, an academician and a professor in clinical-oriented regional anatomy, has advocated that teachers should guide students to learn human anatomy in clinical settings, especially with an aim to cope with issues occurring in surgeries, rather than sheerly describe morphologies and structures. In the 1970s, Zhu Tailai, also my teacher then working at the First Affiliated Hospital of Nanjing Medical University, was challenged by a clinical issue about how to cut the vagus nerves to treat peptic ulcer. He observed 100 cadavers, and published an article "Anatomy of the vagus nerve in the lower oesophagus and stomach: an observation of 100 cadavers," in *Chinese Journal of Surgery*, which further guides clinical practice. This story lays an example in which a clinical issue is resolved by surgeons through deepening their insight into anatomy. New understandings in anatomy have reformed diagnostic and surgical technology. For example, Professor Heald, UK, invented the Total Mesorectal Excision (TME). Professor Büchler of the Heidelberg Surgical Hospital proposed the Heidelberg Triangle Surgery for pancreatic cancer. In 1996, Japanese scholar Shinohara Sho published the book *Illustrated Surgery: Interpretation of Surgical Procedures from Membrane Anatomy*, which refreshed the understanding of traditional mesenteric anatomy, and triggered widespread concern and controversy, causing a frenzy toward "membrane anatomy" among clinicians.

Convened by Prof. Ding Qiang (Nanjing Medical University), a team of experts and professors from renowned medical colleges and universities, and rich in teaching and clinical experience, has compiled this book, which bridges anatomy with clinical surgery and better combines the knowledge of structures and functions. With the advances in computer-aided imaging, endoscopy, intervention, augmented reality, 3D printing, imaging histology correspondence, robotic surgery, telemedicine, among many others, the depth, coverage, and clinical practicability of regional anatomy should be further explored. This book focuses on the integration of anatomical theory with clinical practice, structure description with surgical procedures, anatomy altus with surgical altus. In addition, dissection procedures and summaries are provided, reflecting the new teaching mode of clinical-oriented regional anatomy. At last, the chapters, concepts, words, and the significances of regional anatomy in clinical scenarios are better illustrated.

This book is praised for its innovation in polishing the thinking mode and consolidating the knowledge of learners, which further deepens their understanding of regional anatomy and clinical practice in an era of ever-updating medical sciences. I sincerely recommend this book for medical students and clinical workers.

Nanjing, China
May 2025

Yi Miao

Preface

Regional anatomy and surgery, as two subjects, show their own characteristics in terms of teaching time, contents, and staff that vary across the medical universities and colleges of China. In addition, traditional regional anatomy often fails to provide knowledge that stands at the frontiers of clinical medicine, and the key issues and concerns in clinical medicine are seldom discussed in the teaching of regional anatomy. As a consequence, it is common to see that medical students, after graduation, are often incapable of employing knowledge of regional anatomy to guide their clinical practice.

To culture medical students in an era of modernizing medicine and integrating their anatomy-related knowledge into clinical practice, an experts' team has been convened to compile this textbook, headed by Prof. Ding Qiang, vice president of Nanjing Medical University, and formed by professors from Shenzhen University, Zhejiang University, Southeast University, Shandong University, Central South University, Fudan University, and Hebei Medical University, all renowned for their experience in the teaching and practice of clinical medicine. In this textbook, the fundamentals and frontiers in regional anatomy and surgery are melded into 12 chapters (in more than 150,000 words) with 364 illustrative figures, suitable for the culture of medical undergraduates, medical graduates in clinical medicine or anatomy, as well as resident physicians in training.

This textbook is based on *Regional Anatomy*, a textbook previously published by the Department of Human Anatomy, Nanjing Medical University, and enriched by a wealth of anatomy knowledge for clinical purposes. After rounds of revision, this textbook is unveiled, paying off the sweat and intelligence of all its authors.

The Chinese and English terms in this textbook are defined according to the *Nomenclature of Human Anatomy* (second and Definitional Edition) (2014) published by the National Committee for the Verification of Scientific and Technical Nomenclature. Some parts of the book take references from *Clinically Oriented Anatomy* (fourth edition) edited by Keith L. Moore and Arthur F. Daly and translated by Li Yunqing, *Regional Anatomy* (ninth edition) edited by Cui Huixian and Li Ruixi, and *Regional Anatomy* (second edition) edited by Zuo Guoping. Some of the illustrations in the book refer to the Colour Atlas of Human Anatomy (second edition) edited by Guo Guangwen and Wang Xu. All figures are drawn and revised by Dou Xiaokang, and reviewed by Zhang Yongjie and Qin Chao.

Special thanks to professors who have retired from the Department of Human Anatomy, the Teaching Office of Surgery, and the Basic Surgery Teaching and Research Office for their constructive advice, Academician Shen Hongbing, Prof. Wang Shui, Prof. Yu Rongbin, and Prof. Ji Mingjun for their work in revising, as well as Prof. Miao Yi, Prof. Zuo Guoping, and Prof. Han Qunying for their work in checking.

Great thanks to Prof. Miao Yi for writing the preface.

Limited by our knowledge and schedule, this textbook surely has room for improvement. We will weigh and consider any suggestions from readers and write them into future editions.

Nanjing, China — Qiang Ding
Nanjing, China — Yongjie Zhang
Nanjing, China — Chao Qin
May 2025

Contents

Chapter 1
Introduction

Qiang Ding, Yongjie Zhang, Yizhi Zuo, and Chao Qin

1.1 Clinical Oriented Regional Anatomy

Human anatomy sprouts various branches, each of them closely linked to clinical medicine. Modern science and technology have promoted the integration and interaction of these discipline branches with clinical medicine. In this setting, clinically oriented regional anatomy is established by fusing clinical medicine with regional anatomy, a crucial branch of human anatomy. This science investigates human morphology and structure through the lens of regional anatomy. It explores the layered architectures of various human body parts from superficial to deep, the complex interrelationships among organs within each anatomical region, and the distribution patterns of blood vessels and nerves. It also focuses on the localization of specific organs on the surface.

Regional anatomy is rooted in systematic anatomy but takes on a distinct profile. Systematic anatomy focuses on the organs and their functions in the nine systems of the human body. Regional anatomy is mainly involved in the layered structures and spatial relationships of different anatomical regions. To make a good mastery of regional anatomy, learners should have a strong competence in hands-on dissection, on-site observation, and summarization. These practical skills, along with the knowledge of systematic anatomy, are essential to establish a solid foundation for studying other medical courses.

Q. Ding · Y. Zhang (✉) · Y. Zuo · C. Qin
Nanjing Medical University, Nanjing, China
e-mail: dingqiang@njmu.edu.cn; zhangyongjie@njmu.edu.cn;
zuoyizhi@njmu.edu.cn; qinchao@njmu.edu.cn

Q. Ding et al. (eds.), *Clinically Oriented Regional Anatomy*,
https://doi.org/10.1007/978-981-95-9888-5_1

1.2 Regions of the Human Body

The human body is divided into four anatomical regions, including the head, neck, trunk, and limbs. The trunk consists of the back, chest, abdomen, and pelvis. The back is the posterior wall of the chest and abdomen. The body wall (covering the chest wall, abdominal wall, pelvic wall, and perineum) and the body cavities (thoracic, abdominal, and pelvic cavities) form the chest, abdomen, and pelvis. The limbs refer to the upper and lower limbs.

1.3 Basic Concepts of Human Structures

In the teaching and learning of Regional Anatomy, it is necessary to dissect a human body, which we respect as a "teacher of the human body." The morphological characteristics of the basic structures of the human body should be mastered before carrying out correct dissections and discriminating different structures.

1.3.1 Skin

Serving as a defense barrier, skin envelopes the whole human body, except for several apertures. It is the largest sensory organ for external stimuli, such as pain, temperature, touch, and pressure. Furthermore, skin plays critical roles in regulating body temperature and balancing water and electrolytes. Skin thickness varies across different body parts, typically thinner on the ventral side and thicker on the dorsal side, but vice versa on the hand palm and foot sole. Skin color shows variations among races and individuals. Skin around the nipples, perineum, external genitalia, and anus presents heavier pigmentation. Connective tissue fiber bundles are aligned non-uniformly in the dermis, leading to various dermatoglyphs (dermal ridges) across the body parts. An incision aligning with the dermatoglyph can leave a less evident scar post-surgery.

1.3.2 Superficial Fascia

Superficial fascia, also referred to as subcutaneous tissue or subcutaneous fascia, is distributed beneath the whole body's skin. It consists of loose connective tissue. Superficial fascia contains varying amounts of adipose tissue, except in the eyelids and scrotum. The thickness and content of adipose tissue in the superficial fascia vary significantly across body parts. Even within the same area, they change with sex, age, and occupation. The superficial fascia is lined with honeycomb-like bundles of fibers connecting the skin to the deep fascia, the strength and tightness of which affect the mobility of the skin.

Cutaneous nerves, superficial blood vessels, superficial lymphatic vessels, and lymph nodes are distributed in the superficial fascia. Cutaneous nerves pass from deep fascia into superficial fascia and distribute extensively over the skin. Sizable cutaneous nerves in constant positions are often chosen for nerve transplantation and repair. The superficial arteries are generally small, appearing in the form of a direct branch from the deep artery or a branch from the muscular branch of the deep artery. Care should be taken to protect the deep artery (axial artery) when selecting a flap to ensure flap viability. The superficial veins are thicker, anastomosis-rich, and usually do not accompany the superficial arteries. The superficial veins of the extremities are usually used for venipuncture. Superficial lymphatic vessels are small, thin-walled, transparent, and difficult to identify. The lymph nodes cluster along the lymphatic vessels.

1.3.3 Deep Fascia

Deep fascia (also known as fascia propria) is deep to the superficial fascia and composed of dense connective tissue. In the extremities, the deep fascia forms deep intermuscular septa to separate the muscle groups and attaches to the bone, forming an osteofascial sheath. The deep fascia also envelops blood vessels and nerves, forming a neurovascular sheath (Fig. 1.1). Deep fascia can also serve for muscle attachment, and as an origin or insertion for muscles; in the wrist and ankle joint, deep fascia thickens into a restraining band called retinaculum that constrains tendons passing through its deep portion and serves as a pulley around which the tendons may move. A fascial space is formed between deep fasciae, or between the deep fascia and the periosteum, allowing blood vessels and nerves to pass through. In pathological cases,

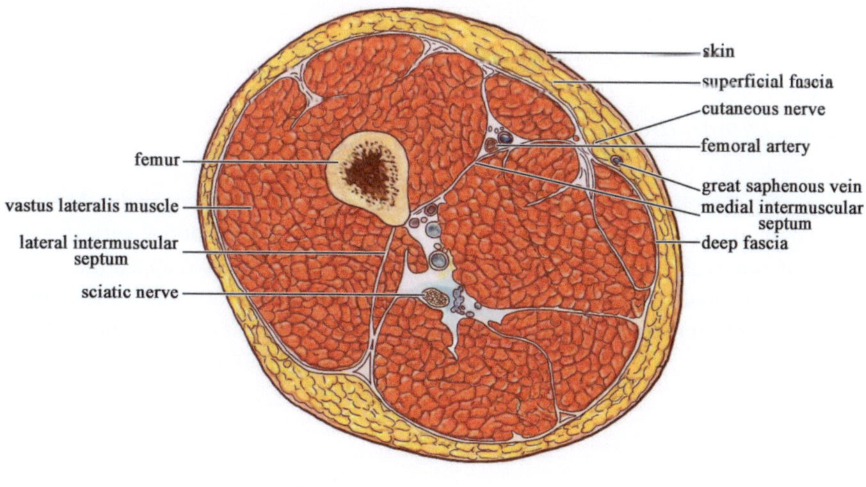

Fig. 1.1 Cross-section of the mid-thigh (mainly deep fascia)

the deep fascia restricts the spread of inflammation, but the connectivity of the fascial interstices makes it easy for inflammatory exudates to spread.

1.3.4 Muscles

The distribution of skeletal muscles takes on different profiles across body parts. Trunk muscles are layered, facial muscles are distributed around the foramen, and limb muscles are distributed according to the action of the joint. The intermuscular space is formed between muscles, and that in the limbs serves as the passage of blood vessels and nerves. Some of the intermuscular spaces on the body wall are weak areas and may be prone to forming a hernia when hypertension appears in the body cavity. The vessels and nerves always enter and exit from a certain area of the muscle, and during dissecting or freeing the myocutaneous flap, it is really important to avoid injuries to the vessels and nerves at the above area.

1.3.5 Blood Vessels and Nerves

Arteries are cylindrical, with a thick elastic wall and a reddish color. Veins are thin-walled, with a diameter larger than that of the accompanying arteries. Veins often collapse and show clots in the lumen. Veins can be divided into superficial and deep. Superficial veins travel in the superficial fascia, while deep veins travel with the arteries. The medium-sized deep arteries in the limbs are often accompanied by two veins, one on each side. The nerves are white or yellowish and shiny striated cords. With the exception of the cutaneous nerves, most nerves are accompanied by blood vessels and wrapped by deep fascia to form the neurovascular tracts (bundles) that often travel within the intermuscular spaces.

1.3.6 Lymphatic Vessels and Lymph Nodes

Lymphatic vessels are typically slender, with thin and transparent walls. Most of the lymphatic vessels are not apparent in the cadaver. Lymph nodes vary in size, with flat and oval shapes. Furthermore, they present a gray-brown appearance with palpable firmness. Lymph nodes are often located along the veins, distributed within the intermuscular spaces, near the portals of organs, and at the flexor aspect of limbs.

During development, variation and malformation may arise in an individual. Variation refers to the individual differences that occur at a low rate and have little effect on appearance or function, such as those in the location and shape of organs, as well as the origin, course, branching, and distribution of blood vessels and nerves. Malformation refers to the abnormalities that occur at a very low rate and affect appearance or function, such as cleft lip and palate, congenital heart malformations, and situs inversus viscerum. The human body is in constant development after birth, and acquired dispositions can also affect the morphological structure of the human body and cause individual differences. When studying Regional Anatomy, variation and malformation should be kept in mind.

1.4 Application of the Essential Anatomical Dissection Tools

1.4.1 Scalpel

The belly of a scalpel is usually used to section the skin, separate and lift the skin flaps, and cut muscles. The tip of the scalpel is used to trim the muscles, blood vessels, and nerves. The handle or back of the scalpel is used to bluntly dissect tissues. There are two styles of holding the scalpel (Fig. 1.2). (1) Violon bow-holding: the scalpel is held with the thumb and middle finger, and it is adequate for sectioning the skin. (ii) Pencil-holding: the scalpel is held by the thumb, index finger, and middle finger. It is used to cut, separate, or trim tissues.

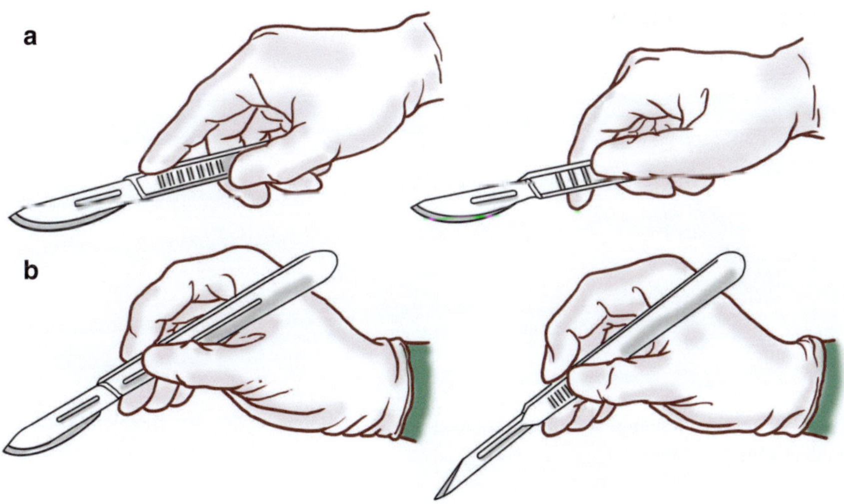

Fig. 1.2 Scalpel-holding styles. (**a**) Violin bow-holding style; (**b**) Pencil-holding style

1.4.2 Forceps

Forceps vary in length and are divided into two types as toothless forceps and toothed forceps. Toothless forceps are used to hold soft tissues and to separate blood vessels, nerves, and muscles; toothed forceps are only used to hold skin or harder tissues. Forceps are also held in a pencil-holding style (Fig. 1.3). During dissection, the scalpel is usually held in the right hand and the forceps in the left.

1.4.3 Surgical Scissors

Surgical scissors are categorized into straight-bladed and curved-bladed, with each type further divided into pointed-tip and blunt-tip. Surgical scissors are used for cutting or separating soft tissues.

1.4.4 Other Instruments (Figs. 1.1, 1.2, 1.3, and 1.4)

1. Vascular clamp: Either straight or curved, used for tissue separation and fixation.
2. Bone shears: Used for cutting bone and cartilage.
3. Bone saws: Divided into flat type and arc-shaped type. The former is mainly used for sawing cylindrical bones, while the later for sawing recessed bones.
4. Bone chisel: Used for chiseling bone.
5. Probe: Used in exploring tissue.

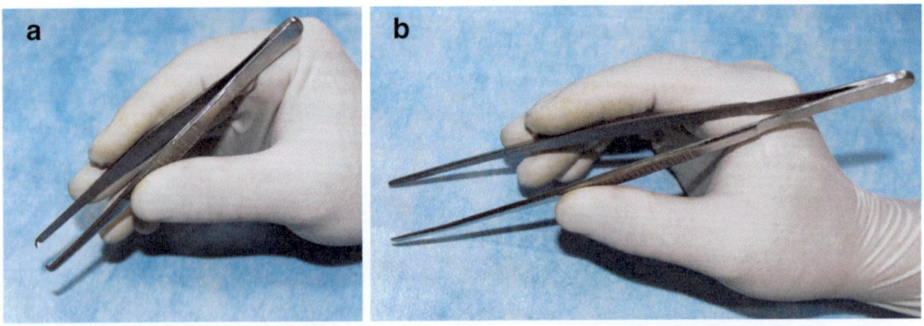

Fig. 1.3 Forceps-holding style. (**a**) Toothed forceps-holding style; (**b**) Toothless forceps-holding style

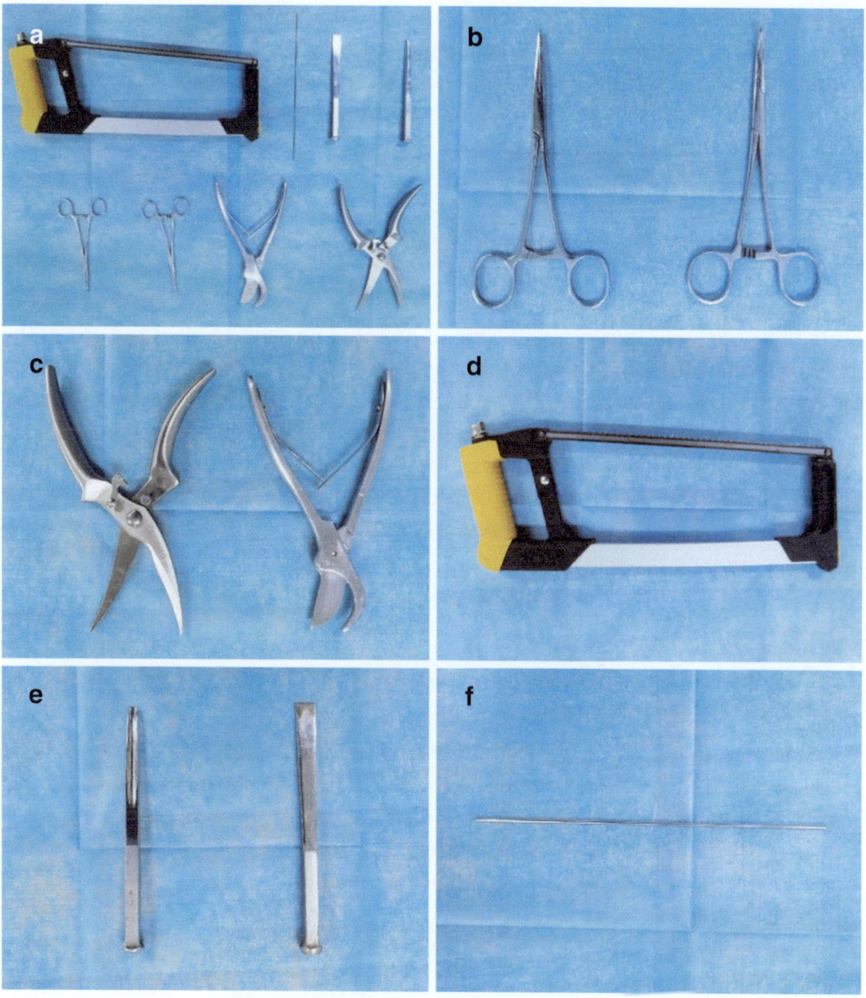

Fig. 1.4 Other instruments. (**a**) Overview of all instruments (vascular clamp + bone shears + bone saws + bone chisels + probes); (**b**) Vascular clamp; (**c**) Bone shears; (**d**) Bone saws; (**e**) Bone chisels; (**f**) Probes

1.5 Techniques for Dissection

1.5.1 Dissection of Skin

1.5.1.1 Approach for Skin Incision

The incision is determined according to the guidance of a "schematic diagram of skin incision" provided in each chapter, gently delineated using a marker pen. Subsequently, the scalpel tip is vertically inserted into the origin point of the incision, and then the scalpel's belly is pressed downward, forming a 45-degree angle to the skin surface. A longitudinal incision is made from the upper down, and a transverse incision from left to right. A moderate and consistent force should be exerted during skin incision. Heavy force should be avoided to prevent deeper incisions that may damage underlying structures.

1.5.1.2 Approach for Peeling and Flipping Skin

For a unilateral skin incision, the skin should be flipped to both sides of the incision. For a cross skin incision, the skin should be lifted up with toothed forceps at the junction of each incision, so as to keep the skin under a sufficient tension, and then the connective tissues attached to the skin in the superficial fascia are cut off with a scalpel at an angle of 45° to the deep surface of skin; and then, the skin is turned over from inside to outside following the "schematic diagram of skin incision." During flipping the skin, it is important to protect the superficial blood vessels and cutaneous nerves in the superficial fascia (Fig. 1.5), especially the expression muscles when flipping the skin of the head, face, and neck.

1.5.2 Dissection of Subcutaneous Fascia

Subcutaneous fascia, also known as superficial fascia, contains abundant superficial blood vessels and cutaneous nerves. When dissecting the subcutaneous fascia, we should be familiar with the courses and distributions of these vessels and nerves. During dissection, the blade should advance in the direction consistent with the

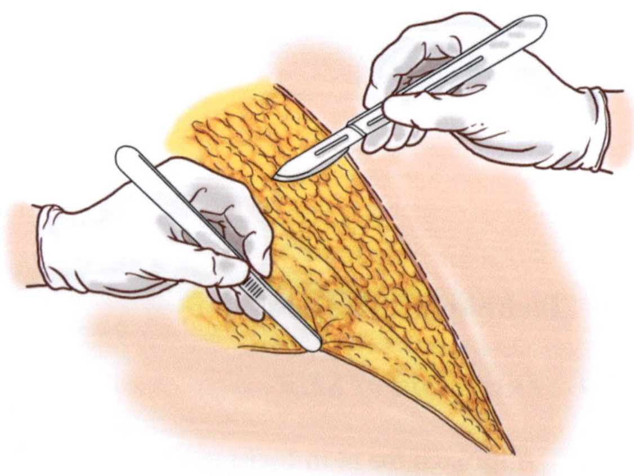

Fig. 1.5 Schematic diagram of peeling and flipping skin

courses of vessels and nerves; otherwise, vessels and nerves would be damaged. These vessels and nerves should be traced retrogradely or anterogradely. Blood vessels and cutaneous nerves within the superficial fascia can be exposed just in the subcutaneous tissue, and should not be traced too deep, in order to avoid damaging the deeper structures.

1.5.3 Dissection of Proper Fascia

Following complete exposure of blood vessels, nerves, and lymph nodes within the superficial fascia, the residual connective and adipose tissues are excised to better explore the superficial layer of proper fascia. Focus should be placed on the derivative structures of deep fascia in the limbs, such as retinacula.

1.5.4 Dissection of Muscles

For dissecting muscles, their edges, origins, and terminations should be clarified. Before cutting the muscle, it is necessary to reach the handle of the scalpel or fingers into the deep side of the muscle to separate the muscle from the deep structures, and then cut the muscle at 0.5–1 cm away from its origin or termination. During turning over the muscle, attention should be paid to the vessels and nerves in the deep surface of the muscle. Only one endpoint of a muscle is allowed to be cut off, and it is strictly prohibited to cut off innocent muscles. Except for very few muscles needing to be cut off, most vessels and nerves can be visualized after exposing the spaces between muscles.

1.5.5 Dissection of Vessels and Nerves

The dissection of superficial blood vessels and cutaneous nerves has been described previously. Deep blood vessels and nerves generally travel in the intermuscular spaces, interfascial spaces, and tissues surrounding the organs. Therefore, the dissection of deep blood vessels and nerves should not be performed before careful navigation. Similar to the dissection of superficial blood vessels and cutaneous nerves, the courses and locations of deep blood vessels and nerves should be clarified first, and then the blood vessels and nerves in the above spaces are exposed and traced. This approach can ensure the integrity of blood vessels and nerves and their interrelationships to the surrounding muscles and organs.

1.5.6 Dissection of Organs

Except in special circumstances, the organs in body cavities cannot be dissected with a sharp scalpel but bluntly separated with the handle of a scalpel or forceps. The dissection of organs should start from superficial to deep. As superficial organs can be observed, they are then turned superficially or to the opposite side to expose the deeper structures. Particular attention should be paid to the hila of the organs, such as the pulmonary, hepatic, and renal hila, etc. The positions and arrangements of the ducts should be carefully clarified.

1.6 Requirements of Regional Anatomy Practice

1.6.1 Competent Operational Skills

Regional anatomy practice mainly involves the operations on the bodies of donors. Operations help deepen students' understanding of regional anatomy. Only through hands-on operation can a student perceive the tissues and organs in a certain region of the body, and their spatial, morphological, and structural characteristics. Hands-on operation is an efficient means to sharpen the basic operation skills of medical students.

1.6.2 Autonomic Learning in the Previous Lesson

Regional anatomy is rooted in systematic anatomy. Before learning this course, it is necessary for students to review the relevant content of systematic anatomy, such as the morphological characteristics of organs, the distributions of vessels and nerves, etc. A careful preparation before class will yield much more in the classroom. However, the students should not consider regional anatomy as a review or complement of systematic anatomy. Autonomic learning in the previous lesson benefited much from the theoretical learning and operational training of students.

1.6.3 Stringent Adherence to the Operational Protocols

Dissection of the donor body should strictly adhere to operational protocols. Guided by a principle of scientificity and precision, a "continuous hierarchical dissection method" should be performed to minimize damage to the specimens, thereby facilitating repeated observational study. Therefore, it is crucial to strictly standardize dissection procedures according to the instructions outlined in each chapter of the regional anatomy and teachers' instructions to achieve successful dissection practice. Each step during dissection must be purpose-driven. Blind practice or over-dissection range must be avoided to prevent damage to structures. Each practice group should collaborate effectively during dissection practice. Active participation and communication are needed. After practice, specimens should be properly wrapped to prevent drying.

1.6.4 Careful Observation and Identification

The dissection of specimens is a crucial step, but not the ultimate goal. In order to master this subject, careful observation is necessary after the dissection is completed. Each student should adhere to the principle of "dissect, examine, identify, and ascertain." "Dissect" refers to specimen dissection. "Examine" represents observation and investigation. "Identify" means accurately identifying and distinguishing the main structures. "Ascertain" refers to locating important structures and determining their interrelationships in a certain region.

1.6.5 Cultivation of a Sense of Gratitude

Dissection courses in medical universities and colleges cannot be established without the contribution of donor bodies. It is essential to cultivate a true sense of gratitude in medical students. This sense should be embodied in the dissection courses through various activities, such as a ceremony of silence prior to dissection procedures (Fig. 1.6) and engagement in volunteer services.

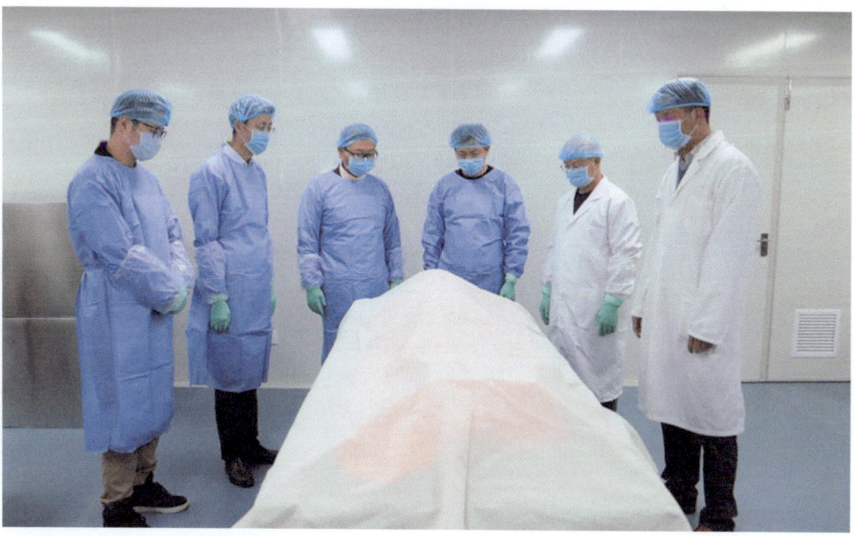

Fig. 1.6 Before body dissection, teachers and students held a ceremony of silence

Chapter 2
Anatomy of the Back Region and Its Clinical Application

Peidang Liu, Yongxin Ren, and Min Zhu

2.1 Anatomy of the Back Region

2.1.1 Boundary

The back has an upper border bilaterally extending from external occipital protuberance, along the superior nuchal line, to the mastoid process; two lateral borders extending from the mastoid process, along the anterior margin of the trapezius, to the acromion, then vertically along the midaxillary line to the iliac crest; and a lower border extending from the middle of the posterior and upper margin of the sacrum, externally along the iliac crest to the inferior end point of the lateral border. According to C7 (vertebra prominens), the spinous process and the 12th rib, the back region is divided into the nucha, back, and lumbar-lower parts.

2.1.2 Anatomical Landmarks

2.1.2.1 Superficial Landmarks

External Occipital Protuberance

A protuberance in the middle of the outer side of the occipital bone. Its internal side is called the sinus confluence.

P. Liu
Southeast University School of Medicine, Nanjing, China

Y. Ren · M. Zhu (✉)
Nanjing Medical University, Nanjing, China
e-mail: zhumin@njmu.edu.cn

Q. Ding et al. (eds.), *Clinically Oriented Regional Anatomy*,
https://doi.org/10.1007/978-981-95-9888-5_2

Vertebral Spinous Process

It is located at the posterior midline. Vertebra prominens has a long spinous process, and its end does not bifurcate. The landmark is often referred to as the number of the vertebra.

Spine of Scapula

It is a transverse high bone bridge at the back side of the scapula. The line connecting the bilateral spines of the scapula is at the level of the spinous process of the third thoracic vertebra.

Inferior Angle of the Scapula

An acute angle between the axillary border and the vertebral border of the scapula, at the level of the seventh rib or the seventh intercostal space. This angle is also used to number the rib.

The 12th Rib

The angle between the 12th rib and the lateral border of the erector spinae produces an area called the renal area. Percussion pain in this area is common in patients with nephropyelitis. To set a lumbar approach for renal surgery, the upper end of the incision is often marked by the 12th rib.

Iliac Crest

It is the upper side of the ilium wing. The line between the highest points of bilateral iliac crests is at the level of the spinous process of the fourth lumbar vertebra. Lumbar puncture is usually performed in the space between the third and fourth, or the fourth and fifth lumbar vertebrae.

2.1.2.2 Anatomical Lines

Posterior Median Line

It is an imaginary line running vertically along the median of the back and connecting the tips of all vertebra processes.

Scapula Line

A vertical line passing by the inferior angle of the scapula.

Anterior Axillary Line

A vertical line passing through the junction between the anterior axillary wall and the lateral chest wall.

Posterior Axillary Line

A vertical line passing through the junction between the posterior axillary wall and the lateral chest wall.

Midaxillary Line

A vertical line passing through the midpoint of the axilla.

2.1.3 Hierarchical Structures

2.1.3.1 Skin

The skin on the back is thick and tight, with low mobility but rich hair follicles and sebaceous glands.

2.1.3.2 Superficial Fascia

Superficial arteries contain the branches of the occipital artery, dorsal scapular artery, posterior intercostal artery, and lumbar artery. Superficial veins are those running along the arteries. Among these vessels, the occipital artery has a larger diameter and runs across the surface of the trapezius origin at the superior nuchal line. The branches of the posterior intercostal and lumbar arteries are finer and distributed on the bilateral sides of the spine.

The nucha region has the branches of the posterior cervical nerve, mainly the greater and third occipital nerves. The greater occipital nerve is the branch of the second posterior cervical nerve, beneath the superior nuchal line and at the origin of trapezius, out of the occipital nerve, and underneath the occipital skin. The thoracic and lumbar regions are distributed with branches of the posterior thoracic and lumbar nerves. Each branch runs out by the spinous processes. All the upper branches stretch laterally and almost horizontally, and the lower branches stretch laterally and downward. The branch of the 12th posterior thoracic nerve can reach the hips. The external branches of the first-third posterior lumbar nerves make up the superior cluneal nerves, which run through the lumbar region, out of the thoracic and lumbar fascia, over the iliac crest, and into the upper part of the hip region. They run out from the upper part of the iliac crest and concentrate within an area 2 cm inside the outer margin of the erector spinae. Therefore, a sudden twist of the waist may injure these nerves.

2.1.3.3 Superficial Layer of the Deep Fascia

The superficial layer of the deep fascia in the back is thin and adherent to the surface of the trapezius and latissimus dorsi, serving as the sheath of trapezius. This fascia migrates in a direction opposite to those in the cervical, thoracic, and abdominal regions.

2.1.3.4 Muscles, Vessels, and Nerves

The muscles in the back are clearly layered, while the vessels and nerves are segmented.

Dorsal Muscles

Dorsal muscles are stratified into three layers.

First Layer

This layer is superficial, containing the trapezius, latissimus dorsi, and the posterior part of obliquus externus abdominis. The trapezius, a triangular platysma, is located in the superior neck region, extending from the external occipital protuberance, the 1/3 of the upper nuchal line, the nuchal ligament, C7, to the spinous process of the 12th thoracic vertebra and supraspinous ligament. Its upper bundles are directed externally and downward, up to the posterior margin of the outer 1/3 clavicle. Its medial bundles run horizontally and laterally to the inner side of the acromion and the upper side of the spine of the scapula. Its lower bundles turn external and upward to the inner side of the spine of the scapula. The latissimus dorsi, the largest broad muscle located at the lumbar back and both sides of the posterior chest, extends from its aponeurosis at the lower sixth spinous process and supraspinous ligament, the posterior layer of thoracolumbar fascia (covering all lumbar vertebra spinous processes, sacral median ridge, and posterior iliac crest), and connecting through its muscular teeth with the outer side of the lower third-fourth ribs. Occasionally, a small number of bundles originate from the dorsal part of the inferior angle of the scapula.

Second Layer

This layer is made of levator scapulae, rhomboideus, serratus posterior inferior, etc. The former two are located deep beneath the trapezius, and the latter deep beneath the latissimus dorsi (Fig. 2.1).

Third Layer

This layer is composed of erector spinae and splenius. The former is the longest among all the dorsal muscles, longitudinally arranged in the back creases on both sides of the spine. The splenius is located beneath the trapezius and rhomboideus (Fig. 2.1). The erector spinae are broad, long, corded, and paraspinous, running

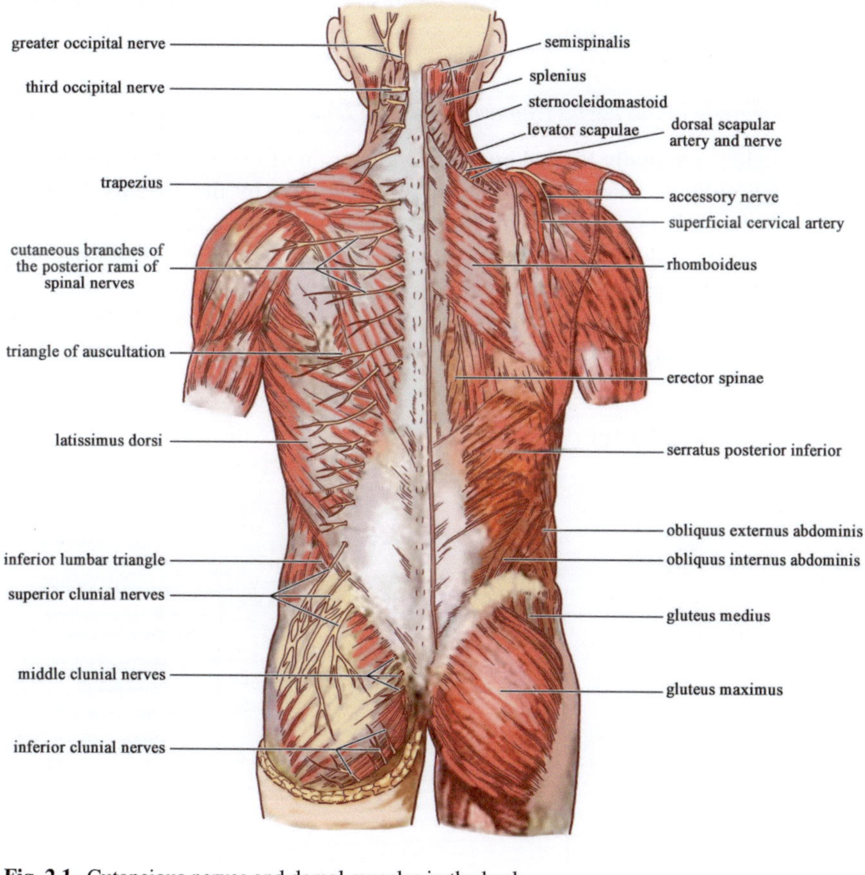

Fig. 2.1 Cutaneious nerves and dorsal muscles in the back

from the sacrum up to the occipital bone. They connect with the dorsal sacrum, posterior iliac crest, lumbar vertebra spinous process, and thoracolumbar fascia through tendons and bundles, and are divided into three longitudinal columns (lateral, middle, and medial). The lateral column attaching to the rib is called the iliocostalis, the middle column attaching to the transverse process is called the longissimus, and the medial column attaching to the spinous process is called the spinalis and has the least power.

Intermuscular Structures

Triangle of Auscultation

This region is superiorly bounded by the outer and lower margin of trapezius, externally by the medial margin of the scapula, and inferiorly by the superior margin of the latissimus dorsi. This triangle is based on adipose tissue, deep fascia, and the sixth intercostal space and covered by skin and superficial fascia. In auscultation, breath sounds from this triangle are the clearest. As the scapula moves forward or outward, this triangle expands.

The Quadrangle of the Levies (Superior Lumbar Triangle)

This triangle is internally limited by the lateral margin of the erector spinae, inferiorly by the obliquus internus abdominis, and superiorly by the serratus posterior inferior. If the latter two pieces of muscles are not interconnected at the 12th rib, this rib can serve as a fourth side to make up a quadrangle, which is called the quadrangle of the Levies. The quadrangle of the Levies (the superior lumbar triangle) is based on the aponeurosis at the origin of the transvers abdominal muscle. Subcostal, iliohypogastric, and ilioinguinal nerves run deep through the triangle (Fig. 2.2).

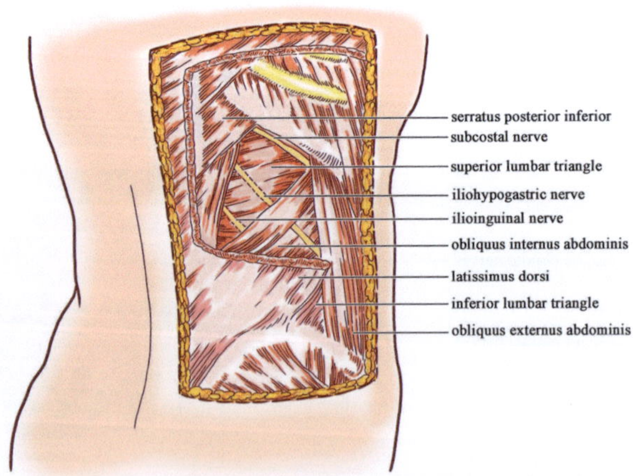

Fig. 2.2 Superior and inferior lumbar triangles

During renal surgery, an extraperitoneal approach can be planned to pass through this triangle, thus necessitating the protection of the three nerves.

The 12th rib is anteriorly close to the pleural cavity. To expand the surgical field view, the lumbocostal ligament is often cut to elevate the 12th rib, during which the pleura should be protected to prevent pneumothorax. In the case of a perinephric abscess, this triangle can be incised for drainage. Besides, this triangle is less powerful, and a lumbar hernia may develop as abdominal content protrudes backward into this triangle. In addition, the retroperitoneal abscess can be punctured through it.

Inferior Lumbar Triangle

This triangle is made of the iliac crest, the posterior margin of the obliquus externus abdominis, the anterior inferior margin of the latissimus dorsi, based on the obliquus internus abdominis, and covered by skin and the superficial fascia. This triangle is another weak area on the posterior abdominal wall. Lumbar hernia may develop here, but with a lower possibility than that in the superior lumbar triangle.

Vessels and Nerves

The back is supplied by the occipital artery, vertebral artery, dorsal scapular artery, thoracodorsal artery, posterior intercostal artery, subcostal artery, and lumbar artery. Synonymous veins run along with these arteries. The nerves in the back include the posterior branches of the spinal nerves, the accessory nerve, the thoracodorsal nerve, and the dorsal scapular nerve. Among them, the accessory nerve enters the trapezius through two points at the middle and lower 1/3 of its anterior margin. The thoracodorsal nerve runs parallel with the thoracodorsal artery, along the outer margin of the scapula, into the latissimus dorsi through its deep surface. The dorsal scapular nerve parallels the dorsal scapular artery, downward along the inner margin of the scapula, to control the levator scapulae and rhomboideus.

2.1.3.5 Deep Fascia

This layer adheres deep to the muscles, vessels, and nerve trunks, including the endothoracic fascia, transverse fascia, and thoracolumbar fascia (Fig. 2.3).

Thoracolumbar fascia envelopes the erector spinae and the quadratus lumborum, consisting of the superficial, middle, and deep layers. The superficial layer, also called the posterior layer, covers the surface of the erector spinae, as well as the deep surfaces of the quadratus lumborum, latissimus dorsi, serratus posterior inferior, and extends superiorly into the nuchal fascia, attaches inferiorly to the iliac crest and the lateral sacral crest, medially to the spinous processes of the thoracic and lumbar vertebrae, the supraspinous ligament, and the median sacral crest, and externally in the thoracic dorsal region to the costal angles of the ribs and the intercostal fascia; in the lumbar region, the thoracolumbar fascia spreads into the tendon membrane where

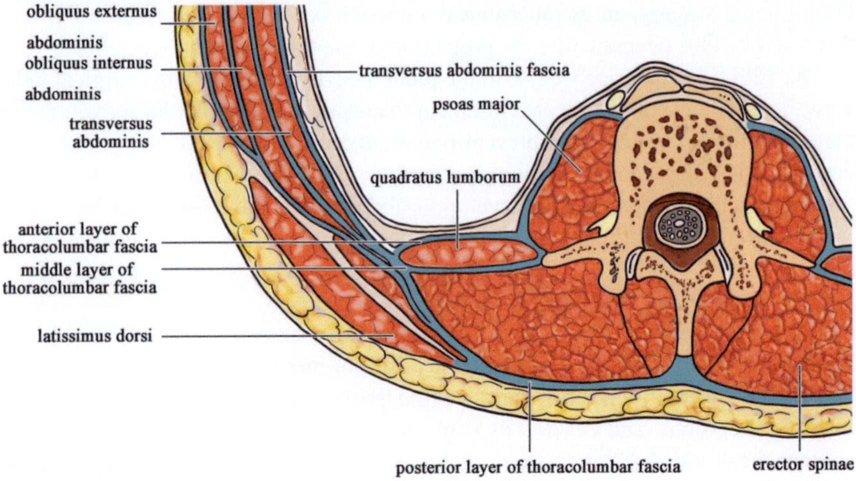

Fig. 2.3 Thoracolumbar fascia

the transversus abdominis begins, and extends into the lateral aspect of the sacrospinous muscle and the deep layer of thoracolumbar fascia (lumbar dorsal fascia).

The middle layer of the thoracolumbar fascia separates the erector spinae from the quadratus lumborum, attaches upward to the inferior border of the 12th rib, downward to the iliac crest, medially to the transverse processes of the lumbar vertebrae, and laterally to the superficial layer of the thoracolumbar fascia to form the lumbocostal sheath. Also called the lumbocostal ligament, the upper part of this layer of fascia is significantly thickened between the 12th rib and the transverse process of the first lumbar vertebra. The deeper (anterior) layer of the thoracolumbar fascia covers the anterior aspect of the quadratus lumborum, attaches medially to the tip of the transverse process of the lumbar vertebrae, and downward to the iliolumbar ligament and posterior part of the iliac crest. The upper part of this layer thickens distally to form the lateral arcuate ligament and continues with the medial arcuate ligament. The three layers of fascia meet at the lateral border of the quadratus lumborum, forming the tendon membrane of the obliquus internus abdominis and the origin of the transversus abdominis.

2.1.4 Anatomy of the Back

2.1.4.1 Objectives

To dissect the back at different levels, to be familiar with the structural characteristics of each layer of the back, to understand the distribution of superficial blood vessels and cutaneous nerves in the superficial fascia, and to master the intermuscular structure.

2.1.4.2 Position

Prone position.

2.1.4.3 Examination of Body Landmarks

The signs of the body surface can be copied onto live bodies. The clinical significance of each landmark should be understood.

2.1.4.4 Procedures

Step 1: Make a skin incision according to the lines shown in Fig. 2.4. In the posterior midline, at the junction of each skin incision line, lift the skin with forceps, pull it apart with force, and gently cut off the subcutaneous connection with a scalpel.

Step 2: Remove the superficial fascia. When removing the subcutaneous fat, preserve the blood vessels and nerves within the superficial fascia as much as possible. On the surface of the beginning of the occipital part of the trapezius, examine the occipital artery, the great occipital nerve and the occipital lymph nodes; on the surface of the trapezius and the latissimus dorsi, find out one or two posterior branches of the thoracic nerve; on the lateral edge of the lower part of the erector spinae, pick out the superior clunial nerve on the superior part of the iliac crest, and observe the direction and distribution of the above mentioned superficial blood vessels and the cutaneous nerves.

Step 3: Repair and clear the contour of the trapezius and latissimus dorsi, examine the circumference of the auscultatory triangle and the inferior lumbar triangle, and observe the shape of the posterior layer of the thoracolumbar fascia and its connection with the surrounding structures.

Step 4: Starting from the outer inferior border of the trapezius, use the back of the scalpel to gradually separate the trapezius and its deeper structures from the bottom upwards. Insert the forceps into the deep surface of the trapezius, hollow out the trapezius, and sever the trapezius from below upward at a position approximately 1 cm lateral to the posterior midline, and then outward to the spine of the scapula. Observe the upper edges of the splenius capitis, splenius cervicis, levator scapulae, rhomboideus, and latissimus dorsi on the deep surface of the trapezius, and examine the paracrine nerves that are located on the deep surface of the trapezius and penetrate into it.

Step 5: Separate the outer lower edge of the latissimus dorsi by severing the beginning of the latissimus dorsi on the iliac crest, then sever the muscle at the lateral 1 cm of the thoracolumbar fascia, turn it over onto the outer upper surface, and examine the thoracodorsal nerve and thoracodorsal artery (which are located on the deep surface of the latissimus dorsi) in close proximity to the

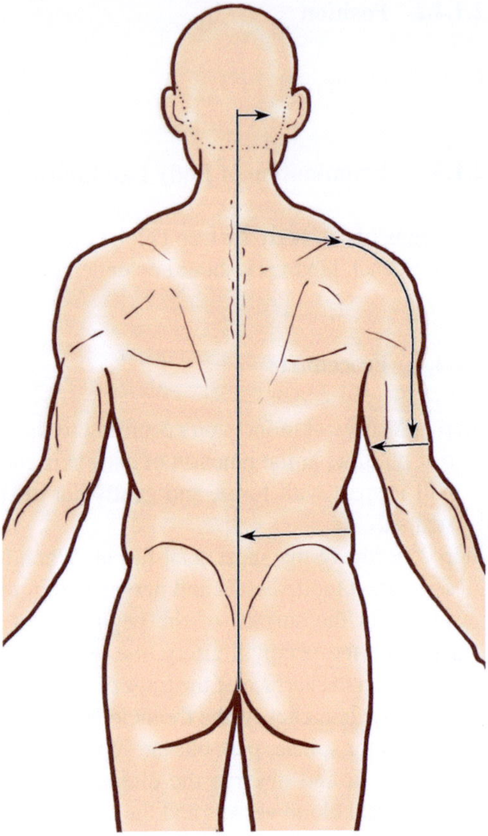

Fig. 2.4 Skin incision lines on the back

axillary region. Observe the shape and circumference of the suprasternal triangle.

2.1.5 *Summary*

2.1.5.1 Hierarchy of the Back

The back comprises the dorsal lateral wall of the trunk, which is divided from top to bottom into the neck, back, and lumbar region. This part is also separated into five layers, including the thick and dense skin; superficial fascia with superficial blood vessels and cutaneous nerves; the thin superficial layer of the intrinsic fascia, forming the sheath of trapezius; underneath is three layers of muscles; the auscultatory triangle is where respiratory sounds are most clearly heard; the quadrangle of the Levies and the lower lumbar triangle are the weak areas of the lumbar region; the intrinsic fascia is well developed at the lumbar region, forming the thoracolumbar fascia.

2.1.5.2 Lumbar Renal Surgery Entrance

The lumbar oblique incision is commonly used in clinical renal surgery. The incision starts from the midpoint of the lower edge of the 12th rib and ends 2 cm above the anterior superior iliac spine. The incision passes through layers of skin, superficial fascia, latissimus dorsi, and obliquus externus abdominis in sequence, and through the superior lumbar triangle (upward to cut the lateral border of the serratus posterior inferior, and downward to cut the obliquus internus abdominis for enlarging the surgical field). If further enlargement of the incision is required, the 12th rib needs to be raised or excised. When cutting through the superior lumbar triangle, care should be taken to protect the subcostal nerve and ilioinguinal nerve.

2.1.5.3 Latissimus Dorsi Flap

The latissimus dorsi is the superficial triangular broad muscle of the back, located in the lower half of the back and the posterolateral chest. Its nutrient is mainly provided by the thoracodorsal artery. The advantages of the free latissimus dorsi flap include: large coverage area, long and constant vascular tip, high rate of vascular anastomosis, rich blood supply of the flap, strong resistance to infection, and no impact on the function of the donor area after resection. It is suitable for the repair of oral and maxillofacial soft tissue defects, large soft tissue defects of limbs, etc. It can also be used as the kinetic muscle for various functional reconstruction. Now, it is widely used in clinical practice.

2.1.5.4 Lumbar Puncture (Subarachnoid Space Puncture)

Clinically, a lumbar puncture to the subarachnoid space can be performed to extract cerebrospinal fluid or inject drugs for the diagnosis or treatment of certain neurological diseases. This method also realizes the injection of anesthetics for lumbar anesthesia. It is usually performed in the side-lying knee-thoracic position and through the following levels: skin, superficial fascia, deep fascia, supraspinous ligament, interspinous ligament, ligamentum flavum, spinal dura mater, and arachnoid membrane.

2.2 Clinical Application of Key Anatomical Structures of the Back

The anatomical structure of the back can be divided into five layers: skin, superficial fascia, superficial layer of the deep fascia, muscles, vessels and nerves, and deep layer of the deep fascia. In clinical surgery, it is often necessary to pay attention to the hierarchy and adjacency of important anatomical structures, such as the superficial layer of the deep fascia, muscles, vessels, and nerves and the deep layer of the deep fascia. In this section, the clinical application of the important anatomical structures of the back will be described according to the intraoperative observation of lumbar spine fracture incision and internal fixation by posterior median approach.

1. Position

The patient is placed in a prone position on a radiographically permeable operating table, with cotton pads placed under the chest and iliac crests to ensure abdominal suspension and minimize epidural bleeding. The thoracic and iliac pads are adjusted to restore the sagittal sequence of the lumbar spine by gravity (Fig. 2.5a).

2. Surgical Path

The line connecting the highest points of the iliac crests on both sides parallels the spinous process of the fourth lumbar vertebra. According to this line, the lumbar vertebra, if fractured, can be determined by its sequential number. A posterior median skin incision of about 12 cm can be made, centered on the fractured lumbar vertebrae, and the skin and superficial fascia are incised to reveal the superficial layer of the intrinsic fascia. The superficial layer of the intrinsic fascia is cut open to observe the supraspinous ligament. The muscles are stripped along both sides of the supraspinous ligament on the bony surface until the spinous processes, vertebral plates, and articular synovial joints are exposed. The muscles near the lumbar spine mainly include the superficial latissimus dorsi and the deep paravertebral muscles, which can be divided into the superficial erector spinae, deep multifidus, and rotator spinae. It should be noted that the paraspinal muscles are often stripped as a whole for surgical visualization, so their layers are not apparent intraoperatively (Fig. 2.5b, c).

The lumbar artery, a segmental artery supplying blood to the lumbar spine, originates from the posterior wall of the abdominal aorta and splits into two branches adjacent to the pedicles, one supplying the spinal cord and the other supplying the paravertebral muscles posteriorly. Usually found between the transverse processes adjacent to the articular synovial joints, these vessels are often prone to injury and bleeding during surgical dissection. In addition, the branches of the arteries in the paraspinal muscles often form a network of blood supply; however, no blood vessels run across the midline, so it is recommended that the dissection be done as close to the midline as possible. If the lumbar fracture is a flexion-distraction fracture (Chance fracture) involving the anterior, middle, and posterior columns, the posterior lumbar structures, such as the supraspinous ligament and spinous processes, can be seen to have been damaged or ruptured during the exposure.

This approach is the easiest to reveal the lumbar spinous processes, plates, and synovial joints.

3. Entry-Point Positioning and Placement of Pedicle Screws

The pedicle of the vertebral arch is a tubular bony structure that connects the anterior and posterior columns of the spine. The medial wall of the pedicle is close

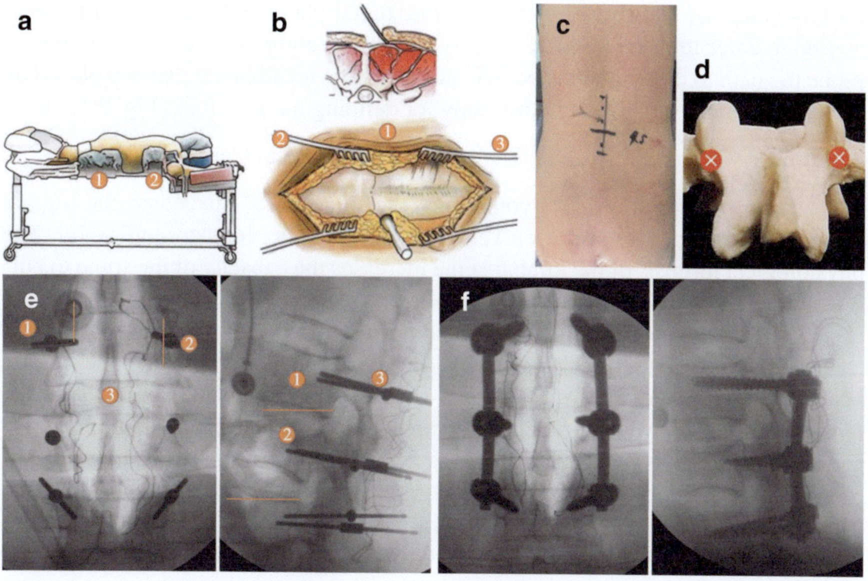

Fig. 2.5 Posterior median approach lumbar spine fracture incision and internal fixation. (**a**) A patient in a prone position (1. iliac crest cushion; 2. thoracic cushion). (**b**) Exposure to the fascial layer (1. transverse process; 2. caudal; 3. cephalad). (**c**) Posterior median incision after marking. (**d**) Entry points of pedicle screws. (**e**) Intraoperative fluoroscopy of the positions of pedicle screw rods (left: 1. left pedicle; 2. right pedicle; 3. spinous process). Right: 1. Normal vertebral body; 2. Fractured vertebral body; 3. pedicle). (**F**) A fluoroscopic image after repositioning and internal fixation

to the dural sac, and the medial wall is close to the nerve roots that travel through the intervertebral foramen. The lumbar nerve roots are usually located in the upper third of the foramen, so it brings more risks to enter the screws from the medial or inferior side of the pedicle than from the lateral or upper side. Both the commissural space and the midpoint of the transverse process are important reference points in the positioning of pedicle screws.

Three methods are commonly used to locate an entry point: the herringbone ridge apex method, the crossover method, and the mastoid process method. Here, the herringbone ridge apex method is illustrated as an example. The lumbar isthmus has an elevated longitudinal ridge, called the isthmus ridge; the superior articular process has an elevated longitudinal ridge, called the paramedian ridge, on the posterior-lateral aspect of the root. The herringbone ridge is composed of the paraspinal and isthmic ridges, with the apex of the herringbone ridge at the confluence (Fig. 2.5d). The paravertebral muscles are stripped through the bony surface to reveal the isthmus of the arch, the upper and lower articular synchondrosis, and the herringbone ridge above the arch isthmus. The opening is made at the apex of the herringbone crest, and the angle of the pedicle screws is adjusted on the horizontal and sagittal planes according to the preoperative pedicle planar CT scanning results and intraoperative plain images, generally with an inward inclination of 5° to 10°

for L1–3 and 10° to 15° for L4–5 on the horizontal plane. Subsequently, an opener is used to enter the pedicle till a sense of "frosted feeling" is felt. A ball is used to probe the path to determine the pedicle position. The localization pins are placed on each side to carry out C-arm fluoroscopy for defining the positions (Fig. 2.5e).

4. Lumbar Vertebra Fracture Reduction and Physiological Curvature Recovery

Under normal physiological conditions, the spine is "S"-shaped on the sagittal plane, with four physiological curves: cervical, thoracic, lumbar, and sacral. The physiological lordosis of the lumbar spine increases the capacity of the spine to buffer external forces, bear weights, and stabilize the vertebrae and pelvis. Its structure is critical for humans to maintain a normal posture.

The titanium rods should be selected according to the space between the screws, bent according to the shape of the lumbar vertebrae, inserted, and fixed. The tail cap of the screws is screwed in order to reset the fractured vertebral body. Intraoperative C-arm fluoroscopy is performed to ensure the accurate positions of pedicle screws, reposition of fractured vertebrae, and normal curvature of the lumbar vertebrae (Fig. 2.5f).

Lumbar lordosis is critical for maintaining the sagittal balance of the spine and is the goal of surgical treatment to correct lumbar deformity.

Chapter 3
Regional Anatomy of the Chest Wall and Its Clinical Application

Haiwei Meng, Qiang Ding, Yi Zhao, Huaxing Huang, and Qiannan Zhu

3.1 Regional Anatomy of the Chest Wall

3.1.1 Boundary

With the thoracic cage as the bony framework, the chest wall is superficially covered by skin, fascia, and muscle and intrinsically linked with the endothoracic fascia. The chest wall connects with the neck superiorly through the jugular notch, the sternoclavicular joint, the supraclavicular margin, and the line connecting the acromion to the spinous process of C7; with the abdomen inferiorly through the xiphoid process, costal arch, the anterior end of the 11th pair of ribs, the inferior end of the 12th pair of ribs and the spinous process of T12; and laterally with the upper extremities through the superior portion of anterior and posterior deltoid muscle, and the line connecting the points where the lower portions of anterior and posterior axillary folds meet the chest wall. It superiorly extends the neck, inferiorly separates the abdominal cavity, and laterally connects the upper extremities. Each side of the chest wall is divided into anterior, lateral, and dorsal regions. The anterior region lies between the anterior median line and the anterior axillary line, the lateral region between the anterior and posterior axillary lines, and the dorsal region between the posterior median line and the posterior axillary line.

H. Meng
Shandong University School of Basic Medical Sciences, Jinan, China
e-mail: hwmeng@sdu.edu.cn

Q. Ding · Y. Zhao · H. Huang (✉) · Q. Zhu
Nanjing Medical University, Nanjing, China
e-mail: dingqiang@njmu.edu.cn; doctorzhaoyi@njmu.edu.cn; huanghuaxing@njmu.edu.cn

Q. Ding et al. (eds.), *Clinically Oriented Regional Anatomy*,
https://doi.org/10.1007/978-981-95-9888-5_3

3.1.2 Anatomical Landmarks

3.1.2.1 Jugular Notch

The jugular notch is at the superior segment of the sternum, and parallels between T2 and T3.

3.1.2.2 Clavicle and Subclavian Fossa

The clavicle is a palpable bone lying on the bilateral sides of the jugular notch. The supraclavicular fossa is an indentation beneath the middle-lateral third of the clavicle, where the axillary blood vessels and brachial plexus run deeply through it. The coracoid process can be palpated at a finger's breadth below.

3.1.2.3 Xiphoid Process

The xiphoid process is at the level of T9, which is superiorly connected to the body of the sternum (known as the xiphisternal joint or xiphisternal symphysis). The superior portion of the xiphoid process articulates with the costal cartilage of the seventh rib, and the inferior portion frees and extends into the superior portion of the anterior abdominal wall.

3.1.2.4 Sternal Angle

The sternal angle is a protrusion formed by the manubrium and the body of the sternum. It is located at the approximate level of the second rib and faces inferiorly to the lower edge of T4. The sternal angle is an anatomical landmark for counting ribs and identifying intercostal spaces.

3.1.2.5 Costal Arch and Substernal Angle

The costal arch is a palpable margin descending externally along the xiphoid process, as a landmark of the liver. The bilateral sides of the costal arch and the xiphisternal joint form the infrasternal angle, where the xiphoid process is palpable. The xiphocostal angle is the angle formed by the xiphoid process and the costal arch. The left xiphocostal angle is a commonly used insertion site for pericardiocentesis.

3.1.2.6 Nipple

Male nipples are generally located at the junction of the midclavicular line and the fourth intercostal space, while female nipples are more inferior and lateral.

3.1.3 Anatomical Lines (Fig. 3.1)

3.1.3.1 Anterior Median Line

The anterior median line is a vertical line running across the midpoint of the sternum.

3.1.3.2 Sternal Line

The sternal line is a vertical line running along the lateral border of the sternum.

3.1.3.3 Midclavicular Line

The midclavicular line is a vertical line running across the midpoint of the clavicle.

3.1.3.4 Parasternal Line

The parasternal line is a vertical line equidistant from the sternal line and the midclavicular line.

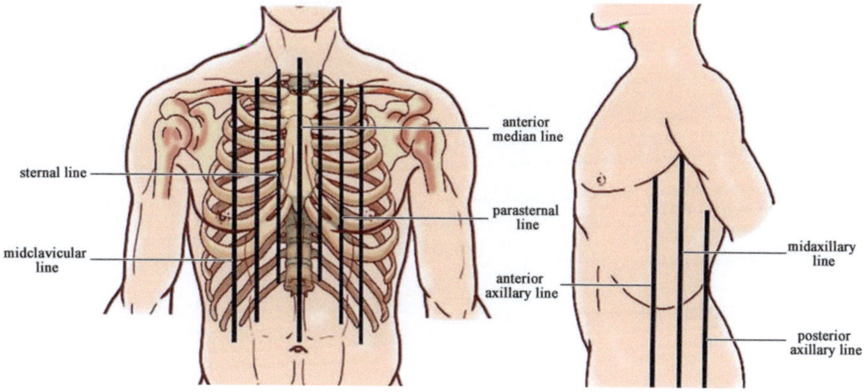

Fig. 3.1 Anatomical lines on the chest

3.1.3.5 Anterior/Posterior Axillary Line

The anterior/posterior axillary line is a vertical line running along the anterior/posterior axillary fold on the chest wall.

3.1.4 Superficial Structures

3.1.4.1 Skin

The skin on the anterior and lateral region of the chest becomes thinner, which can be greatly moved (high mobility), except for that on the sternum.

3.1.4.2 Superficial Fascia

The superficial fascia of the chest wall connects to that of the neck, abdomen, and upper extremities and contains fat tissues, superficial blood vessels, lymphatic vessels, cutaneous nerves, and mammary glands (Fig. 3.2).

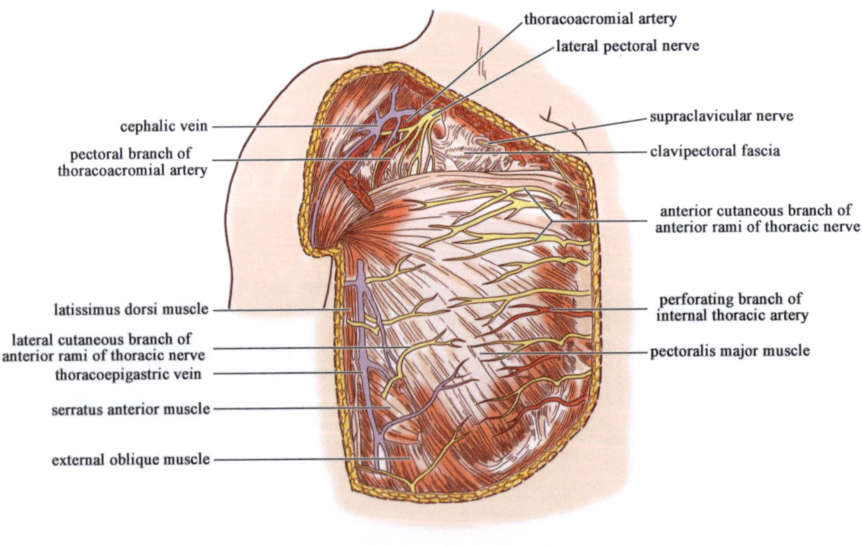

Fig. 3.2 Superficial structures on the anterior region of the chest

Cutaneous Nerves

The supraclavicular nerve arises from the third and fourth cervical nerves and innervates the skin of the anterior region of the chest and the shoulder.

The anterior cutaneous branch of the intercostal nerve derives from the bilateral sides of the sternum and innervates the skin of the anterior region of the chest. The lateral cutaneous branch extends out from the anterior axillary line and then innervates the skin of the lateral and anterior region of the chest.

Superficial Blood Vessels

Perforating branches of the internal thoracic artery are small arteries that run with the anterior cutaneous branch of the intercostal nerve, and pierce out 1 cm from the lateral side of the sternum. They supply the inner part of the anterior chest. The second, third, and fourth perforating branches in women are large and distribute across the breast. Their ligation and hemostasis should be considered during breast surgery.

The dorsal (posterior) and the collateral branches of the posterior intercostal artery run with the corresponding branch of the intercostal nerve and supply the muscle and skin of the anterior and lateral region of the chest, and the breast.

The thoracoepigastric vein arises from the paraumbilical veins, ascends obliquely along the lateral side of the chest wall, and opens into the lateral thoracic vein. It collects venous blood from the superior abdominal wall and the superficial anterolateral region of the chest.

Breast

Location and Structure

The breast of adolescent non-lactating females is hemispherical, vertically overlying the second to sixth ribs and running laterally from the parasternal line to the anterior axillary line. It is composed of skin, mammary glands, and fat tissues. The lactiferous ducts are arranged radially around the nipple and end at the nipple. There are many fiber bundles (Cooper's ligament) perpendicular to the skin in the interlobular connective tissues, which superficially connect to the skin and deeply link with the pectoralis fascia. In breast cancers involving the Cooper's ligaments, the breast skin depresses, resulting in a sign of breast dimpling (Fig. 3.3).

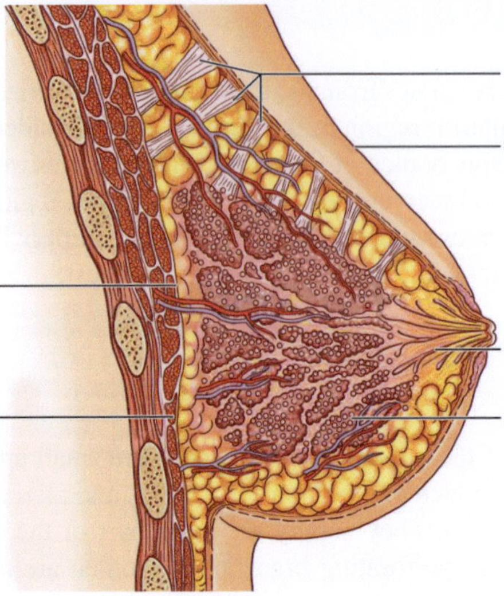

Fig. 3.3 The female breast on the sagittal plane

Arteries and Veins

The blood supply to the mammary gland is rich, mainly from the perforating branches of the internal thoracic artery, the lateral mammary branch of the lateral thoracic artery, and the posterior intercostal artery. Their accompanying veins drain into the internal thoracic vein, axillary vein, and posterior intercostal vein, respectively.

Lymphatic Vessels

The breast has a superficial and a deep lymphatic system. The superficial lymphatic system lies under or inside the skin tissues, and the deep lymphatic system surrounds the lobules of the breast. Extensive communications exist between the superficial and deep lymphatic systems. Lymphatic vessels in the lateral and central parts of the breast drain into the pectoral lymph nodes, which represents the major route of lymphatic drainage into the breast; lymphatic vessels in the upper part of the breast drain into the apical lymph nodes and supraclavicular lymph nodes; lymphatic vessels in the inner part of the breast drain into the parasternal lymph nodes and communicate with those in the contralateral breast; lymphatic vessels in the lower inner part of the breast drain into the superior phrenic lymph nodes and communicate with those draining into the lymphatics in the upper part of the anterior abdominal wall and diaphragm; the deep lymphatic vessels of the breast travel through the pectoralis major to the interpectoral lymph nodes and apical lymph nodes (Fig. 3.4). Breast cancers involving the superficial lymphatic system cause lymphatic obstruction, leading to lymphedema and spot-like depression on local skin. Orange peel, known as the breast peau d'orange, is a vital sign of breast cancer.

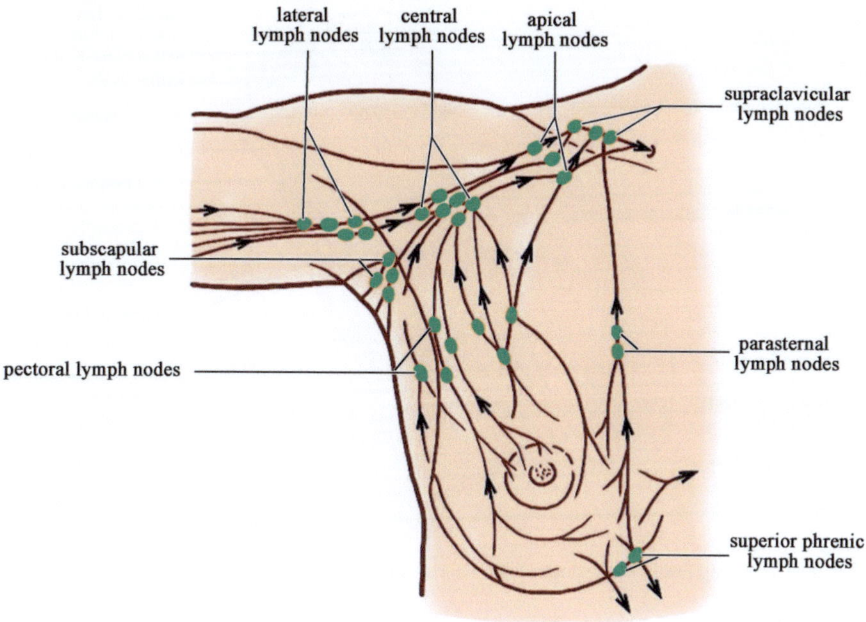

Fig. 3.4 Lymphatic drainage of the breast

3.1.4.3 Deep Fascia

The deep fascia in the anterolateral chest wall consists of the superficial and deep layers. The superficial layer is thinner and covers the surface of the pectoralis major. The deep layer lies on the deep side of the pectoralis major, which superiorly attaches to the clavicle, inferiorly wraps the subclavian muscle and pectoralis minor muscle, and occupies the surface of the serratus anterior muscle. The deep fascia piercing into the coracoid process, subclavian muscle, and the upper portion of the pectoralis minor muscle is known as the clavipectoral fascia. The lateral pectoral nerve and branches of the thoracoacromial artery pierce into the deep layer of clavipectoral fascia and go through the pectoralis major and pectoralis minor muscles. The cephalic vein and lymphatic vessels also run into the deep layer of clavipectoral fascia and into the axillary cavity. The suspensory ligament of the axilla connects the lower portion of the pectoralis minor muscle and the axillary fascia (Figs. 3.5 and 3.6).

3.1.4.4 Muscles

The pectoral muscles and partial abdominal muscles cover the anterolateral region of the chest wall, including four layers from superficial to deep. The outermost layer consists of the pectoralis major, the abdominal external oblique muscle, and the

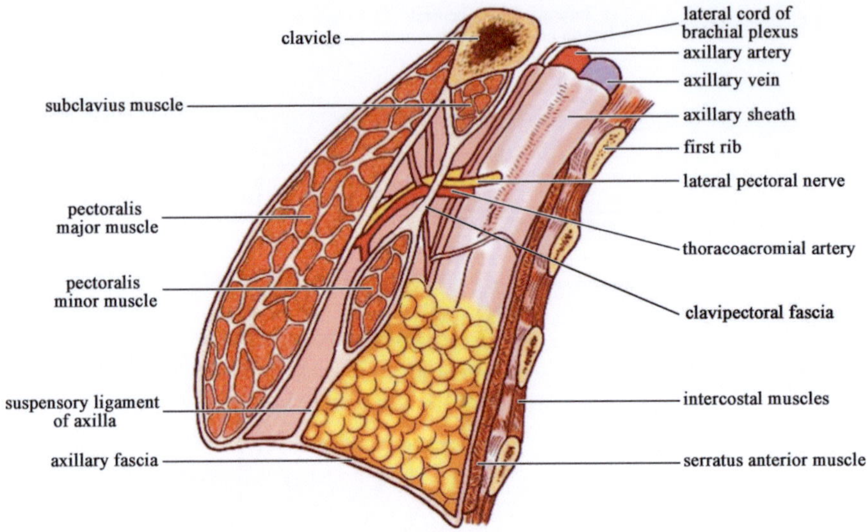

Fig. 3.5 The deep fascia in the anterolateral chest wall

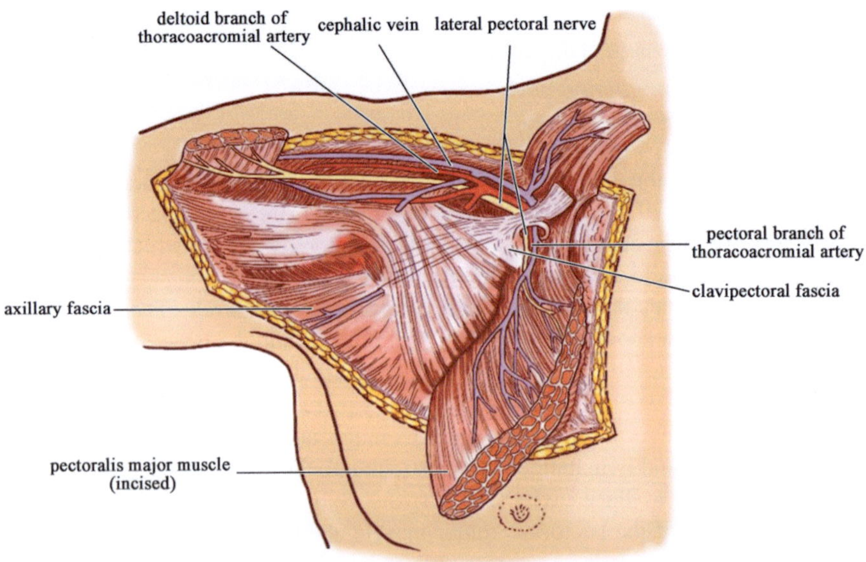

Fig. 3.6 The anterior wall of the axilla

upper portion of the rectus abdominis. The external layer consists of the subclavian muscle, the pectoralis minor muscle, and the serratus anterior. The intercostal muscle and the transversus thoracis muscle, attached to the inner side of the thorax, make up the internal and innermost layers, respectively.

3.1.4.5 Endothoracic Fascia

The endothoracic fascia is a layer of loose connective tissues deeply lining the inner surface of the ribs and intercostal muscles. From thick to thin, the endothoracic fascia lying on the inner surface of the sternum and intercostal space is thicker, and that reaching the bilateral sides of the spine is thinner. There is a layer of loose connective tissues that separates the endothoracic fascia and parietal pleura. Inferiorly, the layer overlies the upper thoracic diaphragm (known as the phrenicopleural fascia) and superiorly overlies the upper pleural dome (known as Sibson's fascia).

3.1.5 Intermuscular Structures

3.1.5.1 Axillary Region

Borders of the Axillary Cavity

The axillary region is an area between the upper portion of the thorax and the upper portion of the arm. When the upper limbs are abducted, an upward shallow fossa located in the axillary region is known as the axillary fossa. The axillary fossa has a thin skin, where underarm hair grows in adults, and contains abundant sebaceous glands and sweat glands. The axillary cavity is the quadrangular pyramid-shaped cavity in the depths of the axillary fossa, through which blood vessels and nerves travel to the neck and upper limbs. It is structurally divided into the apex, base, anterior wall, posterior wall, medial wall, and lateral wall. The pectoralis major, pectoralis minor muscle, subclavian muscle, clavipectoral fascia, and suspensory ligament of axilla make up the anterior wall of the axillary cavity; the subscapularis, teres major muscle, latissimus dorsi muscle, and scapula make up the posterior wall of the axillary cavity; the first to fourth ribs and their intercostal muscles, as well as the serratus anterior, make up the medial wall of the axillary cavity; the medial surface of the proximal segment of the humerus, short head of the bicep brachii, and coracobrachialis make up the lateral wall of the axillary cavity. The base is made up of axillary skin, superficial fascia, and axillary fascia, and can move from the chest wall to the upper extremities. The apex of the axillary cavity, also known as the cervico-axillary canal, is a triangular area surrounded by the outer edge of the first rib, the middle third of the clavicle, and the superior edge of the scapula. The axillary sheath is a fascial sheath enclosing the brachial plexus and axillary vessels at the root of the neck, and these vessels enter the axillary cavity from the apex (Figs. 3.7 and 3.8).

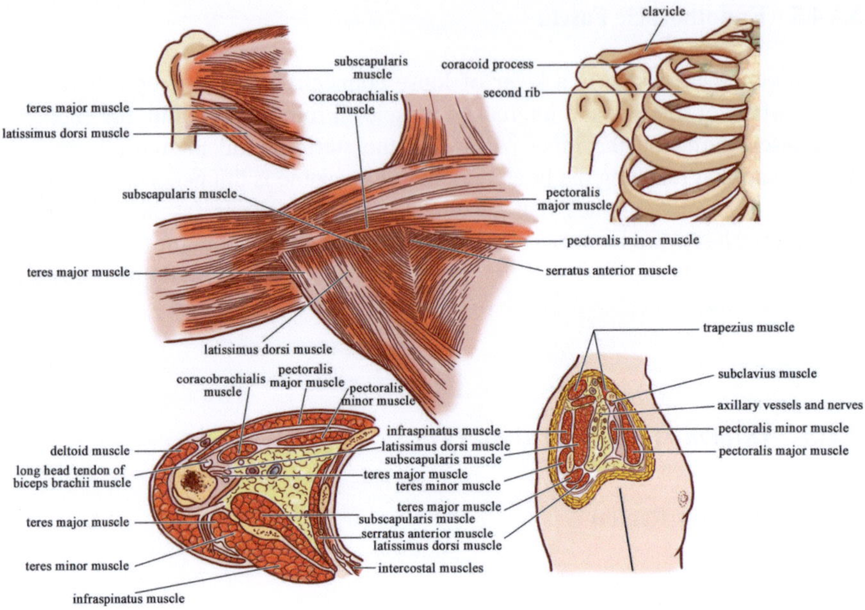

Fig. 3.7 Borders of the axillary cavity

Contents in the Axillary Cavity

Axillary Lymph Nodes

Five groups of axillary lymph nodes present in the axillary cavity, including the lateral group, anterior (pectoral) group, posterior (subscapular) group, central group, and apical group. (1) Axillary lymph nodes in the lateral group lie along the distal side of the axillary vein and receive most of the lymph from the upper extremities. They are initially affected in cases of hand and forearm infections. (2) Axillary lymph nodes in the anterior (pectoral) group lie around the lateral thoracic artery and vein and receive the lymph from the lateral portion and part of the upper portion of the breast, the anterolateral abdominal wall, and the part above the level of the umbilicus. (3) Axillary lymph nodes in the posterior (subscapular) group lie along the subscapular artery and around the thoracodorsal nerve, and receive the lymph from the back, shoulder, and the posterior chest wall. (4) Axillary lymph nodes in the central group lie in the center of the axillary cavity in the axillary fat, which is the largest group that receives the lymph from the above three groups. (5) Axillary lymph nodes in the apical group lie along the proximal side of the axillary vein, are arranged on the upper portion of the pectoralis minor muscle, and extend to the deep layer of the clavipectoral fascia. They receive the lymph in the central group and some part of the upper portion of the breast. Injuries to the long thoracic nerve surrounding the anterior (pectoral) group and the thoracodorsal nerve adjacent to the

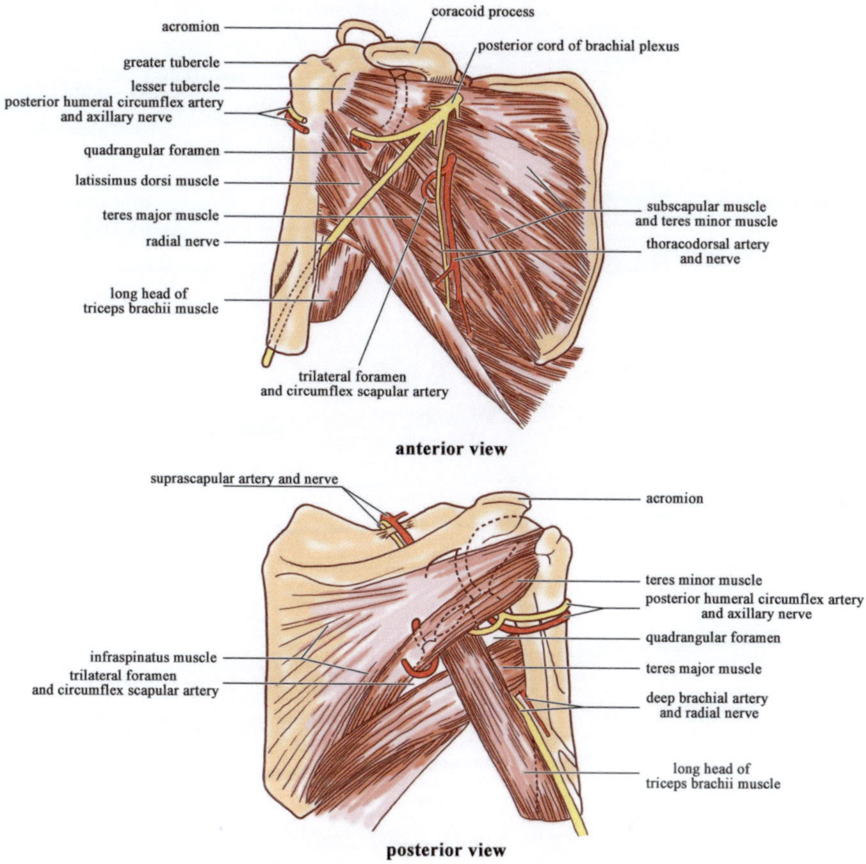

Fig. 3.8 Trilateral foramen and quadrilateral foramen

posterior (subscapular) group should be carefully prevented during the lymph node dissection for radical mastectomy (Fig. 3.9).

Axillary Sheath

The axillary sheath, also known as the cervico-axillary canal, is an extension of the prevertebral fascia in the neck. It encloses the axillary artery, axillary vein, and brachial plexus.

Axillary Artery

The subclavian artery becomes the axillary artery at the lateral border of the first rib, and further the brachial artery after passing the lower margin of the teres major. Marked by the pectoralis minor muscle, the axillary artery is separated into the first, second, and third parts. The first part initiates from its origin to the superior border

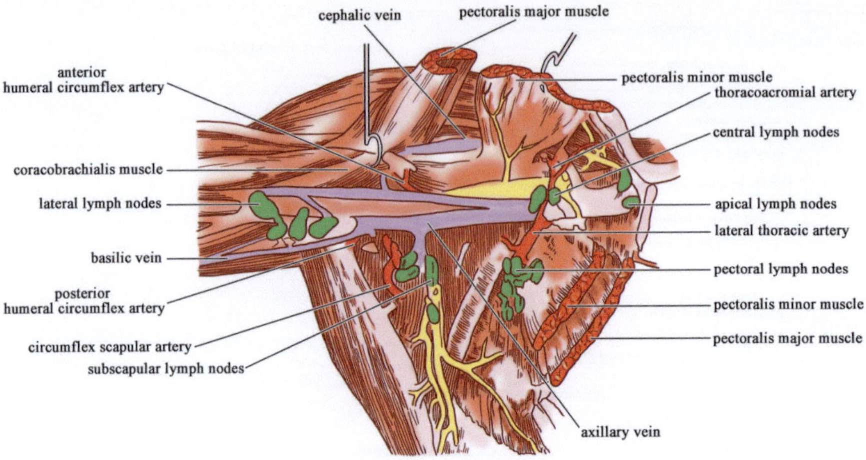

Fig. 3.9 Axillary lymph nodes

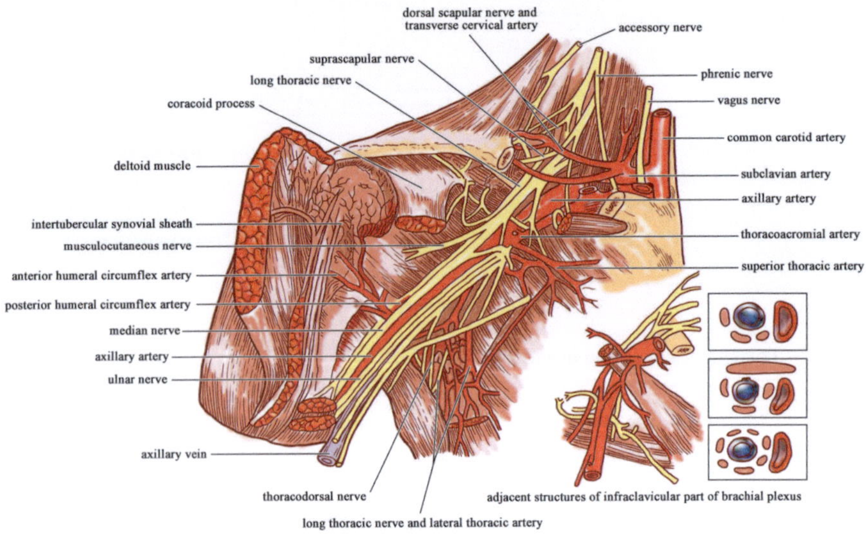

Fig. 3.10 Contents of the axillary cavity and compositions of the brachial plexus

of the pectoralis minor muscle; the second part lies in the deep layer of the pectoralis minor muscle; the third part travels from the inferior border of the pectoralis minor muscle to the inferior border of the teres major. Six branches are given off from the axillary artery during the course, namely the superior thoracic artery, thoracoacromial artery, lateral thoracic artery, subscapular artery, anterior humeral circumflex artery, and posterior humeral circumflex artery (Figs. 3.8 and 3.10).

Axillary Vein

The axillary vein runs anteromedially with the axillary artery. It originates from the brachial vein at the lower border of the teres major and inserts into the lateral border of the first rib, where it becomes the subclavian vein. As the major vein of the upper extremities, the axillary vein conveys the blood from the veins accompanying the axillary artery branches and superficial veins like the cephalic vein and basilic vein.

Branchial Plexus

The branchial plexus starts posterolaterally from the first segment of the axillary artery and then divides into three cords surrounding the second and third segments of the axillary artery. The medial cord is located medial to the axillary artery. It gives off the medial root of the median nerve, ulnar nerve, medial brachial cutaneous nerve, and medial cutaneous nerve of the forearm, all of which supply the upper extremities. The medial pectoral nerve is a branch of the medial cord of the brachial plexus that innervates the pectoralis major and pectoralis minor muscles. The lateral cord is located lateral to the axillary artery and gives off the lateral root of the median nerve, musculocutaneous nerve, and thoracodorsal nerve. The posterior cord is located posterior to the axillary artery and branches into the axillary nerve, radial nerve, and thoracodorsal nerve. The long thoracic nerve is a proximal branch of the brachial plexus and arises from the supraclavicular region (Fig. 3.10).

3.1.5.2 Intercostal Space

The intercostal space, a relatively weak space between two ribs, contains intercostal muscles, intercostal blood vessels, nerves, and connective tissues. The intercostal space varies in width, with a wider upper region and a narrower lower region. Ribs are curved and elastic, and a violent force usually causes rib fractures, especially in the third to eighth ribs due to their large curvatures (Figs. 3.11, 3.12, and 3.13).

The 1st and 2nd intercostal arteries arise from the supreme intercostal artery, a branch of the costocervical trunk of the subclavian artery. The 3rd to the 11th intercostal arteries arise from the posterior intercostal artery. The posterior intercostal arteries arise from the thoracic aorta, with the posterior intercostal veins and intercostal nerves running together in the middle region of the intercostal space. Located in the inner side of the costal angle of the rib, intercostal nerves are surrounded by the posterior intercostal arteries and veins. The posterior intercostal vessels and the intercostal nerves give off smaller branches close to the costal angle of the rib, running forward along the upper edge of the lower rib. The posterior intercostal veins and the corresponding artery and nerves are arranged from superior to inferior in the anterior region of the costal angle of the rib. Intercostal nerves are usually not

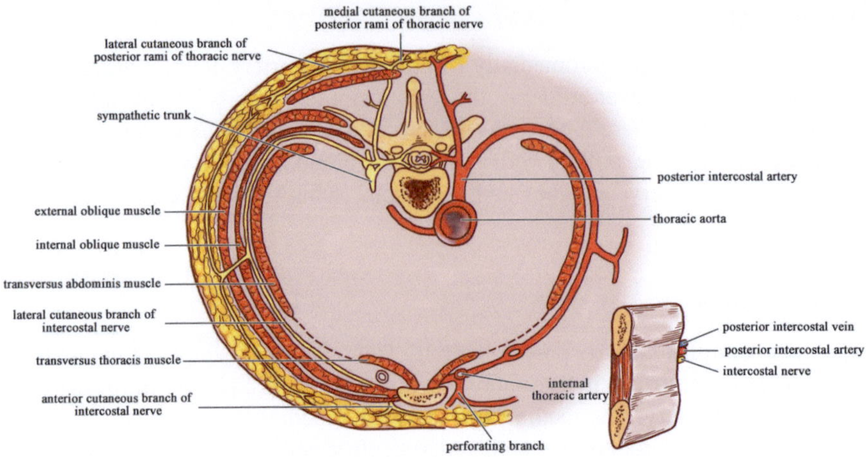

Fig. 3.11 The intercostal space and its contents

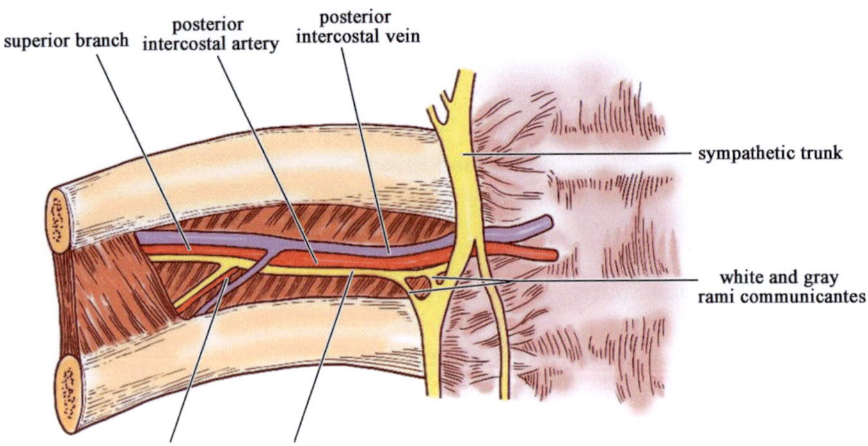

Fig. 3.12 The posterior intercostal vessels and intercostal nerves

covered by the costal groove. The superior and inferior branches of the posterior intercostal arteries (except for the lower three pairs) diverge from the anterior intercostal branches of the internal thoracic artery at the medial third of the corresponding intercostal space. In order to minimize potential injury to the blood vessels and nerves, thoracentesis is most recommended to be performed between the 8th and 9th intercostal spaces in the mid-scapular line at the upper border of the rib. A needle is recommended to be inserted through a point between the upper and lower ribs for anterior thoracentesis (Fig. 3.13).

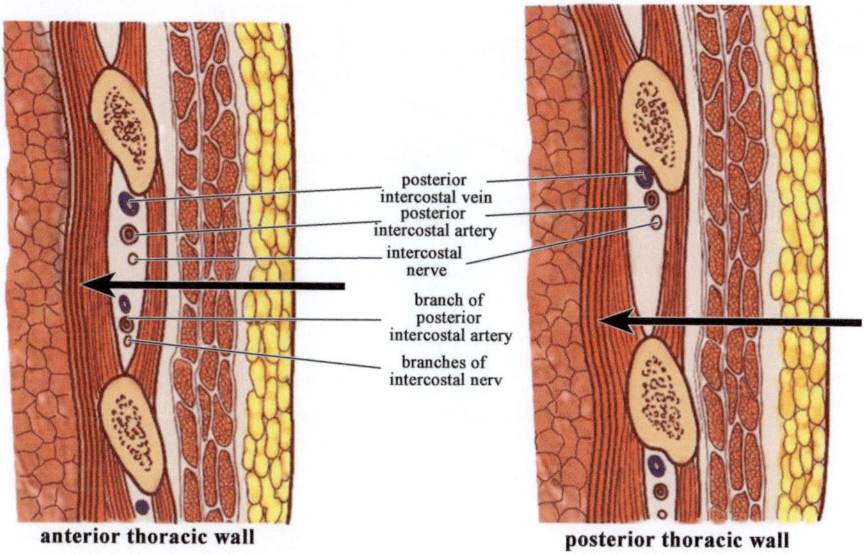

Fig. 3.13 The sectional chest wall showing intercostal structures and a puncture approach (arrow)

3.1.6 Anatomy of the Chest Wall

3.1.6.1 Objective

To dissect the anterior chest wall and axillary region, and to understand the structural characteristics of the chest wall and the borders and contents of the axillary cavity.

3.1.6.2 Position

Supine position.

3.1.6.3 Anatomical Landmarks

To identify anatomical landmarks and lines of the chest wall.

3.1.6.4 Dissection Procedures

Step 1. Remove the skin.

Skin incisions are made as displayed in Fig. 3.14. Lift the skin at the junction of the transverse incision and the median longitudinal incision. Fiber bundles

Fig. 3.14 Skin incisions in the anterior chest wall

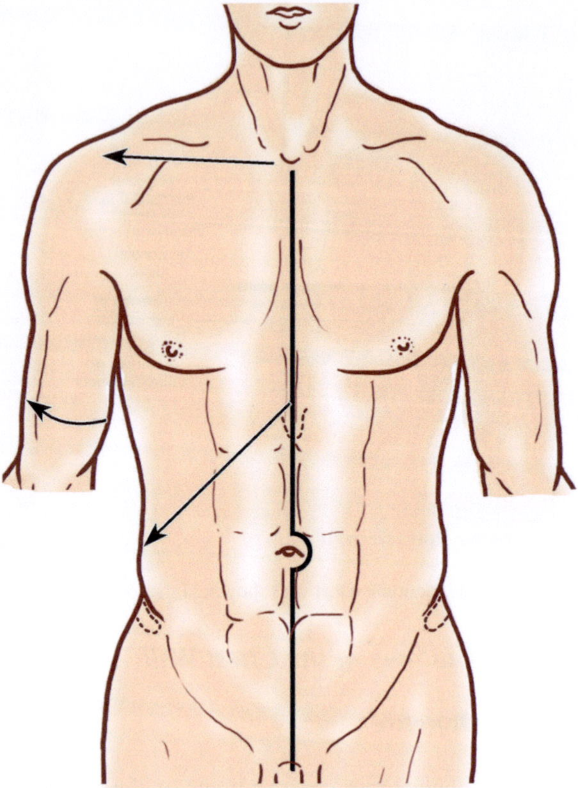

connecting the skin to the superficial fascia are excised. Except for the male nipples and female breast structures, the skin of the chest wall is removed.

Step 2. Remove the superficial fascia.

Dissect one or two branches of the cutaneous nerves and blood vessels at the lateral border of the sternum close to the midaxillary line. The lateral cutaneous branch of the second intercostal nerve is known as the intercostobrachial nerve, which supplies the skin of the axilla and the inner side of the upper extremity. Gently separate the superficial fascia at the deltopectoral groove between the deltoid and pectoralis major muscle using a tweezer, where the cephalic vein passes upwards. The origin of the platysma and several branches of the supraclavicular nerve are observed beneath the clavicle. For the dissection of the female breast, fat tissues are removed radially from the surroundings of the nipples. The mammary gland lobe and its ducts are separated. During their separation from the pectoral fascia, the Cooper's ligaments are observed.

Step 3. Turn the pectoralis major muscle.

Remove the superficial fascia on the surface of the pectoralis major muscle to show its origin and insertion, as well as the orientation of muscle bundles. Insert the fingers into the deep surface of the pectoralis major muscle from the lower edge, and bluntly separate it from the deeply located pectoralis minor. Cut off the pectoralis major muscle at 1 cm away from its origin, while raising up the lower portion. Prevent potential damages to the cephalic vein running between the upper portion of the pectoralis major muscle and the deltoid muscle and blood vessels and nerves piercing into the deep layer of the pectoralis major muscle.

Step 4. Turn the pectoralis minor.

Observe the origin and insertion of the pectoralis minor. The lateral thoracic artery and pectoral lymph nodes are visible near the lower portion of the pectoralis minor. Bluntly dissect the pectoralis minor alongside the deep surface using your fingers. Cut off the origin of the pectoralis minor and raise it up to expose the axillary cavity.

Step 5. Dissect the axillary cavity.

Blood vessels and nerves present in the axillary cavity are surrounded by a large amount of fat tissues and axillary lymph nodes. Identify the location of each group of axillary lymph nodes during the dissection of the axillary cavity.

Identification of the axillary artery and its branches. Marked by the pectoralis minor muscle, the axillary artery is separated into the first, second, and third segments. The first segment gives off the superior thoracic artery, which is a small artery supplying the first and second intercostal spaces. It is occasionally absent. The second segment gives off the thoraco-acromial artery and the lateral thoracic artery. The thoraco-acromial artery gives off several branches that supply the pectoralis major muscle, pectoralis minor, acromion, and the shoulder joint. The lateral thoracic artery descends along the lower portion of the pectoralis minor, is larger in females, and gives off branches to supply the breasts. The third segment gives off the subscapular artery, anterior humeral circumflex artery, and posterior humeral circumflex artery. The subscapular artery is large and descends posteroinferiorly along the lower portion of the subscapularis muscle, where the circumflex scapular artery branches. It courses through the trilateral foramen, within the infraspinous fossa of the scapula. The subscapular artery eventually divides into the thoracodorsal artery and accompanies the corresponding nerve, piercing into the deep layer of the latissimus dorsi. The anterior humeral circumflex artery is a small artery passing anterior to the surgical neck of the humerus in the deep layer of the coracobrachialis muscle. It anastomoses with the posterior humeral circumflex artery and supplies the long head of the biceps brachii and the shoulder joint. The posterior humeral circumflex artery is large and runs across the quadrilateral foramen with the axillary nerve. Horizontally passing medial and posterior to the surgical neck of the humerus, it anastomoses with the anterior humeral circumflex artery in the deep layer of the deltoid muscle and supplies the deltoid muscle and shoulder joint.

1. Identify the axillary vein.

   The axillary vein runs anteromedially to the axillary artery. Most of its branches pass along the corresponding arteries. Remove the axillary lymph nodes in the lateral group lying along the distal side of the axillary vein.
2. Identify the brachial plexus and its branches.

The brachial plexus is formed by the anterior rami of the lower four cervical nerves (C5–8) and the first thoracic nerve (T1). They merge in the lateral cervical area to form the superior, middle, and inferior trunks, and each splits into two divisions. The six divisions regroup in the axillary cavity to become the posterior, lateral, and medial cords that enclose the second part of the axillary artery. Except for the long thoracic nerve, nerves innervating the upper extremities all branch from the three trunks of the brachial plexus. The long thoracic nerve arises from the root of the brachial plexus (the anterior rami of cervical spinal nerves). It descends posteriorly to the brachial plexus, into the axillary cavity, and ends on the superficial surface of the serratus anterior muscle. The lateral cord gives off the musculocutaneous nerve and the lateral root of the median nerve. Passing downwards and laterally, the musculocutaneous nerve passes through the coracobrachialis muscle and finally enters the forearm. The medial cord gives off the medial root of the median nerve, ulnar nerve, medial brachial cutaneous nerve, and medial cutaneous nerve of the forearm from lateral to medial. The medial root of the median nerve joins the lateral root anterolaterally to the third segment of the axillary artery and enters the arm. The ulnar nerve enters the arm medial to the axillary artery. The posterior cord divides into the axillary nerve, radial nerve, subscapular nerve, and thoracodorsal nerve. The axillary nerve runs across the quadrilateral foramen with the posterior circumflex humeral artery and pierces into the deep layer of the deltoid muscle. The radial nerve travels posterior to the axillary artery, courses in front of the teres major muscle and latissimus dorsi, and enters the arm. The subscapular nerves have 2–3 branches travelling in front of the subscapularis muscle and into the subscapularis muscle and the teres major muscle. The thoracodorsal nerve travels along with the corresponding artery and into the deep surface of the latissimus dorsi.

3. Identify the apex and walls of the axillary cavity.

   Separate the blood vessels and nerves of the axillary cavity to expose the components of the medial, lateral, and posterior walls. Observe the anterior wall of the axillary cavity after resetting the pectoralis major and minor muscles. Observe the surrounding of the apex of the axillary cavity.

Step 6. Dissect the intercostal spaces.

Peel off the origin of the external oblique muscle of the fifth and sixth ribs to observe its anatomic interaction with the serratus anterior muscle. In the intercostal spaces, the external intercostal muscles between the costal cartilages are replaced by a membranous layer called the external intercostal membrane. Cut off the origin of the external intercostal muscles along the lower edge of the ribs in the third or fourth intercostal spaces, and note that the dissection should not be made too deep. Insert the plates of the tweezers between the deep layer of the external intercostal muscles and the internal intercostal muscles from the anterior intercostal space, and separate them backward and outward. Dissect the external intercostal muscles, and lift them downwards. Observe the different orientations of the fibers of the internal and external intercostal muscles. Dissect an internal intercostal muscle at the lower edge of the rib, and identify the intercostal nerves and posterior intercostal arteries and veins.

3.1.7 Summary

1. Costal cartilage increases the elasticity of the chest wall and thus protects the sternum and ribs. Rib fractures usually cause damages to the intercostal blood vessels and nerves, or even pneumothorax when the pleura is punctured.
2. Lymphatic drainage of the female breast is of great significance in the metastasis of breast cancer. Considering the extensive lymphatic anastomosis, a thorough examination of lymph nodes in both breasts is necessary.
3. The lymph nodes in the axillary cavity are arranged along the blood vessels and nerves. Be careful of the potential damages to nerves in the axillary cavity during the lymph node dissection. Injury to the long thoracic nerve may paralyze the serratus anterior muscle, resulting in scapular winging. Besides, the thoracodorsal nerve that innervates the latissimus dorsi is also vulnerable and should be carefully protected during the surgery.
4. Identifying the structures of the intercostal space, especially the arrangement and courses of the posterior intercostal arteries and veins, and intercostal nerves, is of great significance to select the insertion sites of the needle for chest drainage.

3.2 Clinical Application of Key Anatomical Structures of the Chest Wall

The breast, an important organ of the chest wall, vertically overlies the superficial surface of the pectoral fascia from the second rib to the sixth rib and runs laterally from the parasternal line to the anterior axillary line. Breasts are one of women's secondary sexual characteristics. Breast cancer is a common malignancy and is usually treated with surgery. The modified radical mastectomy can be divided into two types, in which the pectoralis major and minor muscles are both preserved, or only the pectoralis major muscle is preserved. In the following section, we mainly introduce the clinical applied anatomy of the modified radical mastectomy with preservation of the pectoralis major and minor muscles.

A modified radical mastectomy with preservation of the pectoralis major and minor muscles is a procedure in which the entire breast, ipsilateral axillary lymph nodes, and fat tissues, but not the pectoralis major and minor muscles, are preserved. Free flaps within the range of the inferior region of the clavicle to the superior region of the costal arch (from superior to inferior), and the anterior region of the latissimus dorsi to the lateral region of the sternum (from lateral to medial). During axillary lymph node dissection, fat tissue, lymph nodes, lymphatic vessels, and small blood vessels must be removed, and protect the axillary veins, thoracodorsal arteries and veins, thoracodorsal nerves, and long thoracic nerves.

Anatomical characteristics of the modified radical mastectomy

1. A transverse fusiform incision, vertical fusiform incision, or cloverleaf skin incision is made based on tumor location (Fig. 3.15a). Free flaps as mentioned above (Fig. 3.15b).
2. Remove all breast tissues and pectoralis fascia (Fig. 3.15c).

As mentioned before, five groups of axillary lymph nodes are present in the axillary cavity, including the lateral group, anterior (pectoral) group, posterior (subscapular) group, central group, and apical group. During the axillary lymph node dissection, all five groups of axillary lymph nodes are required to be completely excised. Briefly, remove axillary lymph nodes within the range that is delineated by the superficial layer of the serratus anterior muscle medially, the anterior portion of the latissimus dorsi laterally, and the inferior margin of the axillary vein superiorly (Fig. 3.15d), followed by the excision of fat tissues and the complete breasts (Fig. 3.15e, f).

Keep with following recommendations to prevent damages to the axillary veins, thoracic dorsal nerves, thoracic dorsal arteries and veins, and thoracic long nerves during the modified radical mastectomy.

1. Prevent damages to the axillary vein.

   Dissociate till to the apex of the axilla, and carefully cut through the clavipectoral fascia to expose the axillary vein. Care should be taken to separate along the lower portion of the axillary veins, and transect blood vessels draining into the axillary vein and branches of the axillary artery.
2. Prevent damages to the thoracodorsal arteries, vein, and nerve.

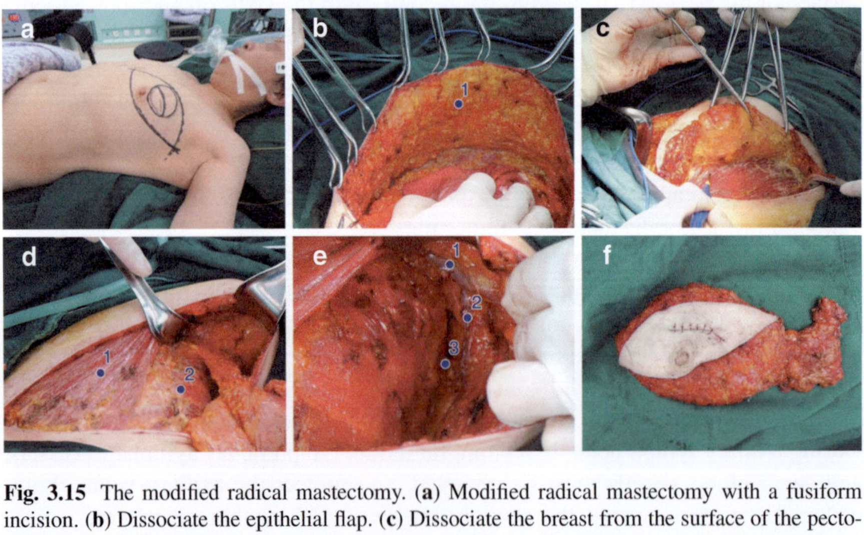

Fig. 3.15 The modified radical mastectomy. (**a**) Modified radical mastectomy with a fusiform incision. (**b**) Dissociate the epithelial flap. (**c**) Dissociate the breast from the surface of the pectoralis major. (**d**) Dissociate axillary lymph nodes and fat tissues (1. the pectoralis major muscle; 2. the serratus anterior muscle). (**e**) Blood vessels and nerves in the axillary cavity after removing the breasts (1. the axillary vein; 2. the thoracodorsal artery, vein, and nerve; 3. the long thoracic nerve). (**f**) Surgical resection specimen

The thoracodorsal artery and vein are branches of the axillary artery and vein, respectively. The thoracodorsal nerve arises from the lateral cord of the brachial plexus and travels along the axillary border of the scapula to the latissimus dorsi. The thoracodorsal artery, vein, and nerve accompany and run along the latissimus dorsi. Be careful to dissociate the lower portion of the axillary vein and expose the thoracodorsal artery, vein, and nerve. Meanwhile, care should be made to dissociate the latissimus dorsi.

3. Prevent damages to the long thoracic nerve.

   The long thoracic nerve arises from the proximal branch of the brachial plexus and descends laterally along the superficial layer of the serratus anterior muscle and innervates it. Care should be taken to identify the serratus anterior muscle during the dissociation along its superficial layer.

Chapter 4
Regional Anatomy of the Abdominal Wall and Its Clinical Application

Shu Han, Mingxin Wen, Lijia Liu, and Yuan Li

4.1 Regional Anatomy of the Abdominal Wall

4.1.1 Boundary

The abdominal wall is superiorly bounded by the xiphoid process and bilateral costal margins; inferiorly by the upper edge of the pubic symphysis, pubic tubercles, inguinal ligaments, anterior superior spine, and iliac crest; and laterally by the midaxillary lines.

4.1.2 Anatomical Landmarks

Bony landmarks for the abdominal wall include the xiphoid process and the costal arch in the upper quadrant, and the iliac crest, anterior superior spine, pubic tubercle, pubic crest, and pubic symphysis in the lower quadrant. The linea alba vertically runs down the deep layer of the midline of the abdomen and separates the rectus abdominis on each side. Fibers of the rectus abdominis are interrupted by 3–5 tendinous intersections. Transverse shallow grooves form when the rectus

S. Han
Zhejiang University School of Medicine, Hangzhou, China
e-mail: han00shu@zju.edu.cn

M. Wen
Shandong University School of Basic Medical Sciences, Jinan, China

L. Liu (✉) · Y. Li
Nanjing Medical University, Nanjing, China
e-mail: drliyuan@njmu.edu.cn

Q. Ding et al. (eds.), *Clinically Oriented Regional Anatomy*,
https://doi.org/10.1007/978-981-95-9888-5_4

abdominis contracts. The umbilicus is located at the midpoint of the anterior midline of the abdomen (at the level of L3–L4).

4.1.3 *Layers*

Layers of the anterolateral abdominal wall vary significantly in different regions. Common surgical incisions on the anterolateral abdominal wall include the upper and lower midline incision, transrectal incision, paramedian incision, Kocher incision, and McBurney incision (Fig. 4.1). It is important to identify the layers and structures of the abdominal wall when performing these incisions.

Generally, there are seven layers of the abdominal wall from superficial to deep, including the skin, superficial fascia (subcutaneous tissue), deep fascia, muscles along with vessels and nerves, transversalis fascia, extraperitoneal fascia (also known as extraperitoneal fat), and peritoneum.

4.1.3.1 Skin

Except for the skin in the umbilical and inguinal regions, the skin of the abdominal wall is thin, elastic, and highly mobile. Sensory nerves of the anterolateral abdominal wall are segmentally distributed. The T6, T8, T10, T12, and L1 nerves supply the skin over the xiphoid process, costal margin, umbilical plane, anterior superior

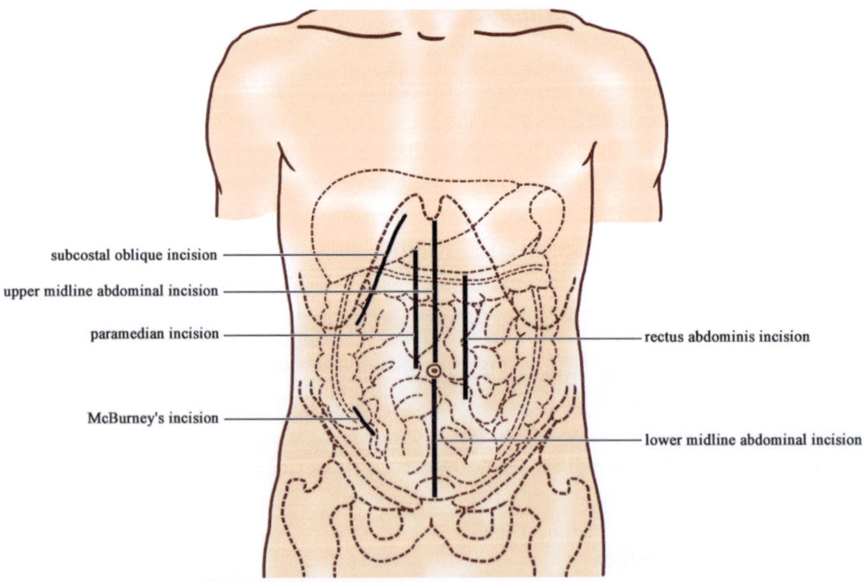

Fig. 4.1 Common surgical incisions on the anterolateral abdominal wall

iliac spine, and pubic symphysis (upper region of the groin), respectively. A sensory disturbance plane in the anterolateral abdominal wall can be identified to assist in determining the location of the thoracic and lumbar spinal cord injuries. In lumbar anesthesia, the plane for nerve block can be identified according to the segmental distribution of sensory nerves.

4.1.3.2 Superficial Fascia (Subcutaneous Tissue)

The superficial fascia of the anterolateral abdominal wall consists of fat and loose connective tissue, and its thickness varies among individuals. The superficial fascia below the umbilicus is divided into the fatty superficial layer (fascia of Camper) and the deep membranous layer (fascia of Scarpa). The fascia of Scarpa attaches to the linea alba in the midline and merges with the fascia lata below the inguinal ligament in the upper thigh. Between the pubic symphysis and pubic tuberosity, the fascia of Scarpa extends downwards with the dartos fascia and the superficial perineal fascia (Colles' fascia). Therefore, urine extravasation, due to the rupture of the urethral bulb, spreads to the ipsilateral anterolateral abdominal wall from inferior to superior but does not cross the linea alba to the contralateral side.

The superficial epigastric artery, superficial epigastric vein, superficial lymphatic vessels, and cutaneous veins pass through the superficial fascia of the anterolateral abdominal wall. The subcutaneous artery, located in the upper quadrant of the anterolateral abdominal wall, is a thin blood vessel that arises from branches of the posterior intercostal artery, subcostal artery, and musculophrenic artery. The superficial epigastric artery and the superficial iliac circumflex artery are two relatively larger subcutaneous arteries found in the lower quadrant of the anterolateral abdominal wall, and they arise from the branches of the femoral artery. The former turns upward from the middle-medial third of the inguinal ligament to the umbilicus, while the superficial iliac circumflex artery runs parallel to the inguinal ligament and extends laterally along the iliac crest.

Superficial veins of the anterolateral abdominal wall are prominent, draining into the periumbilical venous plexus around the umbilical region. Divided by the umbilicus, the superficial veins above it ultimately drain into the axillary vein via the thoracoepigastric vein, and those below the umbilicus drain into the great saphenous vein via the superficial epigastric vein and the superficial iliac circumflex vein, thereby establishing connections with both the inferior vena cava and the superior vena cava. In addition, the paraumbilical veins draining via the periumbilical venous plexus form one of the collaterals of the portal vein by connecting the portal vein, inferior vena cava, and superior vena cava. Dilation of the paraumbilical veins and retrograde flow into the periumbilical venous plexus result in portal hypertension, manifesting as veins radiating around the umbilicus, a condition known as caput medusae (Fig. 4.2).

The superficial lymphatic vessels above the umbilicus ultimately drain into the axillary lymph nodes, and those below the umbilicus drain into the superficial inguinal lymph nodes.

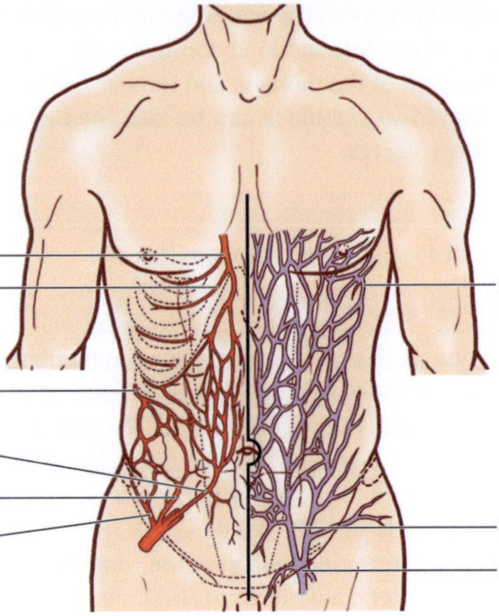

Fig. 4.2 Cutaneous nerves and the superficial veins of the anterolateral abdominal wall

4.1.3.3 Deep Fascia

The deep fascia of the abdomen consists of two layers. The superficial layer is a thin membrane covering the surface of the sarcolemma and aponeurosis of the external abdominal oblique muscle and extending downward to attach to the inguinal ligament. The superficial layer of the deep fascia of the abdomen, together with Scarpa's fascia, helps prevent the extension and displacement of inguinal and femoral hernias.

4.1.3.4 Muscles, Vessels, and Nerves

Based on the anatomical distribution of muscles, vessels, and nerves, the abdominal wall is divided into the rectus sheath, which encloses the rectus abdominis, and the bilateral lateral abdominal walls (Fig. 4.3).

Rectus Sheath

The rectus abdominis sheath is comprised of the anterior wall, rectus abdominis, and posterior wall, arranged in a superficial-to-deep manner.

The anterior wall of the rectus sheath is fused by the aponeurosis of the external abdominal oblique muscle and the anterior portion of the aponeurosis of the internal abdominal oblique muscle. However, approximately 4–5 cm below the umbilicus, it is composed of the aponeurosis of the external abdominal oblique muscle, the

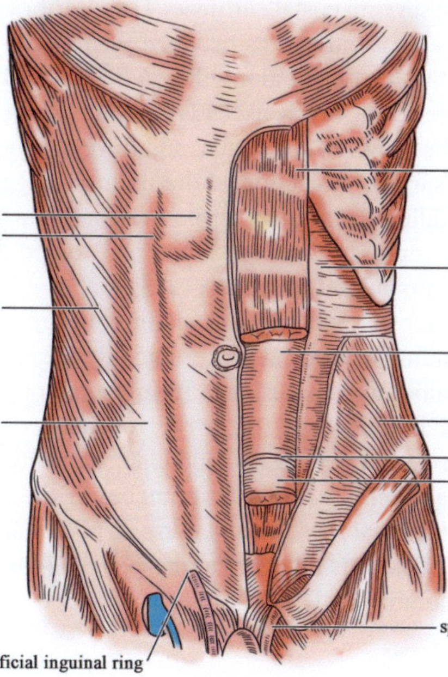

Fig. 4.3 Anatomical structure of the anterolateral abdominal wall

anterior portion of the aponeurosis of the internal abdominal oblique muscle, and the aponeurosis of the transverse abdominis muscle.

The rectus abdominis muscle is a pair of long, flat muscles that widen from inferior to superior. Separated by the linea alba and enclosed by the rectus sheath, the rectus abdominis extends from the pubic symphysis and pubic crest inferiorly and ends at the xiphoid process and costal cartilages of the 5th–7th ribs. Each rectus abdominis muscle is subdivided into four to five muscle bellies by three to four pairs of transverse tendinous intersections. The tendinous intersections are firmly attached to the anterior wall of the rectus sheath but remain unattached to the posterior wall, allowing for free movement of the posterior sheath.

The posterior wall of the rectus sheath is formed by the posterior layer of aponeurosis of the internal oblique muscle and the aponeurosis of transverse abdominis. The anterior wall of the rectus sheath at 4–5 cm above the umbilicus is similarly composed of the posterior layer of aponeurosis of the internal oblique abdominis and the aponeurosis of transverse abdominis. The arcuate line, also known as the semicircular line, is a curved free line situated posterior to the posterior wall of the rectus sheath. Below the arcuate line, the posterior wall of the rectus sheath is absent, leaving the rectus abdominis in direct contact with the transversalis fascia.

The superior epigastric artery ascends, and the inferior epigastric artery descends between the rectus abdominis and the posterior wall of the rectus sheath, which anastomose together at the level of the umbilicus. The superior epigastric artery is a terminal branch of the internal thoracic artery that descends to enter the rectus sheath at the level of the seventh costal cartilage. The inferior epigastric artery arises from the external iliac artery and travels between the transversalis fascia and parietal peritoneum. Traveling vertically along the middle-medial third of the inguinal ligament, the inferior epigastric artery ascends along the medial margin of the deep inguinal ring, pierces the transversalis fascia, and traverses the arcuate line to enter the rectus sheath. The surface projection of the inferior epigastric artery follows a line connecting the middle-medial third of the inguinal ligament to the umbilicus. Damages to the inferior epigastric artery should be avoided during the abdominal paracentesis in the lower quadrant (Fig. 4.4).

The 7th and 8th intercostal nerves travel along the deeper surface of the costal arch from the corresponding intercostal spaces and into the rectus sheath. The 9th to 11th intercostal and subcostal nerves exit from their corresponding intercostal spaces and the inferior margin of the 12th rib, run between the internal oblique abdominis and the transversus abdominis, and enter the rectus sheath from the lateral side of the rectus abdominis. Muscular branches of the 7th to 11th intercostal nerves innervate the intercostal muscles and muscles of the anterolateral abdominal wall, and their anterior cutaneous branches are responsible for the innervation of the skin of the anterior abdominal wall.

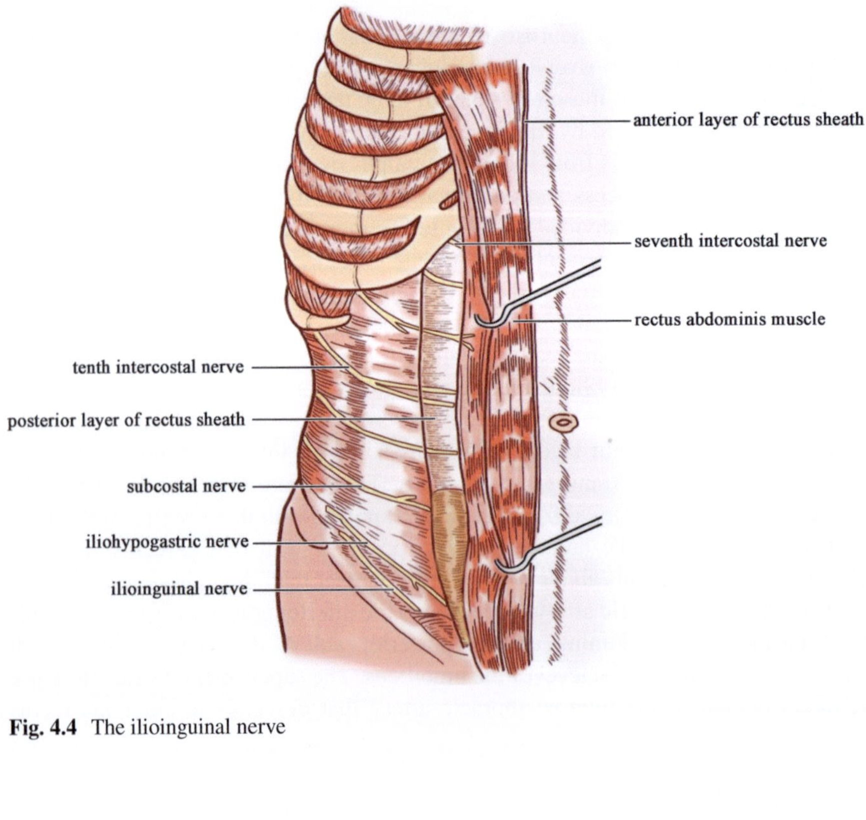

Fig. 4.4 The ilioinguinal nerve

Lateral Abdominal Wall

The lateral abdominal wall is composed of three muscle layers with varying orientations, including external oblique abdominis, internal oblique abdominis, and transverse abdominis (Fig. 4.5). The aponeurosis of three layers of flat muscles forms the rectus sheath at the lateral margin of the rectus abdominis and becomes entwined with the midline of the abdomen, forming the linea alba.

The external oblique muscle is the outermost of the three flat abdominal muscles, with fibers running obliquely downward and medially. It arises from eight fleshy digitations situated laterally to the 5th–12th ribs, and inferiorly and anteriorly runs to end at the superior region of the iliac crest. The superior and posterior portions of the muscle form a thin but firm aponeurosis (Fig. 4.6). The inferior margin of the

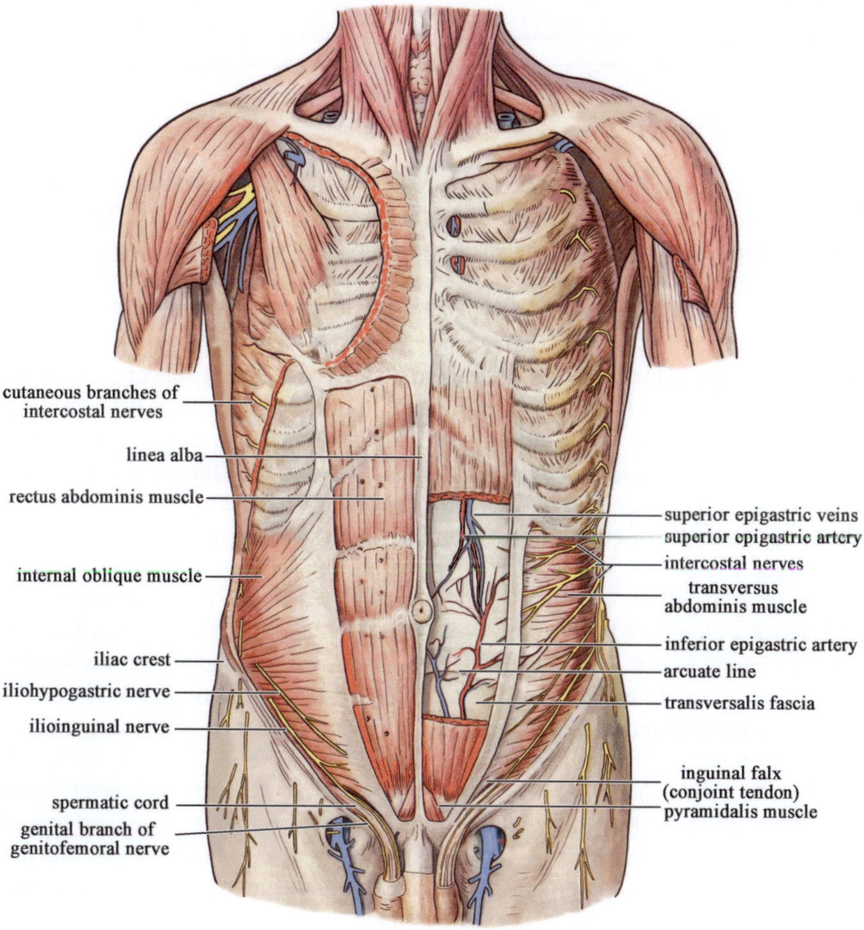

Fig. 4.5 The inguinal ligament

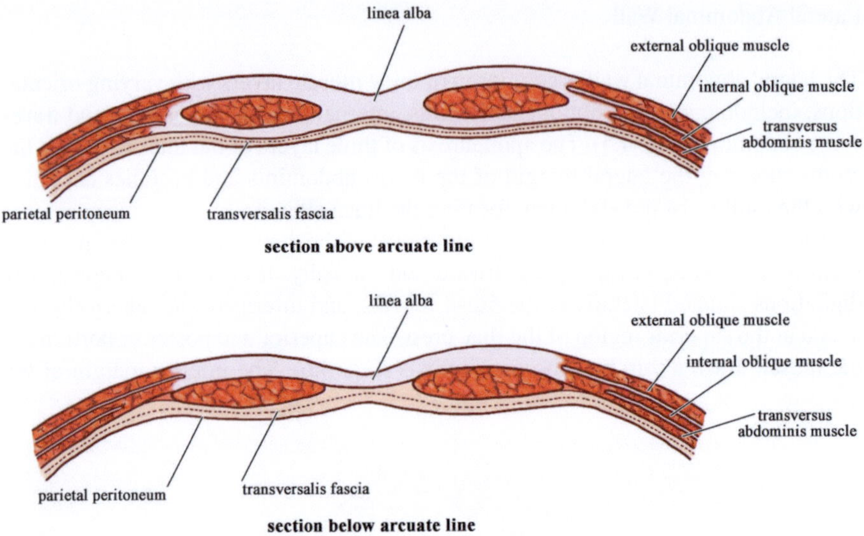

Fig. 4.6 The transversalis fascia

external oblique aponeurosis is thickened and reinforced to form the inguinal ligament between the anterior superior iliac spine and the pubic tubercle. The superficial inguinal ring, also known as the subcutaneous inguinal ring or external inguinal ring, is a triangular opening located superior and lateral to the pubic tubercle. Within the superficial inguinal ring, the medial and lateral crura are attached to the superior portion of the pubic symphysis and the inferior portion of the pubic tubercle, respectively. The reflected inguinal ligament is formed by the inferior reflection of some fibers of the lateral crus, which interlace with the linea alba behind the spermatic cord. The remaining fibers of the lateral crura extend inferiorly and posteriorly and are attached to the pectineal line of the pubis, thus forming the lacunar ligament (also known as Gimbernat's ligament). It extends to connect the pectineal ligament. These ligaments are of great clinical significance in the repair of inguinal and femoral hernias (Fig. 4.7).

The internal oblique abdominis is a flat, fan-shaped muscle extending superiorly and medially alongside the deep surface of the external oblique abdominis. It arises from the lateral half of the inguinal ligament, the iliac crest, and the thoracolumbar fascia, and inserts inferiorly at the lower three ribs. The remaining portion of the internal oblique abdominis extends medially toward the rectus abdominis to form the aponeurosis.

The transversus abdominis is a flat muscle with fibers running transversely from posterior to anterior, deep to the internal oblique. It arises from the inner surfaces of the cartilages of the lower six ribs, the thoracolumbar fascia, the iliac crest, and the lateral third of the inguinal ligament. It forms the aponeurosis lateral to the rectus abdominis.

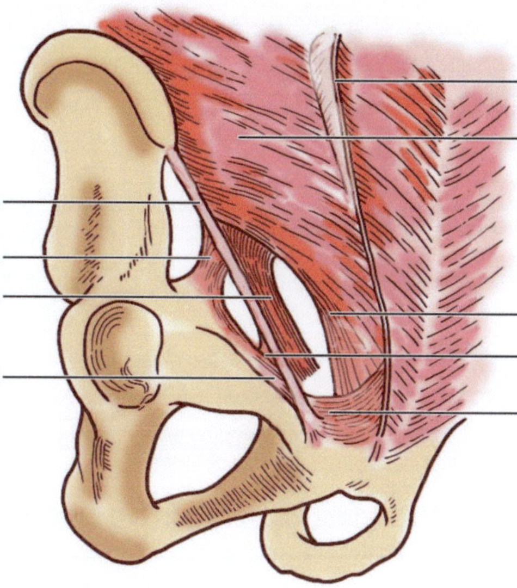

Fig. 4.7 Ligaments in the inguinal region

The internal oblique abdominis and the inferior margin of the transverse abdominis merge to form a convex free margin, known as the arcuate line. The transversus abdominis contributes to the formation of a tendinous structure lateral to the rectus abdominis, called the inguinal falx (or conjoint tendon), which descends to the posterior region of the spermatic cord or round ligament of the uterus. It then descends to the posterior region of the spermatic cord or round ligament of the uterus, inserting into the pectineal line of the pubis, thereby forming the posterior wall of the inguinal canal. When the abdominal wall muscles contract, the free margin of the arcuate line approaches the inguinal ligament to enclose the inguinal canal. Additionally, in males, fibers of the internal oblique contribute to the formation of the cremaster muscle, which surrounds the testis and spermatic cord. The cremaster muscle contracts to raise the testicles (Fig. 4.8).

The posterior intercostal artery and vein, intercostal nerve, deep circumflex iliac artery and vein, iliohypogastric nerve, and ilioinguinal nerve travel between the internal oblique abdominis and the transverse abdominis, both closely contacted via connective tissues. The lower five pairs of the posterior intercostal arteries and subcostal arteries all branch from the thoracic aorta. They anteriorly pass downwards alongside the anterolateral abdominal wall and supply the lateral abdominal muscles. The four pairs of lumbar arteries arise from the abdominal aorta, run laterally to the quadratus lumborum, and enter the lateral abdominal wall. They anastomose with subcostal arteries and then pierce into the lateral abdominal muscles. The deep iliac circumflex artery arises from the external iliac artery, travels superolateral to the anterior superior iliac spine, pierces into the transverse abdominal muscle, and supplies the lateral abdominal muscles, the iliacus muscle, and the psoas major muscle. An incision too large for an appendectomy may damage the deep iliac

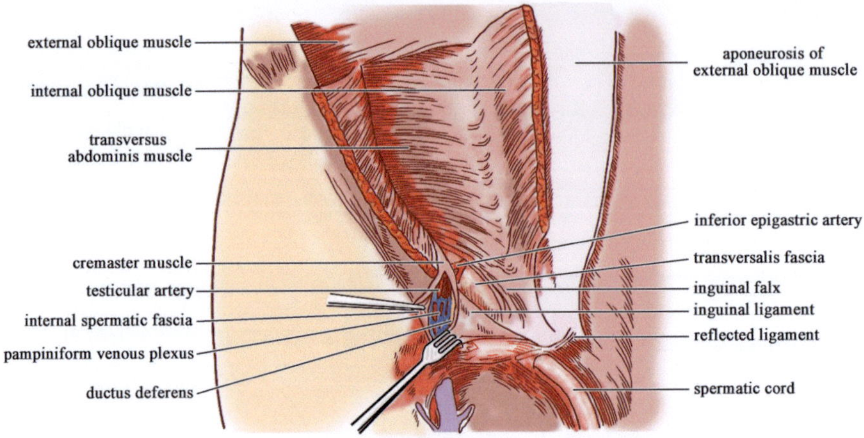

Fig. 4.8 The internal oblique abdominis, transverse abdominis, and inguinal falx

circumflex artery. The arteries supplying the lateral abdominal wall are accompanied by their corresponding veins.

The iliohypogastric nerve and the ilioinguinal nerve originate from the lumbar plexus near the anterior superior iliac spine and penetrate the internal oblique muscle. The iliohypogastric nerve passes into the aponeurosis of the external abdominal oblique muscle 2–3 cm above the superficial inguinal ring. Its anterior cutaneous branch pierces the aponeurosis of the external abdominal oblique muscle to become cutaneous and distributes on the skin above the pubic symphysis. The ilioinguinal nerve travels laterally to the spermatic cord or the round ligament of the uterus through the superficial inguinal ring and distributes on the skin covering the scrotum in males or labium majus in females. In addition, muscular branches sprout from the iliohypogastric nerve and the ilioinguinal nerve that innervate the lateral abdominal muscles. Care should be taken during the inguinal hernia repair to prevent muscle paralysis and/or recurrent hernia due to damage to the iliohypogastric nerve and the ilioinguinal nerve.

4.1.3.5 Transversalis Fascia

The endoabdominal fascia is a layer of deep fascia covering the innermost muscular layer of the abdominal wall and the subphrenic area. It forms the subphrenic fascia beneath the diaphragm, the transversalis fascia situated in the anterolateral abdominal wall, and the fascia covering the quadratus lumborum and the psoas major muscle situated in the posterior abdominal wall. The endoabdominal fascia situated in adjacent areas connect as an integral whole.

The transversalis fascia is a layer of the endoabdominal fascia lining the deep layer of the transverse abdominal muscle. It superiorly connects to the subphrenic fascia and inferiorly expands as the iliac fascia and pelvic fascia. The upper portion of the transversalis fascia is shallow and weak, but thick and strong near the inguinal ligament and lateral to the rectus abdominis muscle. It loosely attaches to the transverse abdominal muscle but tightly connects to the posterior wall of the rectus sheath. The transversalis fascia forms a funnel-shaped protrusion 1.5 cm above the midpoint of the inguinal ligament, that is, the deep inguinal ring (also known as the abdominal inguinal ring or internal abdominal ring). It descends to become the internal spermatic fascia that encloses the spermatic cord.

4.1.3.6 Extraperitoneal Fascia

The extraperitoneal fascia, or extraperitoneal fat, is a loose connective tissue (mainly the fat tissue) situated between the transversalis fascia and the parietal peritoneum. The amount of extraperitoneal fascia is greater in the lower quadrant of the abdomen than in the upper abdomen. The extraperitoneal fascia posteriorly communicates with the loose connective tissue of the retroperitoneal space. The inferior epigastric artery and vein run in this layer, where the testis descends into the scrotum. Due to the loose nature of this fascia, the parietal peritoneum can be easily separated from underlying structures. Therefore, an extraperitoneal approach above the pubic symphysis is usually adopted in bladder surgery and cesarean section to avoid the opening of the peritoneal cavity.

4.1.3.7 Parietal Peritoneum

The parietal peritoneum is the innermost layer of the lateral abdominal wall, which superiorly attaches to the subphrenic fascia and inferiorly connects to the pelvic peritoneum. Below the umbilicus are five longitudinal folds formed by the parietal peritoneum that produce three depressions on the inner surface of the anterior abdominal wall above the groin. (1) The median umbilical fold lies along the midline and extends from the umbilicus to the apex of the urinary bladder, in which the median umbilical ligament (also known as the urachus) is the residue of the allantois obliterated during the embryonic period. (2) A pair of medial umbilical folds line laterally to the median umbilical fold, run obliquely along the inner wall of the pelvic cavity, and extend from the umbilicus to the bilateral sides of the bladder. The ach fold contains the obliterated umbilical artery and is the residue of the umbilical artery obliterated in the embryonic period. (3) A pair of lateral umbilical folds line the outermost surface of the lower anterior abdominal wall, also known as the lateral epigastric folds. They overlie the inferior epigastric artery and vein.

Above the inguinal ligament, the medial and lateral inguinal fossae are situated medially and laterally to the lateral umbilical fold, respectively. They are weak areas in the anterior abdominal wall, where the bulging of the contents forms an inguinal hernia. A pair of supravesical fossae situate bilaterally to the median umbilical fold.

4.1.4 Intermuscular Structures

The linea alba is situated in the midline of the anterior abdominal wall and is a fiber structure formed by the union of the fibers of the bilateral rectus sheath. It extends from the xiphoid process to the pubic symphysis. The width of the linea alba is 1 cm above the umbilicus, but it becomes narrower and thicker below the umbilicus due to its gradual closer contact with the bilateral rectus abdominis. The linea alba is poorly vascularized and innervated, lacks a muscular layer, and thus is usually selected as the approach for abdominal surgeries. However, due to its poor blood supply, incisions in the linea alba tend to be loose and heal more slowly.

4.1.4.1 Umbilicus

The umbilicus, located at the midpoint of the midline of the abdomen, is composed of dense connective tissues, umbilical fascia, and peritoneum. The umbilical region is one of the weak regions of the abdomen. An umbilical hernia occurs when the umbilicus displays developmental dysplasia, or a small gap, if abdominal muscles are not completely fused. Recurrent pregnancy and obesity are the main causes of umbilical hernia.

4.1.5 Inguinal Region

The inguinal region is a triangular area sketched by the line horizontal to the anterior superior iliac spine, the inguinal ligament, and the lateral portion of the rectus abdominal muscle. It contains two vital anatomical structures, namely, the inguinal canal and the inguinal triangle (Hesselbach's triangle). The inguinal canal is formed by the aponeurosis of the external oblique abdominis, where the inferior portions of the internal oblique abdominis and the transverse abdominis cannot connect with the internal part of the inguinal ligament. The spermatic cord in males or the round ligament of the uterus in females penetrates the anterolateral abdominal wall through the inguinal region, where a potential gap is formed to bear a relatively high pressure in the sitting position. Therefore, it is a major weak region in the abdomen.

4.1.5.1 Inguinal Canal

The inguinal canal is a narrow passageway located between muscles and fascia, 1.5 cm above the internal part of the inguinal ligament. In adults, the inguinal canal is usually 4–5 cm long and descends medially and inferiorly. The formation of the inguinal canal in males is linked with the descent of the testes during the embryonic period (Fig. 4.9).

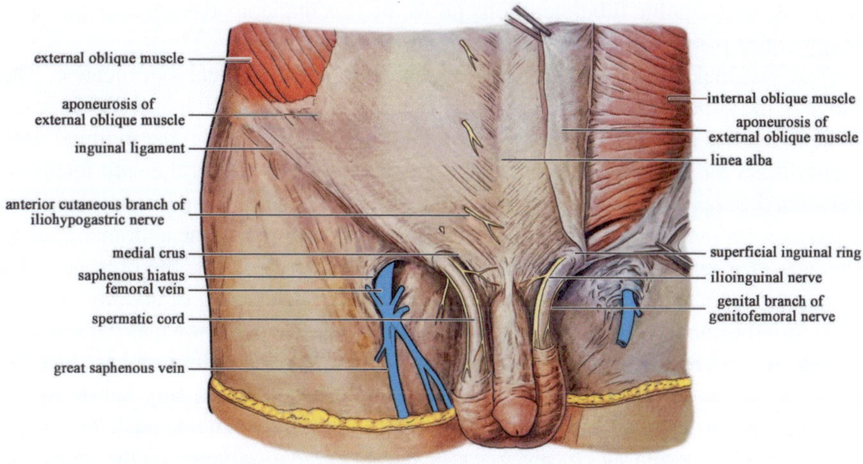

Fig. 4.9 The inguinal canal

The inguinal canal is formed by the deep inguinal ring (internal inguinal ring) and the superficial inguinal ring (external inguinal ring), as well as the anterior wall, posterior wall, and superior wall. (1) The deep inguinal ring is located 1.5 cm above the midpoint of the inguinal ligament and lateral to the inferior epigastric artery. It is a vital structure to include the vas deferens and testicular vessels in males. (2) The superficial inguinal ring is a triangular split formed by the aponeurosis of the external oblique abdominis superolateral to the pubic tubercle. (3) The anterior wall is mainly formed by the aponeurosis of the external oblique abdominis, and fibers of the internal oblique abdominis (lateral third of the inguinal canal only). (4) The posterior wall is mainly formed by the transversalis fascia and conjoin tendon or inguinal falx with varying degrees of development (medial third of the inguinal canal only). (5) The superior wall is mainly composed of the arching fibers of the internal oblique and transversus abdominis muscles. (6) The inferior wall is formed by the inguinal ligament.

The inguinal canal contains the spermatic cord in males or the round ligament of the uterus in females, as well as the ilioinguinal nerve and the genital branch of the genitofemoral nerve. The spermatic cord in males is formed by the vas deferens, vas deferens artery and vein, testicular artery and vein, pampiniform plexus, nerves, lymphatic vessels, and remaining components of the vaginal process (or processus vaginalis). Three layers of sheaths cover the spermatic cord as follows: (1) the internal spermatic fascia that is derived from the transversalis fascia and encloses the spermatic cord at the deep inguinal ring, (2) the cremasteric muscle that is formed by the muscle fibers of the internal oblique abdominis and the inferior margin of the transverse abdominis, and (3) the external spermatic fascia that is derived from the aponeurosis of the external oblique abdominis and encloses the spermatic cord at the superficial inguinal ring. The round ligament of the uterus often fuses with the walls of the inguinal canal and may gradually regress. Alternatively, it may terminate at the pubic tubercle, mons pubis, or subcutaneous tissues near the labia majora after passing through the superficial inguinal ring.

The inguinal canal is an anatomical region of great clinical significance. The range of the superior wall of the inguinal canal (composed of the internal abdominal oblique muscle and the transverse abdominal muscle) attached to the inguinal ligament differs individually. Therefore, the morphology and size of the split localized between the superior and inferior walls of the inguinal canal vary a lot, ranging from 1 cm to 3 cm in height. The inguinal canal is a weak region of the abdomen, due to the lack of a muscular layer in the anterior and posterior walls, the presence of a triangular superficial inguinal ring, and the potential protrusion of abdominal contents into the canal. Hernia often occurs in the inguinal canal, known as the inguinal hernia. An indirect inguinal hernia develops when the abdominal organs, like the intestines or the omentum, protrude through the deep inguinal ring lateral to the inferior epigastric artery and into the inguinal canal. These contents push the peritoneum to form a hernia sac. In severe cases, hernia contents covered by the spermatic fascia may even extend into the scrotum through the superficial inguinal canal.

4.1.5.2 Inguinal Triangle

The inguinal triangle (Hesselbach's triangle) is situated in the medial part of the inguinal region, surrounded by the inferior epigastric artery, the lateral part of the rectus abdominis, and the medial part of the inguinal ligament. The superficial and deep layer of the inguinal triangle is formed by the aponeurosis of the external oblique abdominis and the transversalis fascia and inguinal falx, respectively.

The inguinal triangle is a weak region that can be projected to the superficial inguinal ring in the superficial layer of the anterior abdominal wall. A direct inguinal hernia occurs when the abdominal organs, like the intestines or the omentum, superiorly protrude through the inguinal triangle medial to the inferior epigastric artery, forming a hemispherical, reversible sac in the medial part of the inguinal region. Therefore, the direct inguinal hernia is considered incomplete, as it connects directly through the posterior wall of the inguinal canal, rather than its full-length passage. A direct inguinal hernia protrudes medially to the inferior epigastric artery, and an indirect inguinal hernia protrudes laterally. As a result, the inferior epigastric artery is a landmark for discriminating a direct inguinal hernia from an indirect type.

4.1.6 Anatomy of the Abdominal Wall

4.1.6.1 Objective

To dissect the anterolateral abdominal wall, explore its structures and layers, identify common surgical abdominal incision sites, and understand the rectus sheath, inguinal canal, and inguinal triangle.

4.1.6.2 Position

Supine position.

4.1.6.3 Anatomical Landmarks

Palpate the anatomical landmarks on the human body and observe the anatomical lines of the anterolateral abdominal wall.

4.1.6.4 Dissection Procedures

Removal of the Skin

Three surgical abdominal incisions are made as follows: (1) cut to make a longitudinal incision alongside the midline of the abdomen from the xiphoid process to the upper edge of pubic symphysis; (2) cut to make an incision that descends laterally along the costal arch to the midaxillary line; (3) cut to make an incision alongside the inguinal ligament that ascends laterally from the upper edge of pubic symphysis to the anterior superior spine; (4) remove the abdominal skin laterally along each surgical incision.

Dissection of the Superficial Blood Vessels and the Cutaneous Nerves Situated in the Superficial Fascia

Step 1. Make a transverse incision through the subcutaneous tissue below the level of the umbilicus, and insert your fingers between the fascia of Scarpa and the aponeurosis of the external abdominal oblique muscle to bluntly separate them inferolaterally. Observe the attachment of the fascia of Scarpa to the linea alba, the inguinal ligament, and the fascia lata, and its descent between the pubic symphysis and pubic tubercle to the scrotum.

Step 2. Remove the subcutaneous tissues and dissect the superficial blood vessels and the cutaneous nerves. Identify the anterior and lateral cutaneous branches of the seventh to 11th intercostal nerves on both sides of the midline of the abdomen, and at the extension of the midaxillary line of the anterolateral abdominal wall, respectively. Then, identify the anterior cutaneous branch of the iliohypogastric nerve above the medial crura of the superficial inguinal ring, and be careful to protect the superficial inguinal ring. In the subcutaneous tissues of the lower abdomen, identify the courses and branches of the superficial epigastric artery and vein that ascend medially at the mid-segment of the inguinal ligament, and the superficial circumflex iliac artery and vein that ascend laterally. The groin flaps are primarily supplied by the superficial epigastric artery and the superficial circumflex iliac artery.

Dissection of the External Abdominal Oblique Muscle and the Inguinal Region

Step 1. Using the scalpel handle, carefully separate the inner and outer sides of the spermatic cord at the superficial inguinal ring, exposing its structure. After clearing away the remaining parts of the exposed external oblique abdominis, observe its origin, the orientation of muscle fascicles, and the aponeurosis. Cut off the starting point of the ribs superolateral to the external oblique abdominis, and raise up the external oblique abdominis to the top of the iliac crest. Then, free the aponeurosis of the external oblique abdominis 1.5 cm above the inguinal ligament, and inferiorly, dissect it inward to the outer edge of the rectus sheath. During the dissection, be careful to protect the iliohypogastric nerve and the ilioinguinal nerve. In addition, cut a semi-circular incision above the superficial inguinal ring to carefully preserve its intact structure.

Step 2. Raise up the external oblique abdominis medially, and cut open the anterior wall of the inguinal canal. Observe the origin of the internal oblique abdominis from the inguinal ligament, and its involvement in the formation of the anterior wall of the inguinal canal. Identify the ilioinguinal nerve on the surface of the spermatic cord, and the iliohypogastric nerve superiorly parallel to the ilioinguinal nerve. Examine the superior wall of the inguinal canal, particularly the inferior portions of the internal oblique and transverse abdominis muscles. Subsequently, identify the cremaster muscle originating from the internal oblique abdominis and the transverse abdominis and descending alongside the spermatic cord. Free and raise up the spermatic cord to reveal the inferior and posterior wall of the inguinal canal. Observe the localization of the inguinal falx and the size of the split localized between the superior and inferior walls of the inguinal canal. Reflect the inferior epigastric vessels, exposing the deep inguinal ring lateral to them. Observe the inguinal triangle (Hesselbach's triangle) surrounded by the inferior epigastric artery, the lateral part of the rectus abdominis muscle, and the medial part of the inguinal ligament. Note that the superficial and deep layers of the inguinal triangle are formed by the aponeurosis of the external oblique abdominis, and the transversalis fascia and inguinal falx, respectively.

Dissection of the Muscles, Blood Vessels, and Nerves of the Anterolateral Abdominal Wall

Observe the courses of fan-like fibers of the internal oblique abdominis. Make an incision along the inferior margin of the costal arch. Cut off the attachment of the internal oblique abdominis from the midaxillary line, and downward until the anterior superior spine, where a horizontal incision is made lateral to the rectus sheath. All incisions are superficially made to prevent damage to the transverse abdominis or even the peritoneal cavity. Then, carefully raise up the internal oblique abdominis medially. Above the level of the anterior superior iliac spine, the internal oblique abdominis is closely connected to the transverse abdominis. This region contains nerves and vessels that travel here, including the intercostal nerves, posterior intercostal vessels, and deep circumflex iliac vessels that ascend from the anterior superior iliac spine to the lateral abdominis. Notably, the orientation of the muscle fibers of the internal oblique abdominis differs from that of the transverse abdominis. According to the above anatomical features, identify the internal oblique abdominis and the transverse abdominis, and separate them from the vessels and nerves attached to the surface of the transverse abdominis. Below the level of the anterior superior iliac spine, the internal oblique abdominis is connected to the transverse abdominis more closely. Due to the same orientation of muscle fibers and lack of blood vessels and nerves, the internal oblique abdominis and the transverse abdominis below the level of the anterior superior iliac spine cannot be forcibly separated. Then, observe the courses of the intercostal nerves, posterior intercostal vessels, and deep circumflex iliac vessels, and the orientation of the muscle fibers of the transverse abdominis and those that finally form the aponeurosis.

Dissection of the Rectus Sheath and Rectus Abdominis Muscle

Make a 0.5 cm longitudinal incision on both sides of the linea alba, followed by a 1–2 cm transverse incision at its upper and lower ends. Reflect the anterior layer of the rectus sheath laterally. Carefully dissect the connection between the tendinous intersections and the anterior layer of the rectus sheath, using blunt dissection for any residual attachments. Gently elevate the exposed rectus abdominis muscle and observe the course of the superior and inferior epigastric vessels in the posterior layer, along with the distribution of intercostal nerves penetrating the rectus sheath. At 4–5 cm above the level of the umbilicus, carefully dissect the transversalis fascia to expose the arcuate line in the posterior layer of the rectus sheath. At last, measure the widths of the linea alba above and below the level of the umbilicus.

4.2 Clinical Application of Key Anatomical Structures of the Abdominal Wall

With the widespread adoption of laparoscopic techniques in clinical surgery, laparoscopic inguinal hernia repair has become increasingly common. The anterior approach is conventionally adopted in the dissection of the abdominal wall. Here, we mainly describe the laparoscopic view of inguinal regions using the posterior approach, and the key sites of the inguinal region, serving as landmarks for the laparoscopic surgery of the abdomen, should be carefully identified and protected. Through a detailed introduction to the regional anatomy of abdominal wall, this chapter lays the foundation for performing laparoscopic surgery of the abdomen and planning the anterior approach for conventional abdominal surgery.

Here, we mainly describe the transabdominal preperitoneal (TAPP) repair for inguinal hernias. First, the peritoneal space is observed under the laparoscope, and the five longitudinal folds and three depressions should be identified. The median umbilical fold is the landmark for the linea alba, sided by a pair of medial umbilical folds. The lateral umbilical folds are situated in the outermost surface of the lower anterior abdominal wall (Fig. 4.10a). An overly deep incision in the lateral

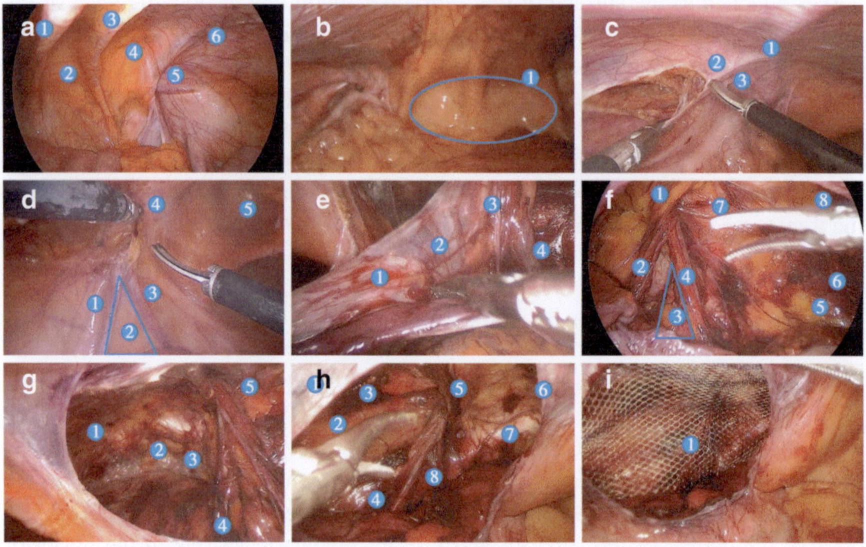

Fig. 4.10 TAPP repair for inguinal hernias. (**a**) Key anatomical structures of the inguinal region as observed laparoscopically (*1*. the median umbilical fold; *2*. the supravesical fossa; *3*. the medial umbilical folds; *4*. the medial inguinal fossa; *5*. the lateral inguinal fossa, with herniation of the right indirect inguinal hernia; *6*. the lateral umbilical folds covering the anteriorly located inferior epigastric artery). (**b**) Laparoscopic view of the supravesical fossa in the inguinal region, highlighting (*1*. the supravesical fossa). (**c**) Laparoscopic view of an indirect inguinal hernia (*1*. the inferior epigastric vessels; *2*. the left indirect inguinal hernia; incise the peritoneum from the intra-abdominal projection of the anterior superior iliac spine to 1–2 cm above the deep inguinal ring, protecting the medially situated inferior epigastric vessels covered by the lateral umbilical folds; *3*. the deep inguinal ring). (**d**) Laparoscopic view of the direct inguinal hernia (*1*. spermatic vessels; *2*. the Triangle of Doom; *3*. the vas deferens; *4*. the inferior epigastric vessels; *5*. the left direct inguinal hernia; a defect of the inguinal triangle, and the protrusion of the peritoneum). (**e**) Laparoscopic view of the sac of the indirect inguinal hernia, the vas deferens and the spermatic vessels (*1*. the sac of the right indirect inguinal hernia, i.e., the peritoneum; *2*. the internal spermatic fascia; *3*. spermatic vessels; *4*. the vas deferens). (**f**) Laparoscopic view of the anterolateral peritoneal space in the inguinal region (*1*. the inferior epigastric vessels; *2*. the vas deferens; *3*. the triangle of doom; *4*. spermatic vessels; *5*. the Bogros space; *6*. the triangle of pain; *7*. the deep inguinal ring connecting the inferior epigastric vessels, the vas deferens, and the spermatic vessels; *8*. the iliopubic tract). (**g**) Laparoscopic view of the anteromedial peritoneal space in the inguinal region (*1*. the Retzius space medial to the inferior epigastric vessels; *2*. the pubis symphysis; *3*. the pectinate ligament; *4*. the umbilicovesical fascia that contains the bladder within the deep layer; *5*. the inferior epigastric vessels). (**h**) The myopectineal orifice (*1*. the inguinal falx; *2*. the iliopsoas muscle; *3*. the indirect inguinal hernia triangle; *4*. the myopectineal orifice; *5*. the direct inguinal hernia triangle; *6*. the lateral part of the rectus abdominis muscle; *7*. the pectinate ligament; *8*. the femoral triangle). (**I**) Placement of a mesh that fully covers the myopectineal orifice and extends to overlap the surrounding tissues

umbilical folds should be avoided to prevent damage to the inferior epigastric vessels running anteriorly. The five folds produce three depressions (fossae) in the pelvic floor, namely the supravesical fossa, the medial inguinal fossa, and the lateral inguinal fossa (Fig. 4.10a, b). The supravesical fossa is situated between the two medial umbilical folds. It is a depression containing the bladder and anteriorly protected by the rectus abdominis muscle. Dissect the peritoneum medially until reaching the site of the medial umbilical ligament, aiming to prevent potential damage to the bladder. The medial inguinal fossa is a depression situated between the medial and lateral umbilical folds, and a direct inguinal hernia often develops here. The lateral inguinal fossa is a depression situated laterally to the lateral umbilical folds, and an indirect inguinal hernia often develops here. The peritoneum is in place, where the spermatic cord in males or the round ligament of the uterus in females can be observed. The anterior superior iliac spine can be palpated here during TAPP repair for inguinal hernias, and its abdominal projection serves as the lateral endpoint of the peritoneal incision.

Second, observe the site, range, and content of the inguinal hernia, and identify a direct or indirect inguinal hernia. Indirect inguinal hernia occurs lateral to the lateral umbilical folds or the inferior epigastric vessels (Fig. 4.10c). The abdominal contents protrude through the deep inguinal ring, which is an oval split in the transversalis fascia conveying the inferior epigastric artery, the vas deferens, and the spermatic vessels. The spermatid cord in males or the round ligament of the uterus in females passes through the deep inguinal ring. The transversalis fascia surrounding the deep inguinal ring descends to combine with the internal spermatic fascia. Direct inguinal hernia develops between the medial and lateral umbilical folds (Fig. 4.10d). Hernia sacs detected both lateral to the lateral umbilical folds, and between the medial and lateral umbilical folds are termed Pantaloon hernia. Femoral hernias occur in the femoral canal, which is bounded by the pectinate ligament and the iliopubic tract. Females are more prone to femoral hernia. Herniated extraperitoneal fat is usually found in the hernia sac, and a part of the iliopubic tract can be dissected if the reduction is challenging. During the repair of a femoral hernia, do not damage branches arising from the femoral vessels. It is necessary to detect any potential abdominal wall defects in the contralateral inguinal region to prevent missed diagnoses of asymptomatic patients. A hidden hernia, often undetectable by preoperative physical examinations or auxiliary examinations, should be repaired as well.

Third, cut open the peritoneum 1–2 cm above the deep inguinal ring and dissect it from the medial umbilical folds to the anterior superior spine. Be cautious to protect the inferior epigastric vessels overlaid by the lateral umbilical folds. Expose the preperitoneal space after freeing the superiorly and inferiorly situated peritoneal flaps. During the repair of a direct inguinal hernia situated medial to the medial umbilical folds, the peritoneum is also cut laterally to prevent damage to the bladder.

Fourth, free the preperitoneal space. After incising the peritoneum to repair an indirect inguinal hernia, the space on both sides of the hernia sac, known as the Bogros space, is then opened (Fig. 4.10e). The Bogros space, located lateral to the inferior epigastric vessels, is easily separated (Fig. 4.10f). Dissect the lateral peritoneal flap inferiorly to the level of the mid-iliopsoas muscle, and taking care to avoid damaging the nerves in the triangle of pain, which is bounded superolaterally by the spermatic vessels and inferiorly by the iliopubic tract (Fig. 4.10f). The lateral femoral cutaneous nerve and the femoral branch of the genitofemoral nerve traverse the triangle of pain. The genitofemoral nerve originates from the lumbar plexus and divides into the femoral and genital branches before entering the deep inguinal ring. The femoral branch pierces the femoral sheath and provides sensory innervation to the superior skin of the thigh. Damage to this branch causes hyperesthesia in the femoral triangle. The genital branch enters the inguinal canal and innervates the cremaster muscle, scrotum, and medial skin of the thigh. Damage to this branch causes ejaculation disorders and painful ejaculation. The lateral femoral cutaneous nerve also arises from the lumbar plexus and runs through the iliacus muscle anteriorly below the iliopubic tract, supplying sensation to the lateral skin of the thigh. It is more easily damaged during the hernia repair due to the superficial anatomic localization. Therefore, in all surgical procedures of hernia repair, it is recommended to attach the peritoneum posterior to the transversalis fascia; meanwhile, the transversalis fascia and the extraperitoneal fat should be protected to avoid postoperative chronic pain.

Fifth, free the anteromedial peritoneal space that is medial to the inferior epigastric vessels. Free the medial peritoneal flap downward and medially to the Retzius space, and expose the pectineal ligament and the pubic symphysis to the contralateral side of the alba linea (Fig. 4.10g). The medial separation should be performed in the loose space between the transversalis fascia and the umbilicovesical fascia. Overly deep dissection may damage the bladder. Carefully protect the corona mortis (or circle of death) during dissection of the Retzius space. This a ring-shaped vascular structure situated on the surface of the pectineal ligament. The corona mortis is a variant vascular anastomosis between the external iliac vessels (either arterial or venous) and the variable and thick obturator vasculature (either arterial or venous). It is situated posteriorly to the superior pubic rami, connects to the inferior epigastric vessels superiorly and the obturator vessels inferiorly. The corona mortis is highly susceptible to injury during the hernia repair, potentially retracting into retraction into the obturator foramen and uncontrollable hemorrhage. If not identified promptly, injury to the corona mortis may result in postoperative massive hematomas or even death.

Sixth, remove the hernia sac. The sac of an indirect inguinal hernia is located lateral to the inferior epigastric artery, with abdominal contents protruding into the inguinal canal through the deep inguinal ring. Subsequently, a laparoscopic high ligation of the hernia sac is performed, a procedure known as the parietalization of the spermatic cord. In summary, the sac of the indirect inguinal hernia is first reduced from the inguinal canal to the deep inguinal ring, followed by the separation of posteriorly located spermatic vessels and vas deferens down to 6 cm below the deep inguinal ring. This step is crucial to ensuring a flat placement of a mesh in a sufficiently large space, thereby preventing mesh curling and subsequent hernia recurrence. The sac of the indirect inguinal hernia is closely connected to the spermatic cord, without a membranous separation. Care must be taken to avoid pulling the spermatic cord during the careful ligation of the sac in the space containing the sac, spermatic vessels, and vas deferens, as this may cause damage to the spermatic vessels or the vas deferens. The Triangle of Doom is an anatomical region bounded by the vas deferens medially and spermatic vessels laterally, which converge at the deep inguinal ring and enter the inguinal canal. This triangle contains the external iliac arteries and veins, and its damage may cause life-threatening hemorrhage. The sac of the direct inguinal hernia is situated in the inguinal triangle. In the absence of posterior localization of the spermatic cord, its reduction is relatively straightforward after separating the peritoneum in the inguinal triangle, extraperitoneal fat, and transversalis fascia. A pseudo-sac may present after the sac of the direct inguinal hernia is reduced, as an obviously thickened transversalis fascia protruding into the preperitoneal space. Reducing a large-volume pseudo-sac creates a sizable peritoneal space where fluid may accumulate to cause hematoma formation that can be prevented by perioperatively stretching the loose transversalis fascia into the abdominal cavity and fixing it with the pectinate ligament or the rectus abdominis muscle.

Notably, the iliopubic tract is a special anatomic structure during the laparoscopic inguinal hernia repair. It is a layer of the transversalis fascia covering the posterior part of the inguinal ligament, and both have the same orientation. The iliopubic tract and the inguinal ligament divide the medial fascial defect into the superior direct hernia and the inferior femoral hernia.

Regardless of whether it is an indirect inguinal hernia, a direct inguinal hernia, or a femoral hernia, the contents in all the sacs protrude towards the body surface through the myopectineal orifice (MPO). The MPO is a congenitally weak area bounded by the rectus abdominis medially, the iliopsoas muscle laterally, the inguinal falx superiorly, and the pectinate ligament inferiorly (Fig. 4.10h). There are no muscle fibers in the MPO, and the pressure from the abdomen is resisted by the transversalis fascia. The laparoscopic inguinal hernia repair is performed under the principle of using a mesh to simulate the role of the transversalis fascia, covering the MPO and overlapping the surrounding tissues (Fig. 4.10i).

Chapter 5
Regional Anatomy of the Limbs and Its Clinical Application

Min Zhu, Huanghe Song, Guqi Hong, and Junjie Zou

5.1 Regional Anatomy of the Limbs

The four limbs, divided into upper and lower, are connected to the trunk. For humans, upright walking and labor have transformed upper limbs into organs, not only providing functional support but also mastering tools. The lower limbs mainly function to support body weight and make movements. Anatomically, the upper limbs consist of lighter bones, thinner and looser joint capsules, and more slender muscles than the lower limbs.

5.1.1 Upper Limbs

5.1.1.1 Boundary

The upper limbs connect the trunk bilaterally. They are superiorly attached to the neck by the line connecting the clavicle, acromion, and the seventh cervical vertebra; anteriorly to the chest by the line connecting the upper border of the anterior margin of the deltoid and the anterior axillary fold; and posteriorly to the back by the line connecting the posterior margin of the deltoid and the posterior axillary fold. The upper limbs are structurally divided into the shoulder, axillary region, arm, elbow, forearm, and hand. In addition, the hand is divided into the palm, back (opisthenar), and fingers. For the convenience of anatomical operation, the regional anatomy of the shoulder and axillary regions is described in the sections of the regional anatomy of the back and chest wall, respectively.

M. Zhu (✉) · H. Song · G. Hong · J. Zou
Nanjing Medical University, Nanjing, China
e-mail: zhumin@njmu.edu.cn

Q. Ding et al. (eds.), *Clinically Oriented Regional Anatomy*,
https://doi.org/10.1007/978-981-95-9888-5_5

5.1.1.2 Anatomical Landmarks and Surface Projections of the Main Blood Vessels and Nerves

Bony Landmarks

The main bony landmarks of the upper limbs include the clavicle, acromion, coracoid process, scapular spine, lateral epicondyle, medial epicondyle, sulcus for ulnar nerve, olecranon, styloid process of radius, styloid process of ulna, pisiform, etc.

Bony landmarks can be based on determining the length of the upper limbs, the location of major blood vessels and nerves, and the lesions of the upper limbs. Under normal circumstances, bony landmarks of the upper limbs are localized in a certain area, and some of them present an evident positional relationship. For example, the upper limb, arm, and forearm lengths are defined as the distance from the acromion to the tip of the middle finger, the distance from the acromion to the lateral epicondyle, and the distance from the lateral epicondyle to the styloid process of the radius, respectively. The superior acromion, inferolateral greater tubercle, and inferomedial coracoid form an isosceles triangle. Their positional relationship alters in the case of dislocation of shoulder. The olecranon and lateral and medial epicondyles are connected into a line during elbow extension, while a posterior cubital triangle forms during elbow flexion. Their positional relationship alters in the case of elbow dislocation. In physical examination, the affected upper limb should be compared with that of the contralateral side (Fig. 5.1).

Muscular Landmarks

Muscular landmarks of the upper limbs mainly include the deltoid, biceps brachii, tendon of the biceps brachii, triceps brachii, brachioradialis, tendon of the flexor carpi radialis, tendon of the palmaris longus, tendon of the flexor carpi ulnaris, tendon of the abductor pollicis longus, tendon of the extensor pollicis brevis, tendon of the extensor pollicis longus, tendon of the extensor digitorum, thenar eminence, hypothenar eminence, etc. The morphology, localization, size, and tension of muscular landmarks of the upper limbs are of great significance in the diagnosis of neurological diseases and the localization of deep blood vessels and nerves.

Surface Projections of Arteries Supplying to the Upper Limbs (Fig. 5.2)

Axillary Artery and Brachial Artery

Keeping the abductive upper limb at a right angle to the trunk and forearms supinated, a straight line is drawn connecting the midpoint of the clavicle to that of the cubital fossa. Surface projection of the axillary artery lies on the upper third of the line, and that of the brachial artery lies in the lower two thirds.

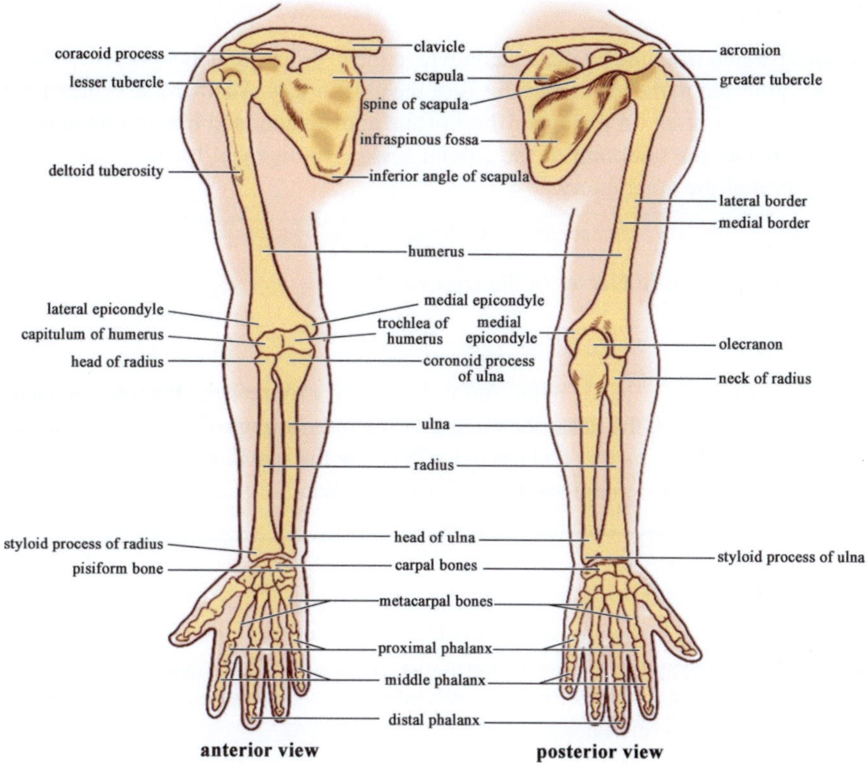

Fig. 5.1 Bony landmarks of the upper limbs

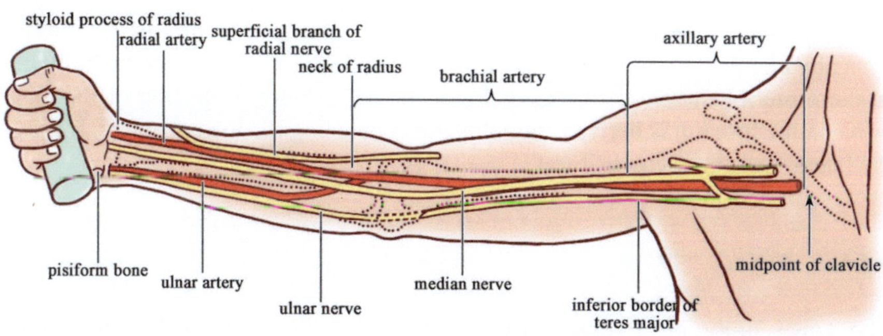

Fig. 5.2 Projections of arteries and nerve trunks of the upper limbs

Radial Artery

A line is drawn from one finger's breadth below the midpoint of the cubital fossa to half one finger's breadth medial to the styloid process of the radius. Deep below this line lies the radial artery.

Ulnar Artery

A line is drawn from the medial epicondyle to the pisiform, and its lower two-thirds can be projected to the lower two-thirds of the ulnar artery. Another line is drawn by connecting the point on the upper third of the abovementioned line to one finger's breadth below the midpoint of the cubital fossa; this line can be projected to the upper third of the ulnar artery.

Surface Projections of Nerves of the Upper Limbs

Radial Nerve

The radial nerve is projected to the surface as a line deriving from the lower third of the posterior deltoid, the posterior margin of the insertion of the deltoid, the posterior margin of the humerus, and the plane between the brachioradialis and the brachialis, to the anterior margin of the lateral epicondyle.

Median Nerve

The median nerve in the arm is projected to the surface as a line identical to that of the brachial artery, which, in the forearm, derives from the line connecting the midpoint of a line joining the medial epicondyle and the tendon of biceps brachii to the midpoint that is slightly lateral to the wrist distal crease.

Ulnar Nerve

The upper segment of the ulnar nerve in the arm is projected to the surface as a line basically identical to that of the brachial artery and the lower segment medially lies in the posterior margin of the medial epicondyle. Surface projection of the ulnar nerve in the forearm is derived from the line connecting the medial epicondyle and the lateral margin of the pisiform.

5.1.1.3 Layers

The upper limbs are cylindrically shaped and centered on bones and joints. Muscles of the upper limbs are arranged based on the axes of joint movement, separated by intermuscular septa and wrapped by deep fascia to form the osteofascial sheath. Generally, the upper limbs have five layers from superficial to deep.

Skin

Skin thickness and mobility vary in different regions of the upper limbs. Except for the palms, the skin on the flexor surface of the upper limbs is thinner and more mobile than that on the extensor surface and more prominent at the joints. The skin on the palmar aspect of hands and fingers is thick and tough, presenting a thick cutinized layer, abundant sweat glands, and a lack of hair, hair follicles, and sebaceous glands. The skin on the palm prints and fingerprints directly connects with the deep fascia, which is less mobile. Nerve endings are especially abundant at the fingertips. The skin on the dorsal aspect of hands and fingers is thin, loose, and highly mobile.

Nail plates lie on the dorsal aspect of distal digits, deriving from the skin through the thickening of the dermis. The nail bed is the dermis beneath the nail plate. Nails grow from the germ layer at the nail root. The cutaneous fold overlapping the nail root and its lateral edges is known as the nail wall.

Superficial Fascia

Except for the central part of palms and the palmar aspect of fingers, the superficial fascia of the upper limbs is thin and loose. The dense superficial fascia in the central part of the palms and the palmar aspect of fingers is intimately bound to the skin and deep fascia, leading to a structure with little skin mobility to favor object-holding. Fibrous septa in the palm hinder the spread of pus to the palm; subsequently, local swelling compresses nerve endings, leading to severe pain.

The superficial fascia is made up of loose connective tissues, superficial veins, superficial lymphatic vessels, superficial lymph nodes, and cutaneous nerves.

Most superficial veins are situated in the palmar aspect of the superficial fascia. Major superficial veins are described as follows.

Cephalic Vein

The cephalic vein originates from the radial side of the dorsal venous network of the hand, ascends along the radial side of the forearm and the anterior surface of the cubital fossa, and superiorly travels along the lateral side of the biceps brachii. Running through the deltopectoral groove, and piercing the clavipectoral fascia, the cephalic vein finally drains into the axillary vein or the subclavian vein. An anastomosis may be observed between the terminal branch of the cephalic vein and the external jugular vein.

Basilic Vein

The basilic vein originates from the ulnar side of the dorsal venous network of the hand, travels up the flexor side of the forearm, and communicates with the median cubital vein in the cubital fossa. It then travels superiorly along the medial side of the biceps brachii, pierces into the deep fascia slightly below the mid-arm, and finally drains into the brachial vein, or the axillary vein by joining the brachial vein.

Median Cubital Vein

The median cubital vein is large and short, with a wide range of anatomical variations. It lies obliquely in the middle of the cubital fossa, bridges the basilic vein and the cephalic vein, and usually receives the blood stream from the median antebrachial vein. The median antebrachial vein sometimes splits and drains into the basilic vein and the cephalic vein, namely, the vena mediana basilica and the vena mediana cephalica, respectively (Fig. 5.3).

Cutaneous nerves are situated in the deep layer of the superficial fascia and close to the deep fascia, most of which are branches of the brachial plexus. Important cutaneous nerves of the upper limbs are described as follows.

Medial Brachial Cutaneous Nerve

The medial brachial cutaneous nerve arises from the medial cord of the brachial plexus and perforates the deep fascia medial to the mid-arm. It distributes in the skin on the medial side of the lower arm.

Lateral Antebrachial Cutaneous Nerve

The lateral antebrachial cutaneous nerve is the terminal of the musculocutaneous nerve and perforates the deep fascia lateral to the tendon of biceps brachii at the elbow. It passes behind the cephalic vein medially and distributes in the skin on the lateral forearm.

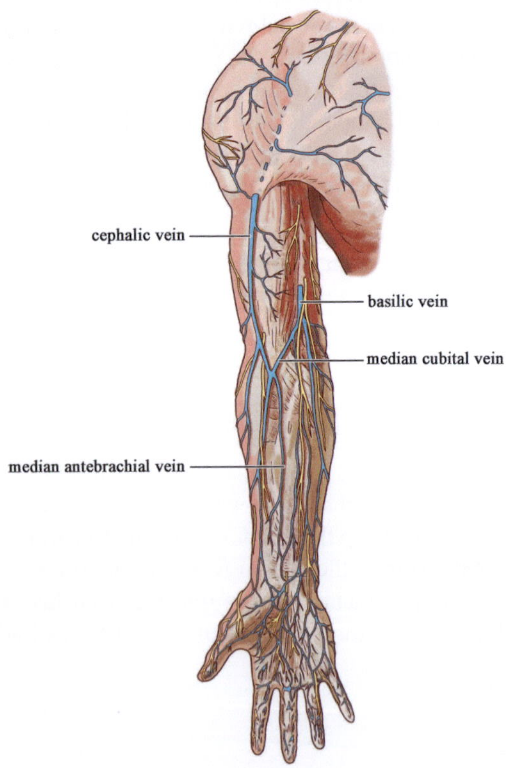

Fig. 5.3 Superficial veins of the upper limbs

Medial Antebrachial Cutaneous Nerve

The medial antebrachial cutaneous nerve arises from the medial cord of the brachial plexus, perforates the deep fascia slightly below the medial side of the arm, and passes alongside the basilic vein. It distributes in the skin on the medial forearm.

Superficial Branch of the Radial Nerve

The superficial branch of the radial nerve is one of the terminals of the radial nerve. It passes along the dorsal aspect of the upper limb to the palmar aspect through the lateral intermuscular septum. Separated by the brachialis, the radial nerve and the lateral antebrachial cutaneous nerve are laterally and medially situated, respectively. The superficial branch of the radial nerve passes alongside the radial artery in the middle third of the forearm and lies on the back of the hand from the superior part of the styloid process of the radius. It is distributed in the skin on the radial side of the dorsal aspect of the hand and the proximal skin on the dorsal aspect of the radial half of fingers (Figs. 5.4, 5.5, and 5.6).

Dorsal Branch of the Ulnar Nerve

The dorsal branch of the ulnar nerve arises approximately 5 cm above the wrist, perforates the deep fascia slightly above the ulnar side of the wrist, and runs alongside the original segment of the basilic vein on the dorsal side of the hand. It distributes in the skin on the ulnar side of the dorsal aspect of the hand, the ulnar side of the dorsal aspect of the little finger and the ring finger, the radial side of the ring finger, and the proximal skin on the dorsal aspect of the radial half of the middle finger (Figs. 5.5, and 5.6).

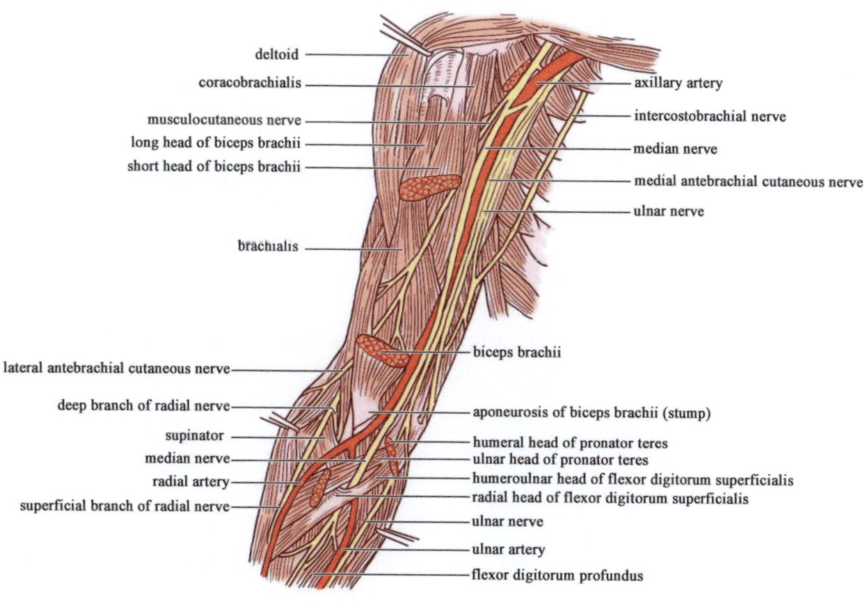

Fig. 5.4 Deep layers of the forearm

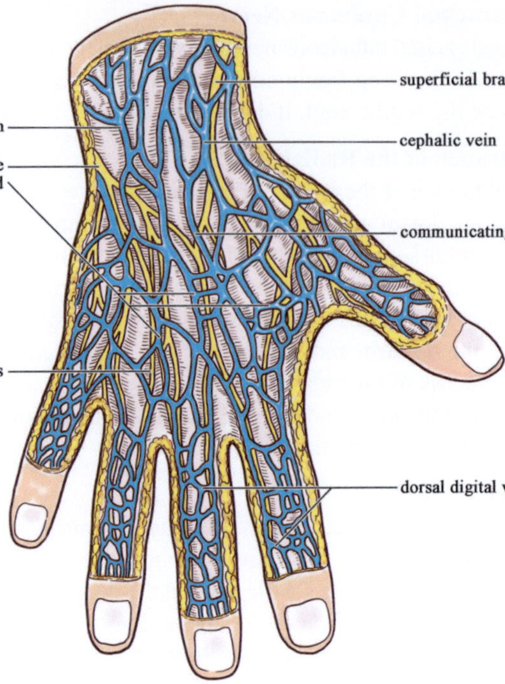

Fig. 5.5 Superficial layers of the dorsal aspect of the hand

Nerves Innervating the Skin on the Palm

Nerves innervating the skin on the palm are derived from the median nerve and the superficial branch of the ulnar nerve. Several branches of the common palmar digital nerves arise from the palm of the hand and split into two proper palmar digital nerves in the web space. The cutaneous branches of the median nerve are distributed in the skin about 3.5 fingers' breadth on the palmar aspect of the radial side and their middle and distal skin on the dorsal aspect. The cutaneous branches of the ulnar nerve distribute in the skin on the ulnar side of the hand and about 1.5 digits on the palmar aspect of the ulnar side.

In addition, the superior and inferior lateral cutaneous nerves of the arm, the posterior cutaneous nerve of the arm, the intercostobrachial nerve, and the posterior antebrachial cutaneous nerve are also important cutaneous nerves of the upper limbs.

Deep Fascia

According to its location, the deep fascia of the upper limbs can be classified into the deltoid fascia, scapular fascia, brachial fascia, antebrachial fascia, and palmar fascia. The brachial fascia covers the muscles of the arm and gives off the medial

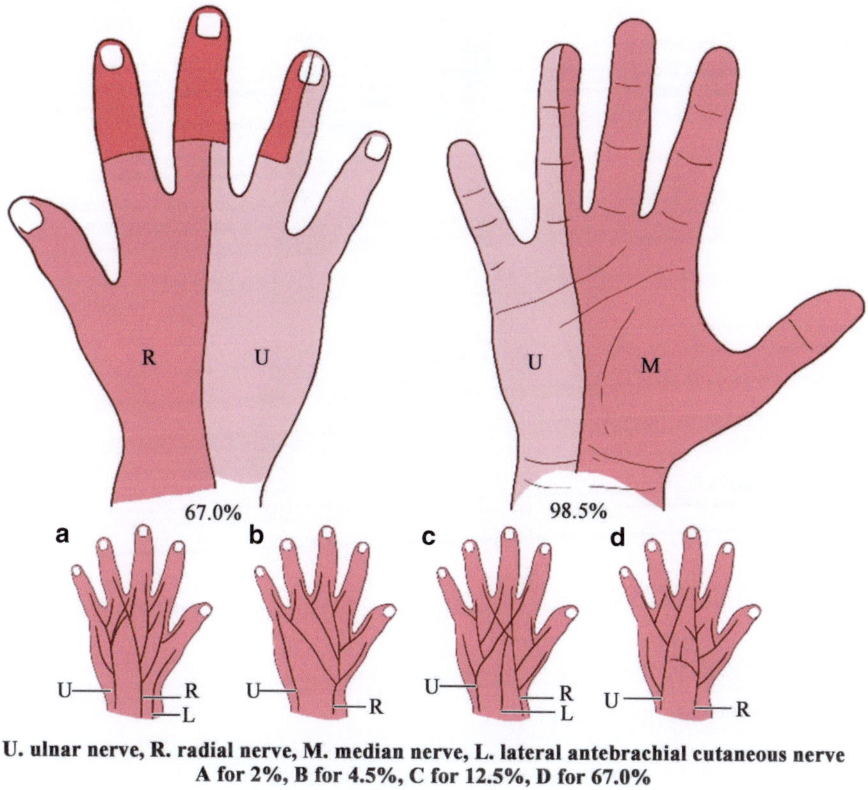

Fig. 5.6 Distribution of nerves in the skin on the hand, and their variations

and lateral intermuscular septa attached to the humerus to separate the flexor and extensor group of muscles in the upper limbs. The anterior and posterior osteofascial sheaths in the upper limbs are enclosed by the medial and lateral intermuscular septa and the humerus. The antebrachial fascia also gives off the intermuscular septum to separate the flexor and extensor group of muscles in the forearm, which is attached to the radius and ulna, and encloses the anterior and posterior osteofascial sheath in the forearms, alongside the interosseous membrane. The antebrachial fascia is especially thickened near the wrist, forming the palmar carpal ligament, flexor retinaculum (also known as the transverse carpal ligament), and extensor retinaculum. The central portion of the palmar fascia is known as the triangular-shaped palmar aponeurosis. Its apex attaches to the flexor retinaculum and is continuous with the tendon of the palmaris longus. Its base is divided into four slips that, respectively, attach the tendon sheath of the index finger, middle finger, ring finger, and little finger. Blood vessels and nerves run alongside the bilateral sides of a finger between two longitudinal slips (Fig. 5.7).

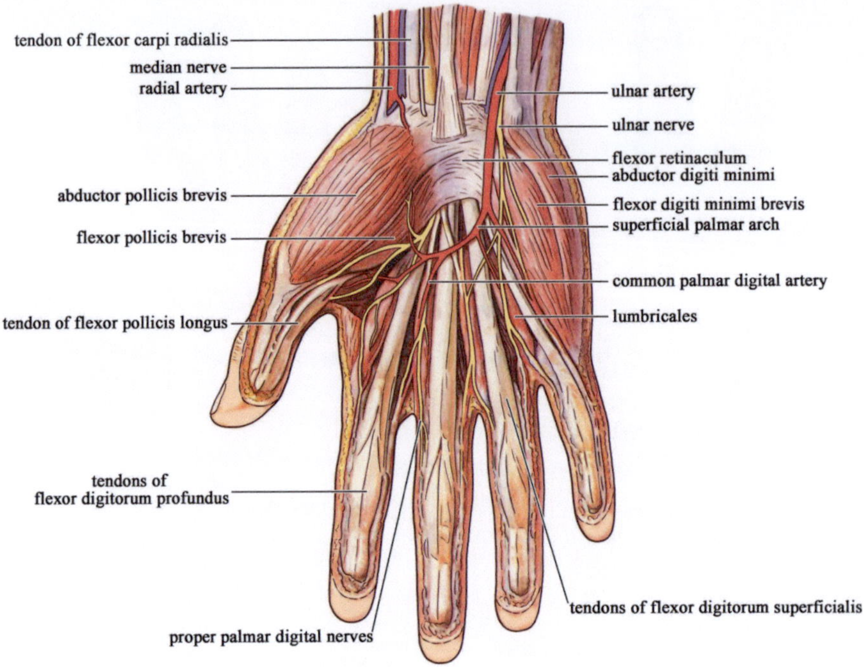

Fig. 5.7 Palmar aponeurosis

Intermuscular Septa and Fascial Sheaths of the Upper Limbs

Muscles in the upper limbs are distributed based on the muscle groups and enclosed by the fascial sheaths formed by the deep fascia, intermuscular septa, and bones. Each sheath contains blood vessels and nerves. Important intermuscular septa and fascial sheaths of the upper limbs are described as follows.

Deltopectoral Groove

The deltopectoral groove is situated between the anterior border of the deltoid and the superolateral border of the pectoralis major, through which the cephalic vein passes.

Medial Bicipital Groove

The medial bicipital groove is situated medial to the belly of the biceps brachii and connects superiorly with the axillary cavity. The brachial artery and vein, the median nerve, and the ulnar nerve pass through the medial bicipital groove. Cubital lymph nodes can sometimes be seen on the inferior portion of the medial bicipital groove.

Humeromuscular Tunnel

The humeromuscular tunnel, also known as the radial nerve canal, is situated between the medial and lateral heads of the triceps brachii and the radial groove of the humerus, through which the radial nerve, deep brachial artery, and vein pass. The radial nerve travels up to the palmar aspect through the posterolateral forearm, runs between the brachialis and the brachioradialis, and descends into the lateral portion of the cubital fossa.

Cubital Fossa

The cubital fossa is a triangular area anterior to the elbow, superiorly bounded by the line connecting the medial and lateral epicondyles, laterally by the medial border of the brachioradialis, and medially by the superolateral border of the pronator teres. The cubital fossa is divided into the skin, superficial fascia, superficial layer of the deep fascia, and bicipital aponeurosis from superficial to deep. The floor of the cubital fossa is bounded by the brachialis, supinator, and the capsule of the elbow joint. The cubital fossa superiorly and medially communicates with the medial bicipital groove, superiorly and laterally connects with the radial nerve extension, and inferiorly joins the intermuscular septum of the forearm. The contents in the cubital fossa, from medial to lateral, include the median nerve, brachial artery, and its branches of the radial and ulnar arteries and veins that accompany them, the tendon of the biceps brachii, and the superficial and deep branches of the radial nerve. The brachial artery is superficial on the cubital fossa and medial to the tendon of the biceps brachii. It is a palpable site to measure blood pressure. The deep cubital lymph nodes are situated near the bifurcation of the brachial artery.

Radial Groove of the Forearm

The radial groove of the forearm is situated in the central and inferior portion of the lateral forearm, between the brachioradialis and the flexor carpi radialis. A neurovascular bundle consisting of the superficial branch of the radial nerve, the radial artery, and the vein passes through the radial groove. The superficial branch of the radial nerve is the direct extension of its main trunk and descends to the lateral border of the radial artery. It lies far away from the radial artery in the medial third of the forearm, travels alongside the radial artery in the middle third, and runs apart from the radial artery in the lateral third. The superficial branch of the radial nerve finally passes to the dorsal aspect of the forearm by traveling through the deep layer of the brachioradialis. Two veins pass alongside the radial artery. The distal third of the radial artery is superficial, where a radial pulse can be palpable. It is the site of pulse diagnosis in traditional Chinese medicine (TCM).

Median Groove of the Forearm

The median groove of the forearm is situated in the middle of the forearm, with the superior portion located between the flexor digitorum superficialis and profundus and the inferior portion located between the plane of the flexor carpi radialis, palmaris longus, and flexor digitorum superficialis. It inferiorly communicates with the carpal tunnel, through which the median nerve passes. The median nerve runs inferiorly into the cubital fossa, perforates the pronator teres, and merges into the median groove of the forearm. The inferior portion of the median groove is only covered by the tendon of the palmaris longus or the palmar aponeurosis on the surface and is susceptible to trauma.

Ulnar Groove of the Forearm

The ulnar groove is situated on the ulnar side of the median-lower forearm, between the flexor carpi ulnaris and the flexor digitorum superficialis, where the ulnar artery, vein, and nerve pass through. The ulnar nerve descends through the groove of the ulnar nerve behind the elbow, enters the origin of the flexor carpi ulnaris, and travels up to the palmar aspect of the forearm. It runs between the flexor digitorum profundus and the flexor carpi ulnaris and continuously descends to the ulnar groove medial to the ulnar artery and vein. The ulnar artery arises from the brachial artery, travels to the palmar aspect of the forearm through the deep layer of the pronator teres, and enters the ulnar groove after passing through the flexor digitorum profundus. Two veins are accompanied by the ulnar artery.

Carpal Canal

The carpal canal is bounded by the flexor retinaculum (transverse carpal ligament) and the carpal groove. Nine flexor tendons pass through this canal, including the tendon of flexor pollicis longus and the encased radial bursa, four tendons of flexor digitorum superficialis, and four tendons of flexor digitorum profundus and the encased radial bursa, and the median nerve (Fig. 5.8).

Fascial Spaces of the Palm

Fascial spaces of the palm are deep in the central part of the palm and filled with loose connective tissues. The thenar space and the midpalmar space are the major fascial spaces lateral and medial, separated by the intermediate palmar septum that connects the palmar aponeurosis and the fascia of the third metacarpal bone.

Thenar Space

The thenar space is deep in the radial side of the palm. It is anteriorly bounded by the anterior portion of the palmar aponeurosis, tendon of index finger, and the first lumbrical and posteriorly bounded by the adductor pollicis muscle and its fascia on

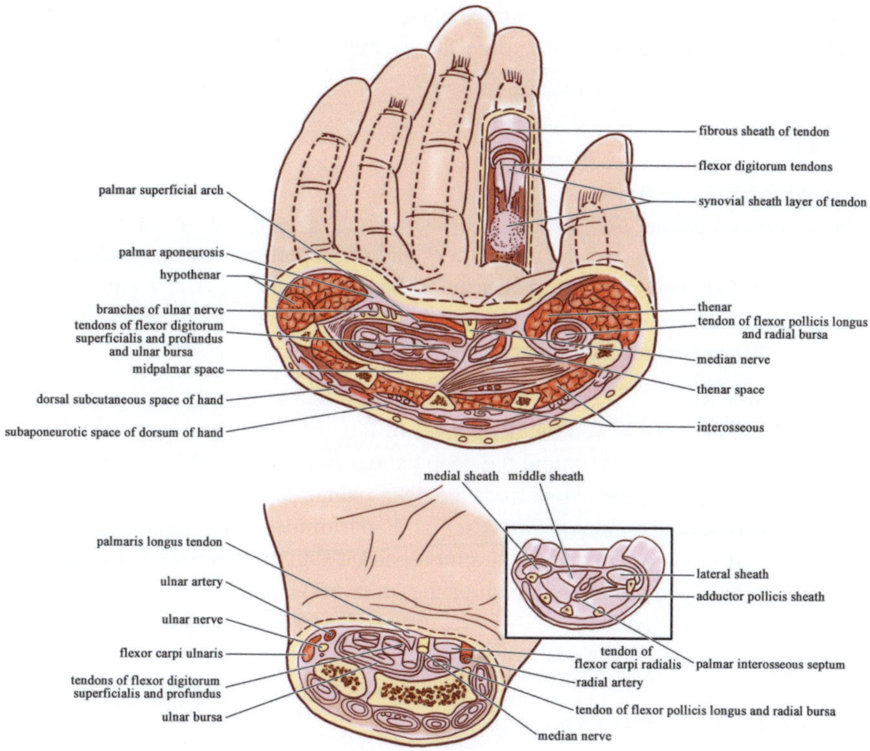

Fig. 5.8 Intermuscular septum of the hand and its contents

the surface. The thenar muscles, tendon of flexor pollicis longus, and its radial bursa (tendinous sheath of flexor pollicis longus) form the lateral border of the thenar space and the posterior portion of the medial palmar aponeurosis. The proximal end of the thenar space is a dead space, and its distal end travels along the first lumbrical canal and communicates with the dorsal side of the index finger. Thenar space infections can be caused by direct puncture, purulent fluid from tenosynovitis of the index finger that overflows upward, or metacarpal osteomyelitis.

Midpalmar Space

The midpalmar space is deep on the ulnar side of the palm, anteriorly bounded by the second, third, and fourth lumbricals and the flexor tendons of the middle, ring, and little fingers, and posteriorly bounded by the posterior portion of the palmar aponeurosis and the third and fourth metacarpal bones. The palmar aponeurosis and the medial intermuscular septum form the lateral and medial borders of the midpalmar space, respectively. Proximally, the midpalmar space narrows down, extends to the deep layer of the common synovial sheath of flexor, and communicates with the posterior flexor compartment of the forearm after passing through the carpal canal. Distally, it runs through the second, third, and fourth lumbrical canals, extends up to the web space between the index and middle fingers and that between the middle and ring fingers, and communicates with the dorsal side of the middle, ring, and little fingers. Similar to that into the thenar space, the pus may spread into the midpalmar space.

Palmar Arch

Superficial Palmar Arch

The superficial palmar arch lies beneath the palmar aponeurosis, as an anastomosis formed by the distal end of the ulnar artery and the superficial palmar branch of the radial artery. Common palmar digital arteries (branches of the superficial palmar arch), the superficial branch of the ulnar nerve, and common palmar digital nerves (branches of the median nerve) run through the deep layer of the palmar aponeurosis.

Deep Palmar Arch

The deep palmar arch lies in the deep layer of flexor tendons and is formed by the distal end of the radial artery and the deep palmar branch of the ulnar artery. Three palmar metacarpal arteries arise from the deep palmar arch, descend alongside the anterior portion of the palmar interossei, and anastomose at the metacarpophalangeal joint with the corresponding common palmar digital artery. The deep palmar arch, its branch, and the deep branch of the ulnar nerve altogether run through the deep layer of flexor tendons.

Bones and Bone Connections

Bones of the upper limb are composed of upper limb girdle bones and free upper limb bones. The upper limb girdle bones include the clavicle and scapula. The free upper limb bones include the humerus, radius, ulna and hand bones. The hand bones include the carpal bones, metacarpal bones and phalanges. Upper limb bone connections consist of upper limb girdle bones connections and free upper limb bones connections. The upper limb girdle bones connections include the sternoclavicular joint, the acromioclavicular joint and the coracoshoulder ligament. Free upper limb bones connections include those of the shoulder joint, elbow joint, the connection between the radius and ulna, and the joints of the hand. The joints of the hand include the radiocarpal joint, intercarpal joints, carpal and metacarpal joints, intermetacarpal joints, metacarpophalangeal joints and interphalangeal joints.

Appendix

Fingers

The metacarpophalangeal joints connect five fingers to the palm. Human fingers are flexible, including the thumb, index, middle, ring, and little fingers. The thumb is short and wide and faces the remaining four fingers, containing only two phalanges.

The thumb carpometacarpal joint is saddle-shaped, with a wide range of motion. Movements of the thumb include flexion, extension, abduction, and opposition, which are of great significance in task performance.

Superficial Structures

Skin

The skin on the palmar side of the finger is thicker and rich in sweat glands and fingerprints but lacks hair, hair follicles, and sebaceous glands.

Superficial Fascia

The superficial fascia on the palmar side of the finger is thick, and subcutaneous fat accumulates beneath the skin into a spherical shape. The fibrous septum connects the skin of the fingers to the flexor tendon sheath. Superficial fascia is absent at the finger creases, where the skin directly connects to the tendon sheath. Therefore, infections in the finger creases usually cause tenosynovitis. The pulp spaces are closed fibrous septa between the skin on the distal 4/5 of the distal phalanx and the periosteum and extend to the subcutaneous area of the distal digital crease and the distal end of the flexor digitorum profundus tendons. The subcutaneous fat of the fingertips is loculated by fibrous septa. Infections in the fingertips cause severe pain and necrosis of the distal phalanges due to the compression of blood vessels and nerve endings. Therefore, a timely decompression of the fingertips via cutting a lateral incision of fibrous septa is necessary to ensure an unobstructed drainage (Fig. 5.9).

Deep Structures

Attachments to the Flexor Digitorum Superficialis and Profundus Tendons

Flexor digitorum superficialis and profundus tendons lie in the tendon sheaths of the index, middle, and ring fingers. The flexor digitorum superficialis tendon covers and wraps the flexor digitorum profundus tendon at the proximal phalanx. Distally, it divides into two branches attaching to the lateral margin of the middle phalanx, where an adductor hiatus forms to allow the passage of the flexor digitorum profundus tendon. The flexor digitorum profundus tendon terminates at the base of the distal phalanx. The flexor digitorum superficialis tendon mainly flexes the proximal interphalangeal joints, and the flexor digitorum profundus tendon flexes both the proximal and distal interphalangeal joints.

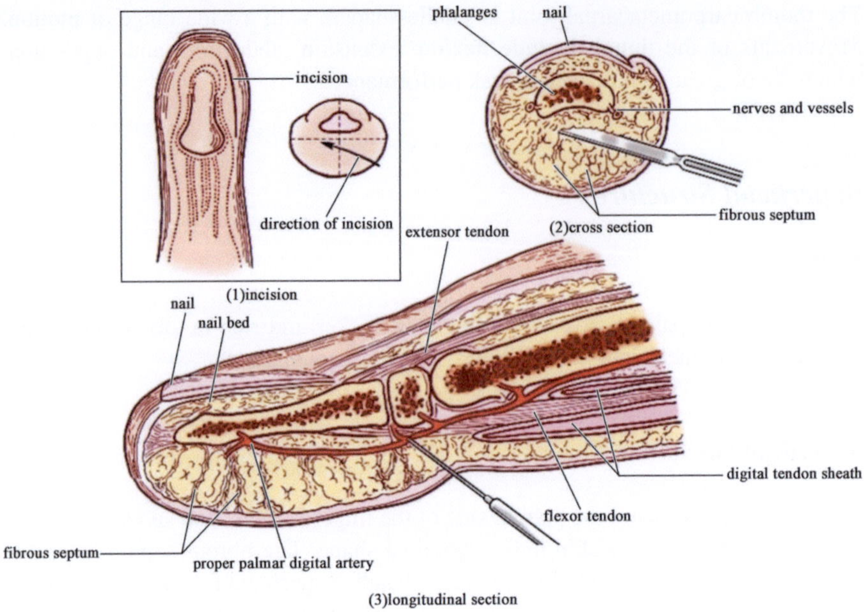

Fig. 5.9 Anatomy of the fingertips

Tendon Sheaths of Fingers

Tendon sheaths of fingers enclose flexor digitorum superficialis and profundus tendons and are composed of fibrous and synovial sheaths. Fibrous sheaths are the thickening of the deep fascia of the fingers and attach on the bilateral sides of the phalanx and joint capsule, forming a tube-like structure responsible for restraining and supporting the tendon. Synovial sheaths are situated in the fibrous sheaths, composed of an inner visceral layer and an outer parietal layer. Those of the index, middle, and ring fingers extend from the base of the distal phalanx to the proximal end via crossing the distal interphalangeal joint and the proximal interphalangeal joint to the proximal end of the metacarpophalangeal joint. Sometimes, synovial sheaths of the thumb and little finger communicate with the radial and ulnar bursa, respectively (Fig. 5.10).

Anatomy of the Upper Limbs

Objectives

To identify bony and muscular landmarks, and surface projections of blood vessels and nerves of the upper limbs.

To dissect major superficial veins (cephalic vein, basilic vein, and median cubital vein) and cutaneous nerves (lateral antebrachial cutaneous nerve, medial brachial

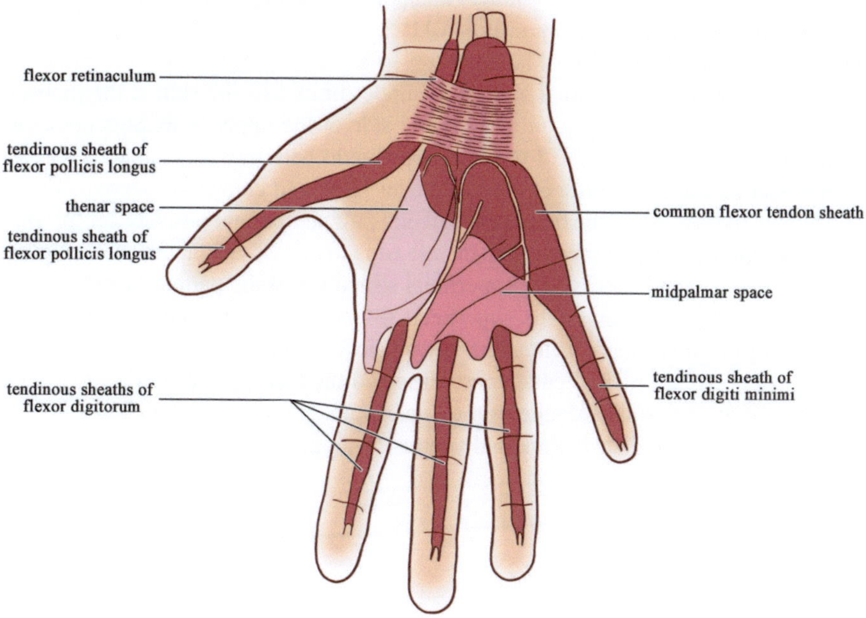

Fig. 5.10 Tendon sheaths and fascial spaces of the palm

cutaneous nerve, and medial antebrachial cutaneous nerve, proper palmar digital nerves, dorsal branch of ulnar nerve, superficial branch of radial nerve, and dorsal digital nerves) of the upper limbs and to localize them.

To dissect the deep fascia of the upper limbs and to observe their characteristics and the main structures.

To observe the distribution of muscles of the upper limbs, their compositions, and connections and the orientation and localization of major nerves and blood vessels in the intermuscular septa.

Dissection Procedures

Dissection of Subcutaneous Superficial Structures of the Upper Limbs

Step 1. Palpate the following bony landmarks of the upper limbs on the human bodies: the clavicle, acromion, scapular spine, lateral epicondyle, medial epicondyle, olecranon, styloid process of radius, styloid process of ulna, pisiform, etc. Palpate the following muscular landmarks of the upper limbs on the human body: the deltoid, tendon of the biceps brachii, tendon of the triceps brachii, brachioradialis, tendon of the flexor carpi radialis, tendon of the palmaris longus and palmar aponeurosis, tendon of the flexor carpi ulnaris, tendon of the abductor pollicis longus, tendon of the extensor pollicis brevis, tendon of the extensor pollicis longus, thenar eminence, hypothenar eminence, etc.

Step 2. In a supine position, anatomical incisions on the upper limbs are cut according to the dotted lines shown in Fig. 5.11.

Step 3. Removal of the skin.

Remove the skin on the palmar side of the upper limb. Lift the skin at the incision site and cut it off laterally until the radial side of the upper limb. Subcutaneous fat beneath the deep layer of the skin flap should be removed as much as possible, and be careful to protect the superficial veins and cutaneous nerves. Do not damage the tendon of the biceps brachii and palmar aponeurosis. Cut off the skin on the middle finger if there is not enough time to cut off that on the other fingers.

Step 4. Clean off and observe the superficial structures of the palmar fascia.

Identify the cephalic vein in the superficial fascia of the anterolateral side of the upper limb, and observe its localization, origin, orientation, and venous drainage.

Identify the medial brachial cutaneous nerve and the basilic vein in the superficial fascia of the anterolateral side of the upper limb, and observe their localization, orientation, nerve distribution, and venous drainage.

Fig. 5.11 Skin incisions on the upper limbs

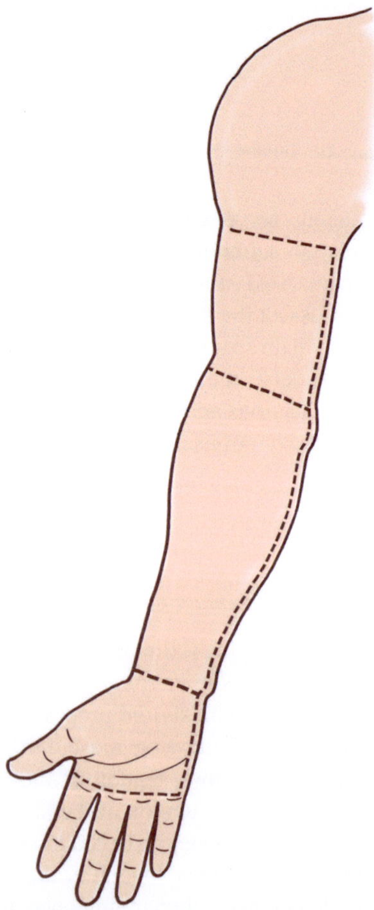

Identify the median cubital vein and the median antebrachial vein in the subcutaneous tissues of the cubital fossa and observe their localization and communication.

Identify the medial and lateral cutaneous nerves of the forearm on bilateral sides of the tendon of biceps brachii in the cubital fossa and the medial and lateral sides of the forearm, observe their localization, orientation, distribution, and anatomic relationship with the cephalic vein and the basilic vein.

Identify the palmar aponeurosis and its margin and the proper palmar digital arteries and nerves lying on the bilateral sides of the middle finger. Observe their localization, origin, and distribution.

Dissect the superficial fascia of the middle finger to observe the vertical attachment of fibrous septa in the subcutaneous fat tissues on the palmar side of the distal phalanx to the periosteum of the distal phalanx. The fibrous septa form tight, airtight cavities with little flexibility.

Step 5. Cut off the skin on the dorsal side of the upper limbs.

Step 6. Remove and observe the superficial structures of the dorsal fascia.

Identify the posterior cutaneous nerve of the forearm and the posterior antebrachial cutaneous nerve on the dorsal side of the upper limb, and observe its localization, origin, and distribution.

Identify the dorsal venous network of the hand, the superficial branch of the radial nerve, the dorsal branch of the ulnar nerve, and the dorsal digital nerves.

Step 7. Observe the characteristics of the deep fascia of the upper limb, including the thickness, tension, structure, perforation sites by cutaneous nerves, and piercing sites by superficial veins.

Dissection of Muscles, Blood Vessels, and Nerves on the Palmar Side of the Upper Limb

Step 1. Reserve and free the superficial veins and cutaneous nerves.

Step 2. Remove the deep fascia while reserving the superficial veins and cutaneous nerves. Notably, superficial muscular branches are tightly connected with the deep fascia in the upper portion of the forearm; a careful removal of the deep fascia is required to prevent muscular damages. Reserve the bicipital aponeurosis at the elbow, flexor, extensor retinaculum at the wrist, and palmar aponeurosis at the palm.

Step 3. Bluntly dissect the muscular margin and remove the intermuscular septa, aiming to identify muscles on the palmar side of the upper limb (Fig. 5.12).

Step 4. Raise up the pectoralis major with the resected origin. Free the brachial artery, brachial vein, median nerve, ulnar nerve, and medial antebrachial cutaneous nerve situated in the medial bicipital groove, and observe the anatomical regions they pass through, their orientation, communication, branches, and distribution. Observe the medial and lateral intermuscular septum between the brachialis and triceps brachii. Find out the cubital lymph nodes anterior to the inferior portion of the medial intermuscular septum and count their number.

Fig. 5.12 Superficial structures on the palmar side of the upper limb

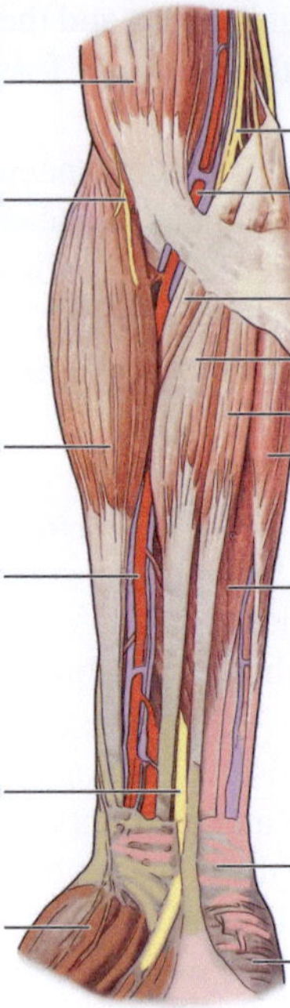

Posterior to the medial intermuscular septum, observe the ulnar nerve passing through the posterior portion of the medial epicondyle.

Step 5. Raise up the medial margin of the biceps brachii laterally, and observe the musculocutaneous nerves in the deep layer, including their origin, orientation, and distribution. They perforate above the cubital fossa and innervate the skin on the lateral forearm.

Step 6. Observe the bicipital aponeurosis and tendon of the biceps brachii in the cubital fossa, and the contents of the cubital fossa after removing fat tissues. Remove the lower part of the radial nerve trunk and its superficial and deep branches, the radial artery and its branch of radial recurrent artery situated in the lateral cubital fossa. Remove the median nerve, lower part of the brachial artery, ulnar artery, and its branches of the ulnar recurrent artery and common interosseous artery in the medial cubital fossa. Observe the communication and accompanying veins running in the cubital fossa.

Step 7. Observe the origin, insertion, and orientation of superficial muscles of the forearm, including the brachioradialis, pronator teres, flexor carpi radialis, palmaris longus, and flexor carpi ulnaris.

Step 8. Observe the branches and distribution of the radial artery, radial vein, and superficial branch of the radial nerve situated in the radial groove composed of the brachioradialis and the flexor carpi radialis (Fig. 5.13).

Step 9. Raise up the pronator teres, flexor carpi radialis, and palmaris longus laterally, and observe the origin, insertion, and orientation of the flexor digitorum superficialis situated in the deep layer.

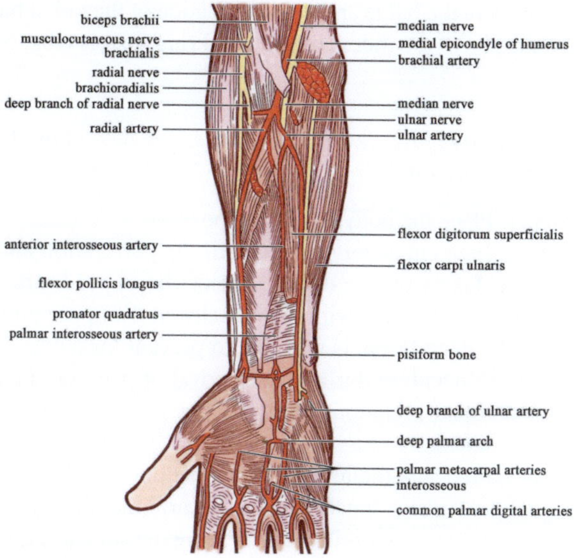

Fig. 5.13 Deep structures on the palmar side of the upper limb

Step 10. Observe the deeply situated flexor digitorum profundus and flexor pollicis longus after, respectively, raising up the flexor digitorum superficialis laterally and medially. Observe the median nerve located between the flexor digitorum superficialis and profundus, especially the derived muscular branches, muscles perforated by them, and the anatomical region where the lower part of it courses through the palm.

Step 11. Observe the origin, insertion, orientation, branches, and innervation of the ulnar artery, ulnar vein, and the main trunk of the ulnar nerve situated in the ulnar groove of the forearm, composed of the flexor digitorum superficialis and flexor carpi ulnaris.

Step 12. Peel off the palmar aponeurosis close to the deep layer from inside on the palmar side of the wrist. Protect the deep superficial palmar arch. Cut off the four slips at the distal end of the palmar aponeurosis that are attached to the tendon sheaths of four fingers. Subsequently, raise up the palmar aponeurosis toward the wrist, and observe the formation of the superficial palmar arch and its branches, recurrent branch of the median nerve, common palmar digital nerve (orientation and branches), and lumbricals (localization and innervation) arising from the ulnar nerve and median nerve.

Step 13. The tendinous sheath of flexor pollicis longus (also known as the radial bursa) and the common synovial sheath for the flexor tendons (also known as the ulnar bursa) are two important tendon sheaths of the palm. The former encases the tendon of flexor pollicis longus, and the latter encases the tendons of flexor digitorum superficialis, the palmar side of flexor digitorum profundus, and the little finger. Flexor tendons of the index, middle, and ring fingers are encased by other sheaths that are usually not communicated with the ulnar bursa. Inject water or light-colored fluid using a syringe into the above tendon sheaths to observe the bulge and communication of the radial bursa, ulnar bursa, and tendon sheaths of the index, middle, and ring fingers (Fig. 5.10).

Dissection of Muscles, Blood Vessels, and Nerves on the Dorsal Side of the Upper Limb

Step 1. Place the body in a prone position.

Step 2. Free cutaneous nerves until the perforation and cut off the superficial and deep fascia on the dorsal side of the upper limb. Notably, the deep fascia is tightly connected with the muscles in the upper portion, where careful removal of the deep fascia is required to prevent muscular damages. Reserve the extensor retinaculum during the removal of deep fascia at the wrist, and observe its anatomical relationship with the extensor tendon and corresponding tendon sheath.

Step 3. Free superficial muscles on the dorsal side of the upper limb, including the deltoid, triceps brachii, extensor carpi radialis longus and brevis, extensor digitorum, extensor digiti minimi, and extensor carpi ulnaris. Observe their localization and arrangement (Fig. 5.14).

Step 4. Cut off the origin of the deltoid on the scapular spine, raise up the posterior portion of the deltoid, and identify the deeply situated long head of triceps brachii. Observe the triangular and quadrangular space formed by the medial and lateral intermuscular septum. The former transmits the scapular circumflex vessels, and the latter transmits the posterior humeral circumflex artery and axillary nerve. Bluntly dissect the long and lateral heads of the triceps brachii, and observe the deep brachial artery and radial nerve traveling through the carpal tunnel. Dissect the brachioradialis and lateral margin of the brachialis, and

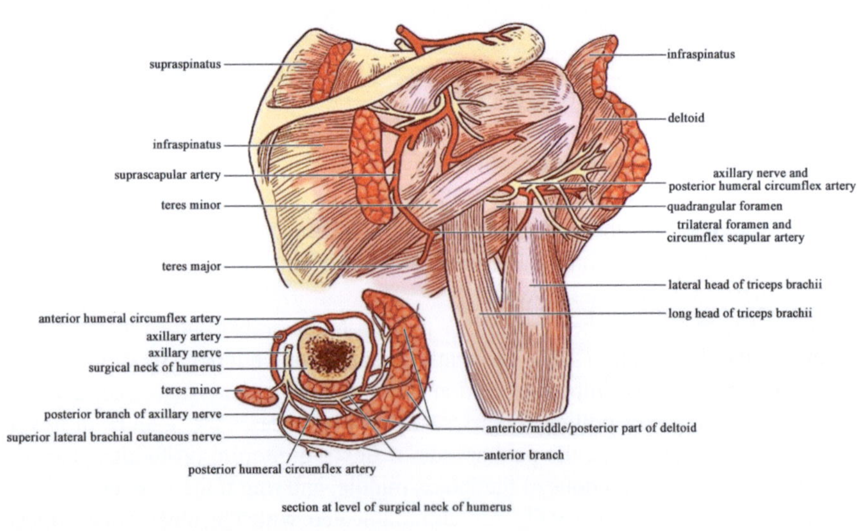

Fig. 5.14 Structure of the deltoid and scapular regions

observe the radial recurrent artery arising from the upper segment of the radial artery and the lower segment of the radial nerve (Fig. 5.15).

Step 5. Raise up the extensor digitorum medially. Free and observe the muscles deep beneath the extensor digitorum, including the supinator, abductor pollicis longus, extensor pollicis brevis, extensor pollicis longus, and extensor indicis.

Step 6. Observe the origin, orientation, and innervation of the posterior interosseous artery, vein, and nerve situated inferior to the supinator. Observe the insertion of the pronator teres on the central part of the lateral surface of the radius and that of the supinator on the proximal end of the anterior surface of radius.

Step 7. Observe the extensor retinaculum, tendons, and tendon sheaths (e.g., tendon sheaths of the abductor pollicis longus, extensor pollicis brevis, extensor pollicis longus, and extensor digitorum) situated on the dorsal side of the hand. Identify the anatomical snuff box, which is bounded by the tendon sheaths of the abductor pollicis longus, extensor pollicis brevis, and extensor pollicis longus. The range of each tendon sheath can be clearly visualized by injecting water. A ganglion cyst on the dorsal aspect of the wrist is a swelling caused by the thickened and enlarged tendon sheath. Tendons on the dorsal side of the hand are prone to incised wounds, which must be precisely repaired to recover their functions. Therefore, it is crucial to learn the anatomical arrangement of tendons in the hand, including the tendons of the abductor pollicis longus, extensor pollicis brevis, extensor pollicis longus, extensor digitorum of the four digits, and extensor digiti minimi from lateral to medial (Fig. 5.16).

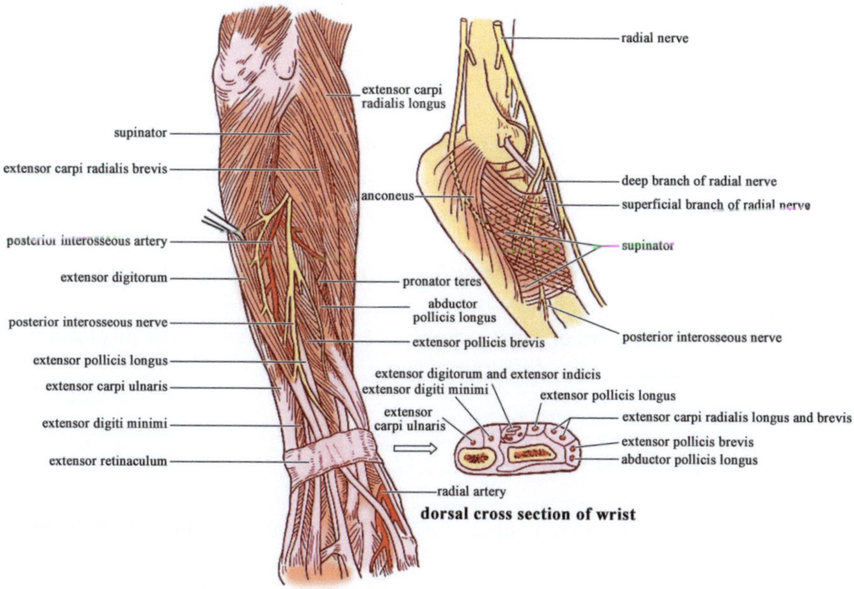

Fig. 5.15 Deep structures of the forearm

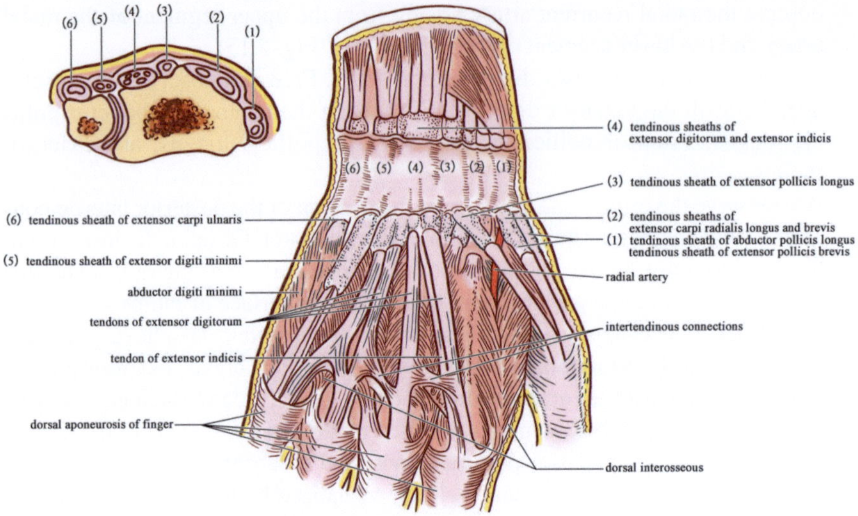

Fig. 5.16 Deep structures on the dorsal aspect of the hand

Summary

Remember the localization and name of major superficial veins of the upper limb, which are the common sites of blood and fluid transfusion.

The cutaneous nerves of the upper limbs lack a segmented distribution. However, they are obviously segmental according to the composition of the nerve trunk from the cervical spinal nerves 4-8 (C4-8) to the thoracic spinal nerves 1-2 (T1-2).

Briefly, C4–8 provide sensation to the shoulder; skin on the radial side of the upper limb; skin on the radial side of the forearm and the thumb, skin on the index, middle, and ring fingers and the palm; and the ulnar side of the forearm and the little finger, respectively. T1–2 provide sensation to the skin on the ulnar side of the upper limb, and the skin on the axillary region, respectively.

Compressions of the nerve roots or damages to the nerve fibers result in skin numbness, tingling, or sensory loss in the corresponding innervated areas of the upper limbs.

Muscle attachments are of great significance to understanding the displacement of fracture fragments and the direction of force.

Cervical Fractures and Displacement

The clavicle is palpable with a superficial localization and attached by the sternocleidomastoid and pectoralis major. Clavicle fractures usually occur in the middle third, or midshaft. The medial end of the fractured cervical is often displaced superoposteriorly due to the traction of the sternocleidomastoid, while the distal end is displaced superoanteriorly due to the traction of the subclavian and pectoralis major, as well as the gravity of the upper limbs (Fig. 5.17).

Humeral Shaft Fractures and Displacement

Humeral shaft fractures can be classified based on the type of fracture line. Those with the fracture line located above the deltoid attachment cause the shortening due to the medial displacement of the proximal end caused by the traction of the pectoralis major, latissimus dorsi and teres major, superolateral displacement of the distal end caused by the deltoid contraction, and the force of the longitudinal muscle group (Fig. 5.18). Humeral shaft fractures with the fracture line located below the deltoid attachment cause the anterolateral displacement of the proximal end due to the traction of the deltoid and the coracobrachialis and the upward displacement of the distal end due to the force from the longitudinal muscle group (Fig. 5.19).

Colles Fracture and the Displacement of the Radius

A fall of the body onto one's outstretched hand leads to consequences varying with the falling position, force, age, etc. The elderly are more likely to suffer from the Colles fracture that occurs 2.5 cm proximally to the radio-carpal joint. It causes posterior (dorsal) displacement of the distal end due to the traction of the brachioradialis, and anterior displacement due to the contraction of the pronator quadratus. A Colles fracture usually results in an impaction on the fractured end (Fig. 5.20).

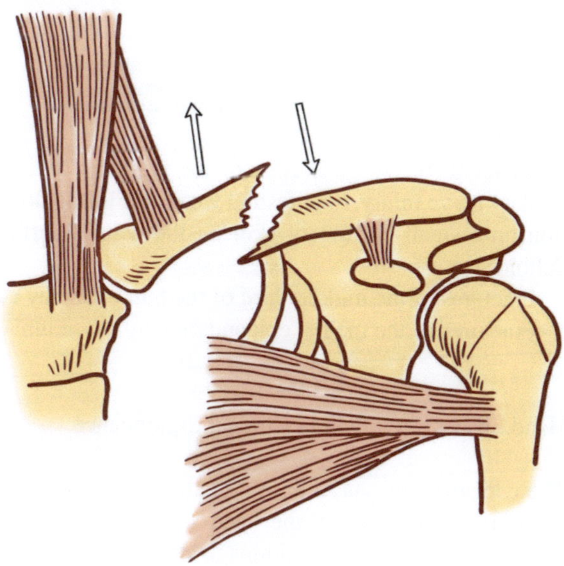

Fig. 5.17 A typical displacement of cervical fractures

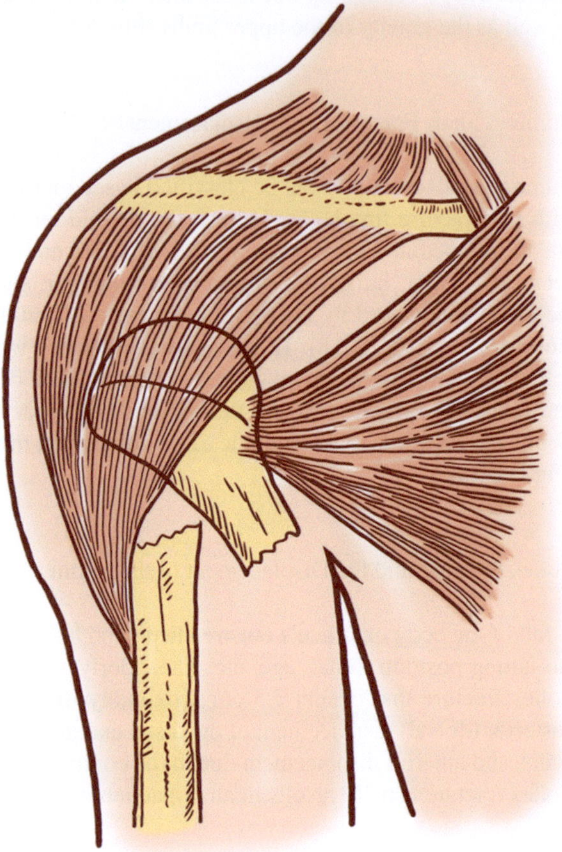

Fig. 5.18 Displacement of the humeral shaft fracture with the fracture line located above the deltoid attachment

Fractures of the Upper Limbs and Nerve Injuries

Fractures of the surgical neck of the humerus or shoulder dislocation may cause axillary nerve injury, manifesting weakness in shoulder abduction and loss of sensation on a small portion of skin on the deltoid surface caused by atrophy of the deltoid.

Fractures of the middle third of the humerus may cause radial nerve injury.

Fractures of the medial epicondyle may cause ulnar nerve injury.

Hand Spaces Are of Great Clinical Significance

Their localization and adjacent anatomical relationship are linked with the purulence after infections in the hand spaces, abscess site, communications between adjacent hand spaces, and drainage site of hand infections.

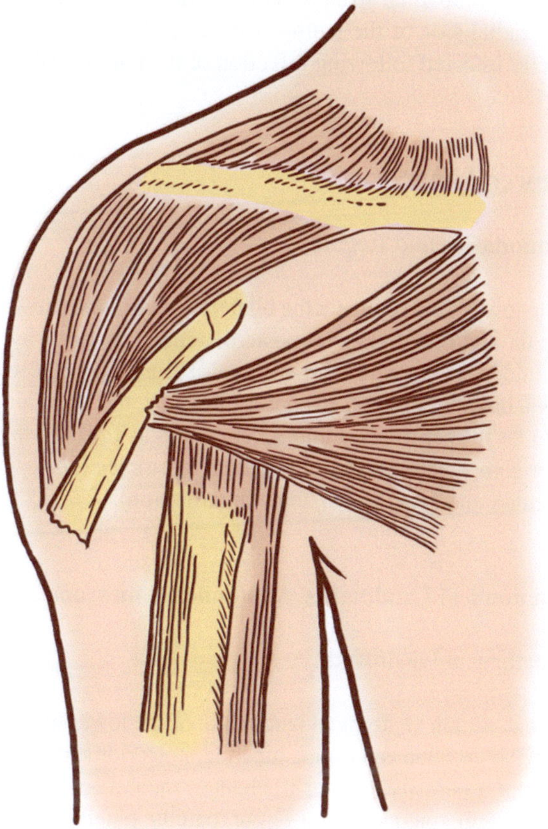

Fig. 5.19 Displacement of the humeral shaft fracture with the fracture line located below the deltoid attachment

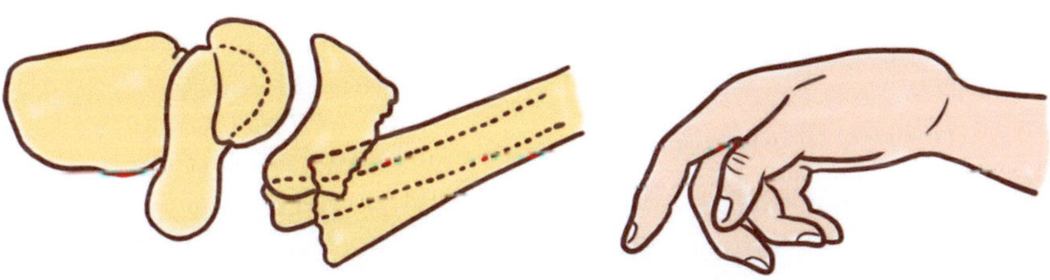

Fig. 5.20 A typical "dinner fork" deformity in a case of Colles fracture

Stab wounds or trauma in the tendon sheaths of the fingers, the tendon sheath of flexor pollicis longus, and the common synovial sheath for the flexor tendons and dactylitis lead to a direct invasion or indirect infection. Infections in the tendon sheath of flexor pollicis longus and common synovial sheath for the flexor tendons can spread to the forearm due to their proximal extension above the wrist.

The midpalmar space situated in the central palm and the thenar space situated in the radial side of the palm can be directly infected by penetrating trauma or indirectly infected following infection of the tendon sheath.

Lower Limbs

Boundaries and Regions

The lower limbs connect the bilateral sides of the trunk. They are anteriorly bounded by the inguinal ligament, posterolaterally bounded by the iliac crest, and medially bounded by the perineum. The lower limbs can be divided into hips, thighs, knees, legs, ankles, and feet. Except for the hips, the remaining regions of the lower limbs can be further divided into several parts as follows: thigh (anteromedial and posterior compartments), knee (popliteal fossa), leg (posterior and anterolateral compartments), and foot (dorsal and plantar region).

Anatomical Landmarks, Anatomical Lines, and Surface Projections

Anatomical Landmarks

The common anatomical landmarks of the lower limbs include the anterior superior iliac spine, iliac crest, iliac tubercle, posterior superior iliac spine, pubic tuberosity, ischial tuberosity, greater trochanter, medial and lateral condyles of femur, medial and lateral epicondyles of femur, patella, patellar ligament, medial and lateral condyles of tibia, tibial tuberosity, adductor tubercle, anterior border of tibia, head and neck of the fibula, lateral and medial malleolus, tendo calcaneus, calcaneal tuberosity, tuberosity of navicular bone, and tuberosity of the fifth metatarsal bone (Fig. 5.21).

Anatomical Lines

Nélaton's Line
In a lateral position with a semi-flexion of the hip, the Nélaton's line is a theoretical line connecting the anterior superior iliac spine, greater trochanter, and ischial tuberosity. In cases of the dislocation of hip joint or femoral neck fractures, the tip of the greater trochanter is above the Nélaton's line (Fig. 5.22).

Shoemaker's Line
In a supine position with the extension of the hip, two lines are projected onto bilateral sides from the tip of the greater trochanter beyond the anterior superior iliac spine and normally extend to meet at the midline at or above the umbilicus, that is,

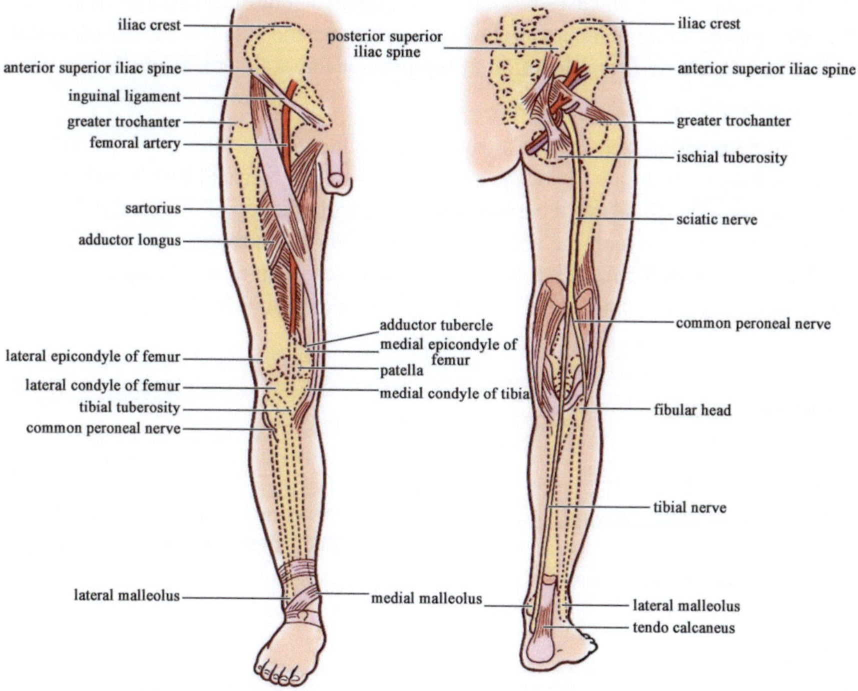

Fig. 5.21 Anatomical landmarks of the lower limbs

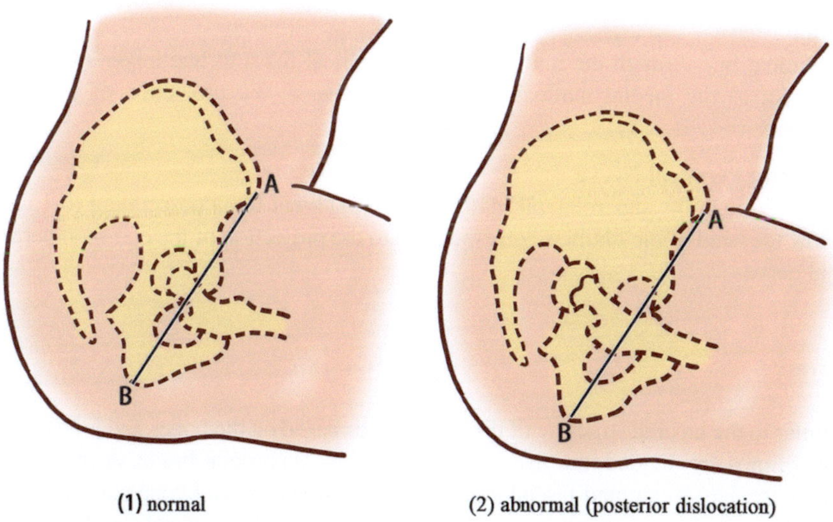

Fig. 5.22 The Nélaton's line

the Shoemaker's line. In cases of an upward displacement of the greater trochanter, the Shoemaker's line is located below the umbilicus and tilts toward the contralateral side, suggesting the dislocation of hip joint or femoral neck fractures.

Bryant's Triangle
In a supine position, the Bryant's triangle is bounded by a line from the anterior superior iliac spine to the top of the greater trochanter, a vertical line from the anterior superior iliac spine, and a perpendicular line from the top of the greater trochanter. The distance between the anterior superior iliac spine to the top of the greater trochanter is about 5 cm, which is shortened in cases of an upward displacement of the greater trochanter and suggestive of femoral neck fractures.

Surface Projections

Femoral Artery
With the hip rotated outward, the upper two-thirds of a line connecting the midpoint joining the anterior superior iliac spine and the pubic tuberosity to the medial epicondyle of the femur (or adductor tubercle) is corresponsive to the projection of the femoral artery.

Sciatic Nerve
The line connecting the upper third joining the posterior superior iliac spine to the ischial tuberosity, the midpoint joining the greater trochanter and ischial tuberosity (or the medial third), and the midpoint joining the medial and lateral condyles of femur is corresponsive to the projection of the sciatic nerve.

Tibial Nerve
A vertical line through the midpoint of the popliteal fossa to one finger's breadth posterior to the medial malleolus is corresponsive to the projection of the tibial nerve.

Common Peroneal Nerve
A line through the superolateral margin of the popliteal fossa descending to 1 cm below the head of the fibula is corresponsive to the projection of the common peroneal nerve.

Layers

Similar to the layered structure of the upper limbs based on the bones and joints, the lower limbs are divided into five layers of the skin, superficial fascia, deep fascia, intermuscular septum and fascial compartments, and bones and bone connections. The lower limbs are mainly responsible for supporting body weight and upright walking; therefore, the lower limbs are characterized by bigger muscles and bones, thicker deep fascia, and less joint mobility than those of the upper limbs.

Skin

The skin on the different regions of the lower limbs varies in thickness and mobility. The skin on the hip is thick, and the skin on the lateral and posterior compartments of the thighs is thicker and less mobile than that of the medial compartment. The skin on the anterior compartment of the legs is thicker and less mobile than that of the posterior compartment. The skin on the plantar region of the feet is thicker and less mobile than that of the dorsal region. The most mobile skin of the lower limb is situated on the flexural surface of the joint.

Superficial Fascia

The superficial fascia of the lower limbs is continuous with that of the adjacent regions, the abdominal region, and the lower back. The superficial fascia of the hip and plantar region of the foot consists of a thick layer of subcutaneous fat and fibrous tissues. The subcutaneous fat is usually thick in the anterior compartment of the thighs. The superficial fascia of the lower limbs contains superficial vessels, cutaneous nerves, superficial lymph nodes, and lymphatic vessels.

Superficial Veins

Dorsal Venous Arch of the Foot
The dorsal digital veins of the foot course on the dorsal region of the foot, where they join the dorsal venous arch of the foot. The great saphenous vein and the small saphenous vein, respectively, merge with the dorsal venous arch of the foot medially and laterally.

Great Saphenous Vein
The great saphenous vein is the thickest and longest superficial vein in the body that originates from the medial end of the dorsal venous arch of the foot. From 1 cm anterior to the medial malleolus, the great saphenous vein travels upward alongside the medial side of the leg, posteromedial side of the knee, and medial side of the thigh, which drains into the femoral vein through the saphenous hiatus at 3–4 cm inferolateral to the pubic tuberosity (Fig. 5.23). The great saphenous vein coursing anterior to the medial malleolus is palpable with an invariant anatomical position, serving as a common site of venipuncture or intubation. It receives the superficial epigastric vein, external pudendal vein, superficial iliac circumflex vein, and superficial medial and lateral femoral veins before joining the femoral vein. They join the great saphenous vein in various ways, forming anastomoses with other tributaries (Fig. 5.24).

As the longest vein in the body, the great saphenous vein has less support from muscles. Congenital weakness of the venous wall, long-term standing work, or other factors (e.g., pregnancy, pelvic tumors) would block venous return in the lower limbs. An obstructed great saphenous vein reflux further causes increased

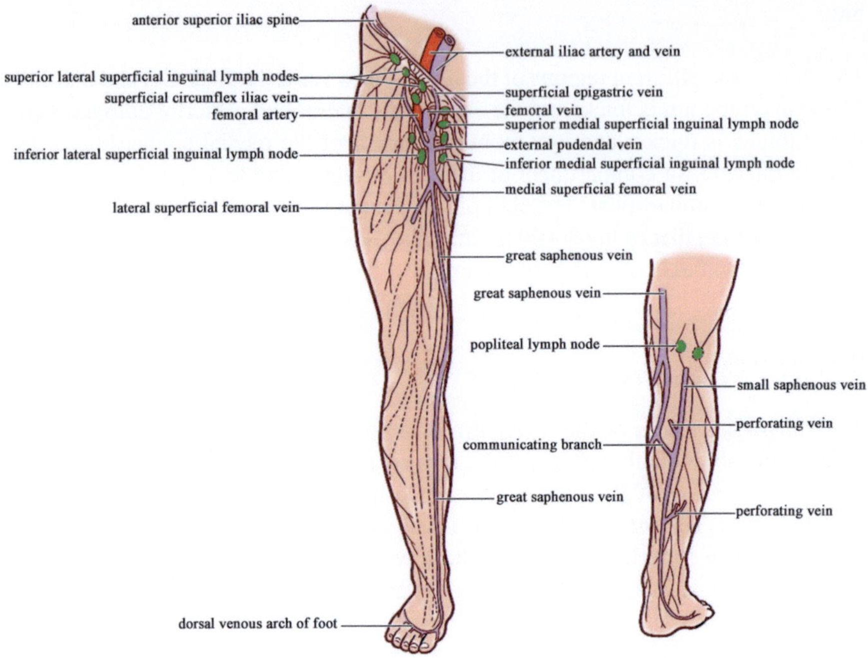

Fig. 5.23 The great saphenous vein and the small saphenous vein and lymphatic drainage in the lower limbs. (1) The superficial iliac circumflex vein, (2) the superficial epigastric vein, (3) the external pudendal vein, (4) the superficial medial femoral vein, (5) the superficial lateral femoral vein

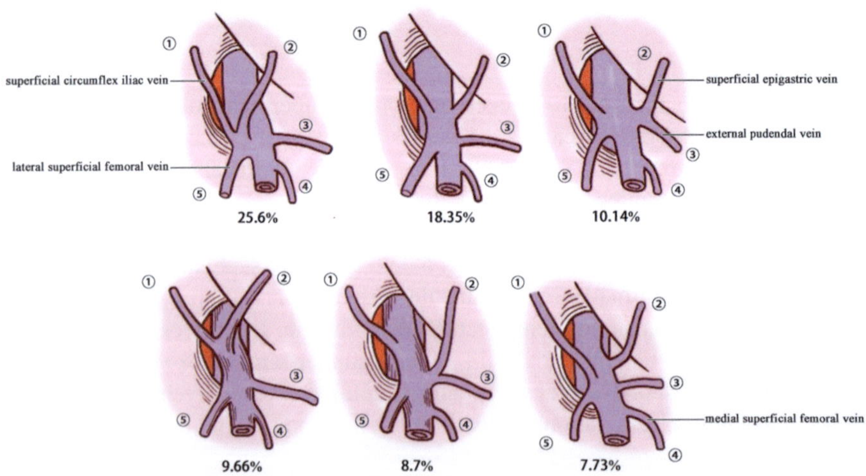

Fig. 5.24 Branches of the great saphenous vein (right side)

pressure, enlarged lumen, valvular insufficiency, and eventually the lower limb varicose veins. During the procedures of high ligation and stripping of the great saphenous vein for lower limb varicose veins, all tributaries of the great saphenous vein should be ligated and cut off at their roots, thus preventing the recurrence.

Small Saphenous Vein The small saphenous vein originates from the lateral side of the dorsal venous arch of the foot, ascends alongside the midline of the posterior side of the leg, and drains into the popliteal vein between the medial and lateral heads of the gastrocnemius (Fig. 5.23).

Superficial Arteries

The superficial epigastric artery arises from the femoral artery at 1 cm below the inguinal ligament and accompanies the superficial epigastric vein after passing through the fascia cribrosa. It ascends to the anterior abdominal wall and supplies the superficial tissue and the skin on the abdomen.

The superficial iliac circumflex artery arises from the femoral artery that is close to the origin of the superficial epigastric artery. It pierces the fascia lata, obliquely runs superolaterally alongside the posterior portion of the inguinal ligament, and supplies the surrounding skin and superficial fascia.

The external pudendal artery arises from the femoral artery that is close to the origin of the superficial epigastric artery and superficial iliac circumflex artery. It pierces the fascia cribrosa and accompanies the external pudendal vein, supplying the skin on the vulva.

Superficial Lymph Nodes

The superficial inguinal lymph nodes are situated in the superior region of the anteromedial groin, which are divided into superior and inferior groups. There are 5.6 superficial lymph nodes situated in the superior group, which are inferiorly parallel to the inguinal ligament. There are 4–5 superficial lymph nodes situated in the inferior group and longitudinally arranged alongside the bilateral sides of the root of the great saphenous vein. Some of the superficial inguinal lymph nodes drain into the deep inguinal lymph nodes, and some drain superiorly into the external iliac lymph nodes around the femoral blood vessels and through the femoral canal.

The superficial popliteal lymph nodes are situated in the popliteal fossa and drain into the popliteal vein through the small saphenous vein (Fig. 5.23).

Cutaneous Nerves

The superior cluneal nerves perforate the superomedial region of the hip and innervate the skin on the superior part of the hip. The inferior cluneal nerves, as branches of the posterior cutaneous nerve of the thigh, pass inferiorly through the inferior region of the gluteus maximus and innervate the skin on the inferior part of the hip. The lateral, intermediate, medial, and posterior femoral cutaneous nerves innervate the skin on the lateral, anterior, medial, and posterior parts of the thigh, respectively. The saphenous nerve accompanies the great saphenous vein in the medial part of the leg. The medial and lateral sural cutaneous nerves innervate the skin on the posterior part of the leg and converge to form the sural nerve in the distal third of the leg and accompany the small saphenous vein. The superficial fibular nerve perforates in the distal third of the anterolateral part of the leg and descends to divide into the lateral and medial dorsal cutaneous nerves of the foot. The deep fibular nerve superficially perforates the foot and innervates the skin between the first and second toes.

Deep Fascia

The deep fascia of the lower limbs is continuous and thick. The superficial layer of the deep fascia covers the surface of lower limb muscles, and the deep layer can be seen in some parts of the lower limbs to separate the superficial and deep muscular layers. The deep fascia of the lower limbs extends with the intermuscular septa that attach to the surfaces of the bones, thus separating muscle groups. It also forms important structures like ligaments.

Deep Fascia of the Hip

The deep fascia of the hip, also known as the gluteal fascia, attaches superiorly to the iliac crest, continues laterally with the fascia lata, and forms the iliotibial tract. It is a thick and dense layer that forms the fibrous septum extending into the gluteus maximus. The gluteal fascia is closely communicated with the muscle. The gluteal aponeurosis is a dense aponeurosis layer on the superolateral part of the hip that overlies the gluteus mediums.

Deep Fascia of the Thigh

The deep fascia of the thigh, also known as the fascia lata, is a layer of tough fibrous membrane that encloses all the thigh muscles. The lateral thickening of the fascia lata forms the iliotibial tract. The upper third of the iliotibial tract is a two-layer structure that encloses the tensor fasciae latae and can be used to repair the anatomical area of weakness or skin defects. The fascia lata forms a weak oval opening in the femoral triangle, namely, the saphenous hiatus. It is covered by a layer of porous loose connective tissue membrane, which is known as the cribriform fascia. The lateral margin of the saphenous hiatus is sharp and falciform, forming the falciform margin. Its superior and inferior ends form the medially arched superior cornu and inferior cornu, respectively. The superior cornu extends medially to attach to the pubic tubercle and communicates with the inguinal ligament and lacunar ligament. The inferior cornu continues medially with the pubic fascia. The saphenous hiatus anteriorly transmits the great saphenous vein, pierces the cribriform fascia, and joins the femoral vein (Fig. 5.23). The deep layer of the fascia lata contributes to forming the medial, lateral, and posterior intermuscular septum of the thigh and attaches to the linea aspera. The lateral intermuscular septum is situated between the vastus lateralis and biceps femoris, and the medial intermuscular septum is between the vastus medialis and adductor muscles. The posterior intermuscular septum is a thin band of fascia between the adductor muscles and the posterior muscles of the thigh. The three intermuscular septa form three osteofascial sheaths alongside the fascia lata and bones of the thigh (Fig. 5.25).

The anterior osteofascial compartment of the thigh contains the muscles of the anterior thigh, femoral artery, femoral vein, femoral nerve, deep inguinal lymph nodes, etc.

The medial osteofascial compartment of the thigh contains the muscles of the medial thigh, the obturator artery, the obturator vein, the obturator nerve, etc.

The posterior osteofascial compartment of the thigh contains the muscles of the posterior thigh and sciatic nerve, which superiorly continues with the deep gluteal space and inferiorly connects the popliteal fossa.

Deep Fascia of the Leg

The deep fascia of the leg can be divided into the superficial layer, the deep layer, and the intermuscular septum. The superficial layer covers the surface of the muscles of the leg, and the thickening of its distal end near the ankle forms retinacula to stabilize tendons, including the flexor retinaculum at the medial side of the ankle, superior extensor retinaculum (transverse crural ligament) at the anterior and slightly superior side of the leg, superior and inferior fibular retinacula at the lateral side of the leg, and inferior extensor retinaculum (cruciate ligaments) at the dorsal side of the foot (Fig. 5.26). The deep fascia of the leg separates the superficial and deep posterior muscles of the leg.

The superficial layer of deep fascia of the leg extends to form anterior and posterior intermuscular septum that attach to the anterior and posterior margin of the fibula, respectively. The anterior intermuscular septum of the leg separates the anterior from lateral muscles of the leg, and the posterior one separates the lateral from posterior muscles of the leg. The superficial layer of deep fascia of the leg,

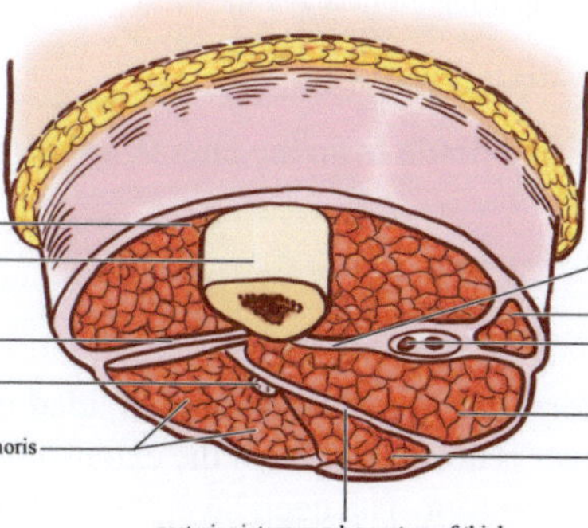

Fig. 5.25 The osteofascial compartment of the middle third of the femur (right side)

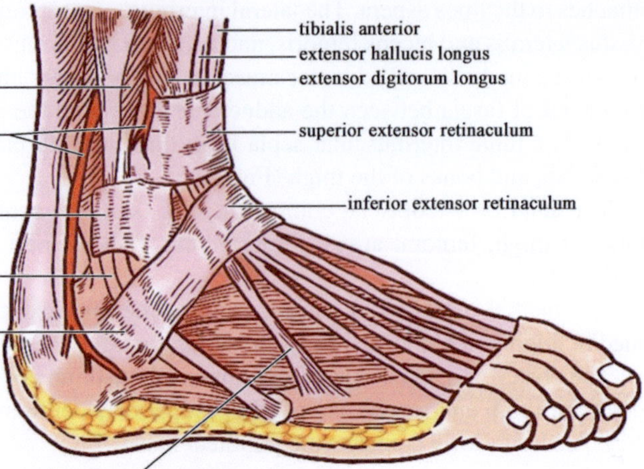

Fig. 5.26 The ankle and the lateral side of the dorsal aspect of the foot

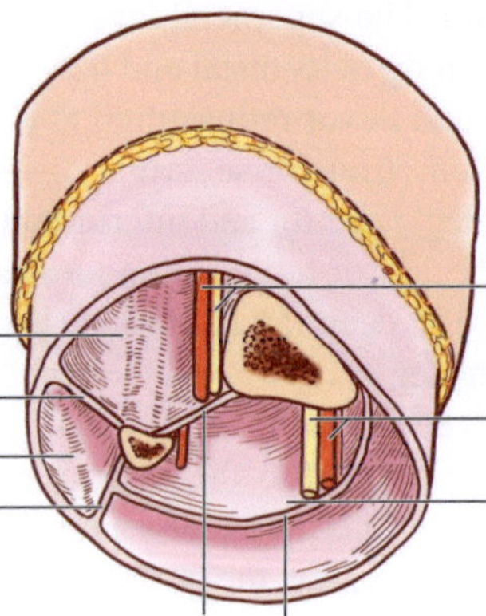

Fig. 5.27 The osteofascial compartment of the middle third of the right leg

intermuscular septa, tibia and fibula form the lateral, anterior and posterior osteofascial sheath (Fig. 5.27).

Deep Fascia of the Foot

The deep fascia of the dorsal aspect of the foot is divided into superficial and deep layers. The superficial layer is the extension of the extensor retinaculum that attaches to the bilateral margins of the foot. The deep layer, also known as the dorsal interosseous fascia, covers the dorsal side of the dorsal interossei and continues with the metatarsal periosteum. The superficial and deep layers enclose the plantar fascial spaces of the foot, where the tendon of extensor digitorum longus, extensor digitorum brevis and its tendon, branches of the deep peroneal nerve, and dorsalis pedis artery and vein pass through (Figs. 5.28 and 5.29). The deep fascia of the plantar aspect of the foot is divided into superficial and deep layers. The superficial layer covers the surface of the plantar muscles. The thickening in the central part is known as the plantar aponeurosis that supports the arch of the foot. The bilateral margins of the plantar aponeurosis extend to form two intermuscular septa that divide the plantar side of the foot into the lateral, intermediate, and medial osteofascial sheath (Fig. 5.29). The deep layer of deep fascia of the plantar aspect of the foot is known as the interosseous plantar fascia.

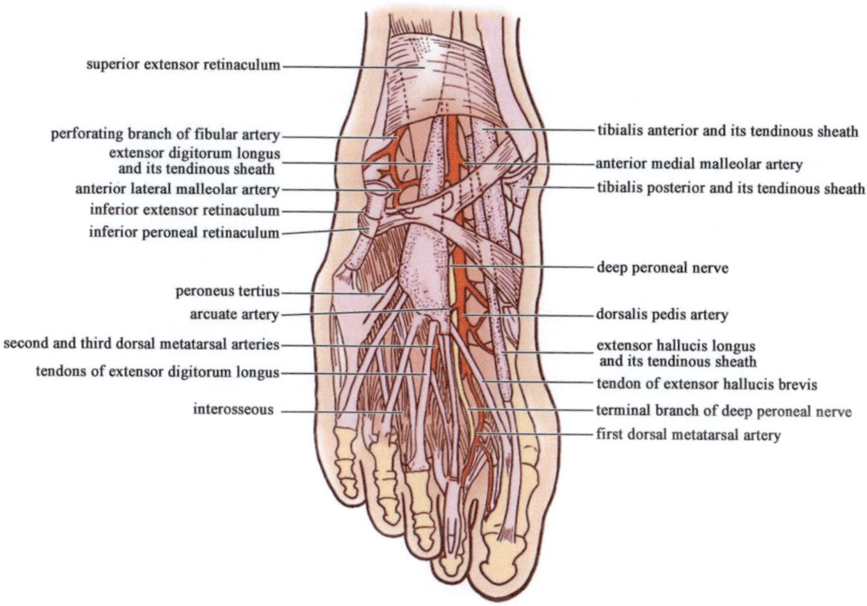

Fig. 5.28 The anterior region of the ankle and the dorsal aspect of the foot

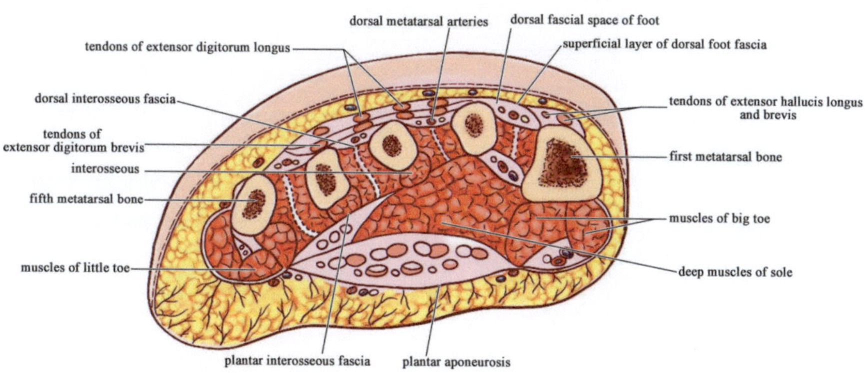

Fig. 5.29 The middle part of the foot in the coronal plane

Intermuscular Septa and Fascial Compartments of the Lower Limbs

Similar to those of the upper limbs, intermuscular septa and fascial compartments exist in the lower limbs and are composed of the loose connective tissues, blood vessels, and nerves. They are communicated with the adjacent intermuscular septum and fascial compartment that allow the spread of the infection. Important intermuscular septa and fascial compartments of the lower limbs are described as follows.

Lacuna Musculorum and Lacuna Vasorum

Separated by the iliopectineal arch between the inguinal ligament and the iliopubic eminence, the space between the inguinal ligament and hip bone is divided into the lateral lacuna musculorum and the medial lacuna vasorum. The lacuna vasorum is anteriorly, posteriorly, medially, and laterally bounded by the inguinal ligament, pectinate ligament, lacunar ligament, and iliopectineal arch, respectively. It contains the femoral artery, femoral vein, and femoral canal and communicates with the retroperitoneal space. The lacuna musculorum is anteriorly, posteriorly, and medially bounded by the inguinal ligament, ilium, and iliopectineal arch, respectively. It contains the iliopsoas and femoral nerve and communicates with the subfascial space of the posterior abdominal wall (Fig. 5.30).

Femoral Triangle

The femoral triangle is a down-pointing triangular area situated in the upper third of the anterior thigh. It is superiorly bounded by the inguinal ligament, medially by the medial side of the adductor longus, and laterally by the medial side of the sartorius.

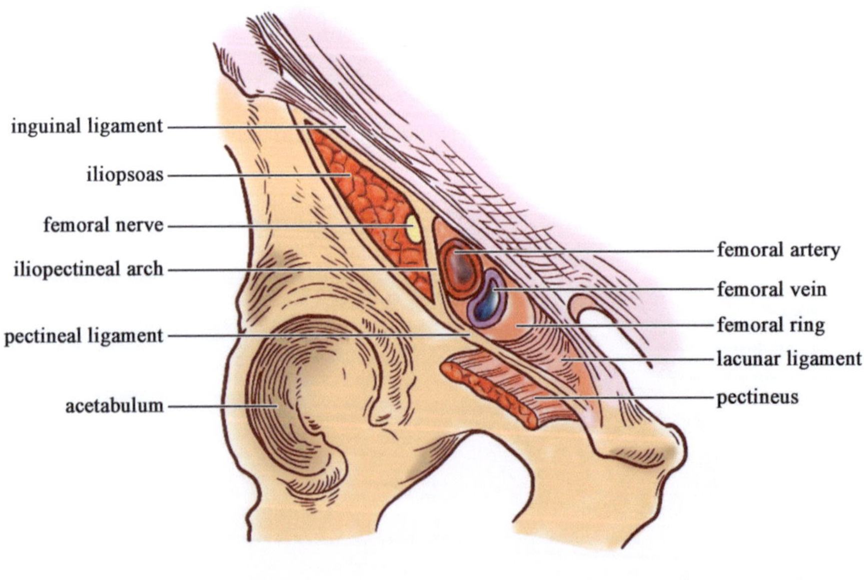

Fig. 5.30 Lacuna musculorum and lacuna vasorum

Its anterior and posterior portions are the fascia lata and a depression, respectively. From lateral to medial, the femoral triangle is formed by the iliopsoas, pectineus, and adductor longus and its tendon. It contains the femoral nerve, femoral artery, femoral vein, and femoral canal from lateral to medial. The femoral triangle is a common site of manual compression for hemostasis, angiography by femoral artery intubation, femoral nerve block anesthesia, and femoral vein puncture (Fig. 5.31).

The femoral triangle superiorly communicates with the subfascial space of the posterior abdominal wall through the lacuna musculorum and inferiorly communicates with the adductor canal. It connects the retroperitoneal space via passing through the lacuna vasorum. In cases of lumbar vertebra tuberculosis, pus can spread inferiorly into the femoral triangle along the psoas major, lacuna musculorum, and lesser trochanter.

Femoral Sheath, Femoral Canal, and Femoral Ring

The femoral sheath is a funnel-shaped aponeurosis 3–4 cm in length. It is the downward extension of the transversalis fascia and iliac fascia that encloses the femoral artery and the upper part of the femoral vein. Its distal end forms the vascular sheath by joining the outer layer (tunica adventitia) of femoral blood vessels. The femoral sheath is divided by two longitudinal fibrous septa into the lateral compartment

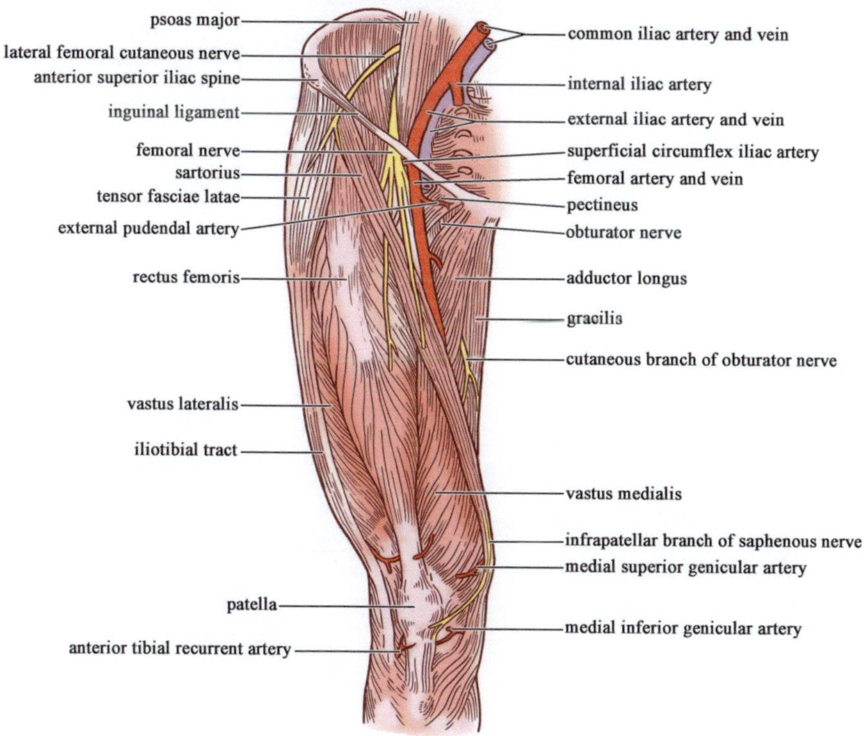

Fig. 5.31 Muscles, blood vessels, and nerves in the superficial layer of the anterior thigh

containing the femoral artery, the intermediate compartment containing the femoral vein, and the medial compartment that is also known as the femoral canal (Fig. 5.32).

The femoral canal is a funnel-like space 1–1.5 cm in length. It is anteriorly bounded by the inguinal ligament and cribriform fascia, posteriorly by the pectinate ligament and pectineus and its tendon, medially by the lacunar ligament and medial margin of the femoral sheath, and laterally by the fibrous septum medial to the femoral vein. The proximal opening of the femoral canal forms the oval-like femoral ring and is bounded by the inguinal ligament, lacunar ligament, pectinate ligament, and fibrous septum medial to the femoral vein. It is superiorly covered by a thin layer of loose connective tissues, that is, the femoral septum. The superior portion of the femoral septum is lined by partial peritoneum, forming a small depression (femoral fossa) that is 1 cm away from the femoral ring. Due to the increased abdominal pressure, abdominal organs may protrude into the femoral fossa. Through the femoral ring and femoral canal, the protrusion exits through the saphenous hiatus and thus forms a femoral hernia (Fig. 5.33).

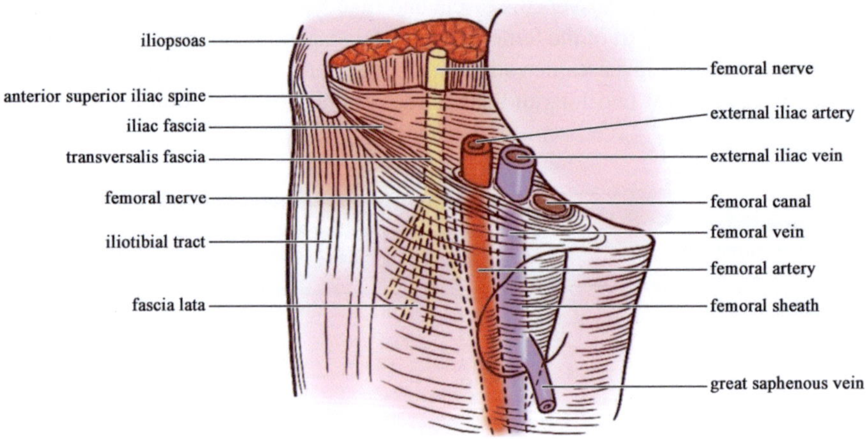

Fig. 5.32 The femoral sheath

Fig. 5.33 A femoral hernia

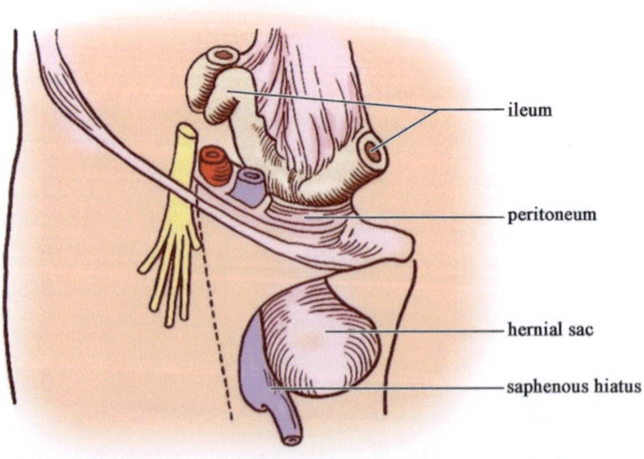

The femoral ring is less extendable because of limitations from ligaments in the anterior, medial, and posterior boundaries. As a result, femoral hernias have a high risk of strangulation. The obturator branch of the inferior epigastric artery, or variant obturator artery, passes around the lacunar ligament and should be protected during the procedures of femoral hernia repair.

Adductor Canal

The adductor canal is situated on the anteromedial side of the middle thigh, serving as a passageway for the muscles of the anterior thigh. Its anterior wall is a strong aponeurosis (lamina vastoadductoria) extending across the vastus medialis, adductor longus, and adductor magnus (Fig. 5.34).

The sartorius lies on the surface of the lamina vastoadductoria. The lateral wall of adductor canal is formed by the vastus medialis, and its posterior wall is bounded by the adductor longus and adductor magnus. The adductor canal superiorly communicates with the apex of the femoral triangle, and its inferior end is the adductor tendinous opening that connects the superior angle of the popliteal fossa. From anterior to posterior, the adductor canal contains the saphenous nerve, femoral artery, femoral vein, and surrounding lymph nodes. The saphenous nerve and the descending genicular artery (a branch of the femoral artery) in the distal end of the adductor canal exit through the anterior wall to the medial side of the knee.

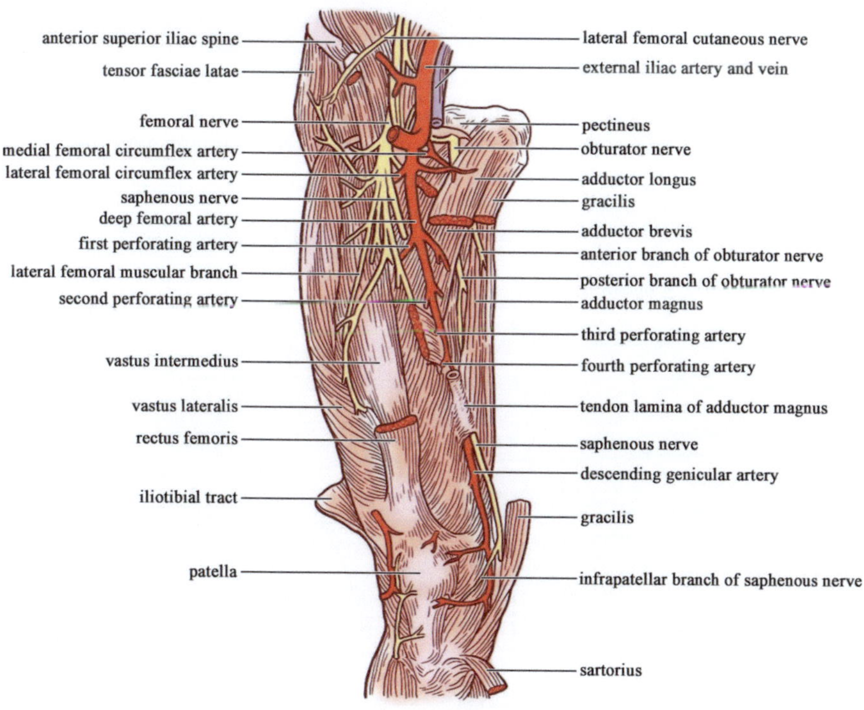

Fig. 5.34 Muscles, blood vessels, and nerves in the deep layer of the anterior thigh

Deep Gluteal Space

The deep gluteal space is situated beneath the gluteus maximus and is especially loose at the greater sciatic foramen. It contains the superior and inferior gluteal blood vessels and nerves, the sciatic nerve, internal pudendal vessels, and the pudendal nerve. It deeply extends to the suprapiriform and infrapiriform foramina and communicates with the pelvic cavity. The deep gluteal space is anteroinferiorly communicated with the inferior portion of the hip, inferiorly with the posterior compartment of the thigh, and inferomedially with the ischioanal fossa after passing through the lesser sciatic foramen. Infections in the deep gluteal space can spread to the pelvic cavity, ischioanal fossa, and posterior compartment of the thigh through the neurovascular bundle or even to the popliteal fossa along the sciatic nerve.

Suprapiriform and Infrapiriform Foramen

The piriformis travels through the greater sciatic foramen and divides it into the suprapiriform and infrapiriform foramina. The former contains the superior gluteal blood vessels and nerve, and the latter contains the sciatic nerve, inferior gluteal blood vessels and nerve, posterior femoral cutaneous nerve, internal pudendal vessels, and pudendal nerve (Fig. 5.35).

The anatomical relationship between the sciatic nerve and piriformis muscle varies (Fig. 5.36).

Posterior Compartment of the Thigh

The posterior compartment of the thigh is situated between the muscles of the posterior thigh and contains the sciatic nerve and inferiorly continues with the popliteal fossa.

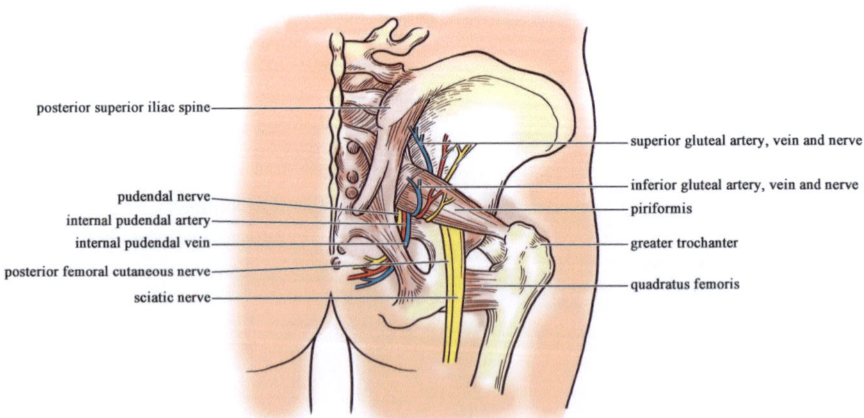

Fig. 5.35 Blood vessels and nerves in the hip

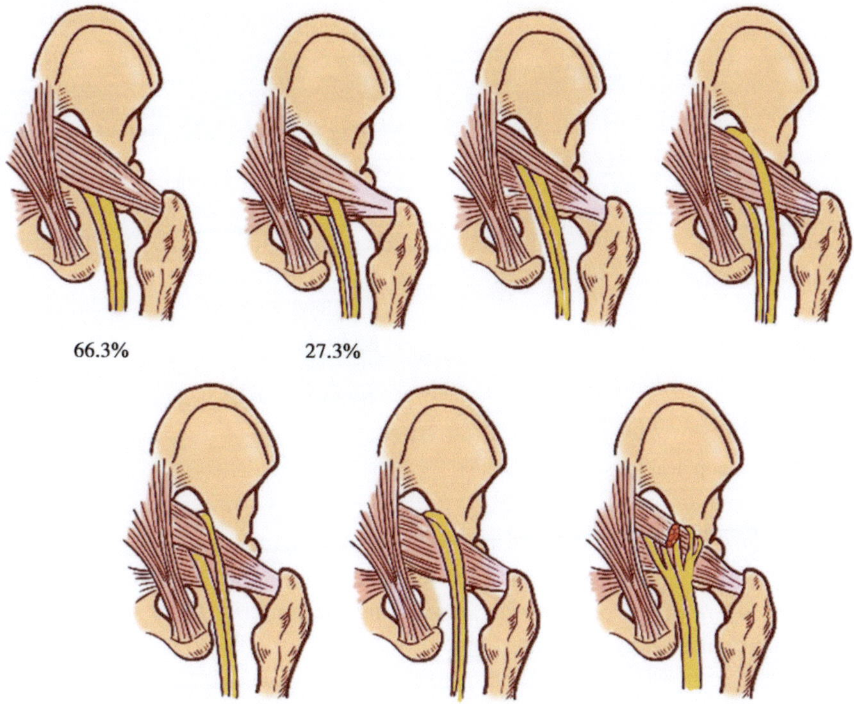

Fig. 5.36 The anatomical relationship between the sciatic nerve and the piriformis muscle

Popliteal Fossa

The popliteal fossa is a diamond-like depression situated posterior to the knee. Superiorly, it is laterally and medially bounded by the biceps femoris and semimembranosus and semitendinosus, respectively. Inferiorly, it is laterally and medially bounded by the lateral and medial heads of the gastrocnemius, respectively. The surface of the popliteal fossa is covered by the popliteal fascia. In addition to massive adipose tissues and popliteal lymph nodes, the popliteal fossa contains the tibial nerve, popliteal vein, and popliteal artery from superficial to deep. The small saphenous vein drains into the popliteal vein through the popliteal fossa. The common fibular nerve descends laterally alongside the tendon of the biceps femoris. Coursing through the lateral head of the gastrocnemius, the common fibular nerve lies below the head of the fibula, winds around the neck of the fibula, and pierces the deep layer of the fibularis longus, where it divides into the superficial and deep fibular nerves. The common fibular nerve is closely attached to the surface of the neck of the fibular and easily damaged in cases of fractures of fibular neck (Fig. 5.37).

The popliteal fossa is superiorly continuous with the adductor canal and posterior compartment of the thigh and inferiorly communicates with the posterior compartment of the leg.

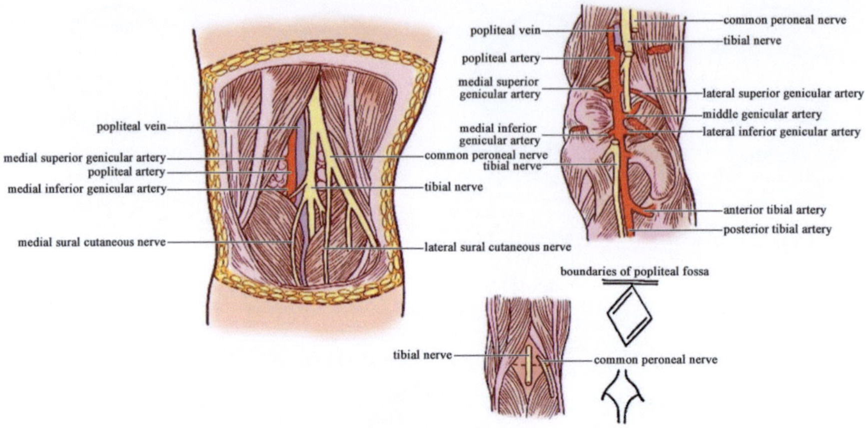

Fig. 5.37 The popliteal fossa and its contents

Posterior Compartment of the Leg

The posterior compartment of the leg is situated between the superficial and deep muscular layers of the posterior leg, containing the posterior tibial vessels, tibial nerve, and fibular artery and vein (Fig. 5.38).

Malleolar Canal

The malleolar canal is formed by the flexor retinaculum, medial malleolus, and calcaneus. The ligaments in the malleolar canal extend deep to divide into four bony fibrous compartments. From anterior to posterior, the malleolar canal contains the posterior tibial tendon and the tendon sheath, the tendon of flexor digitorum longus and the tendon sheath, posterior tibial vessels, tibial nerve, and flexor hallucis longus (Fig. 5.39). The malleolar canal is filled with loose connective tissues, serving as a passageway of the posterior leg to the plantar aspect of the foot. Infections in the leg or plantar aspect of the foot spread through the malleolar canal. Compressions on the tibial nerve in the malleolar canal due to trauma, bleeding, or swelling in the posterior talocrural region result in the tarsal tunnel syndrome.

Bones and Bone Connections

Bones of the lower limb are composed of the lower limb girdle bones and the free lower limb bones. The lower limb girdle bone is the hip bone. The hip bone is composed of the ilium, ischial and pubic . Three bones were combined by hyaline cartilage in childhood and fused with each other around the age of 16. The free lower limb bones include the femur, patella, tibia ,fibula, and the foot bones. The foot bones include the tarsal bones, metatarsals and metatarsals. The connections of lower limb bones consist of lower limb girdle bones connections and free lower

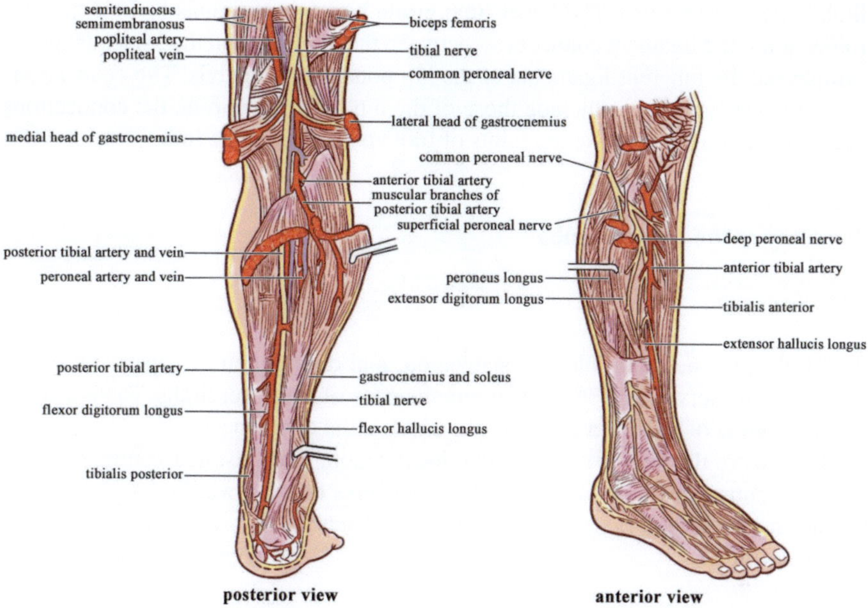

Fig. 5.38 The neurovascular bundle of the leg

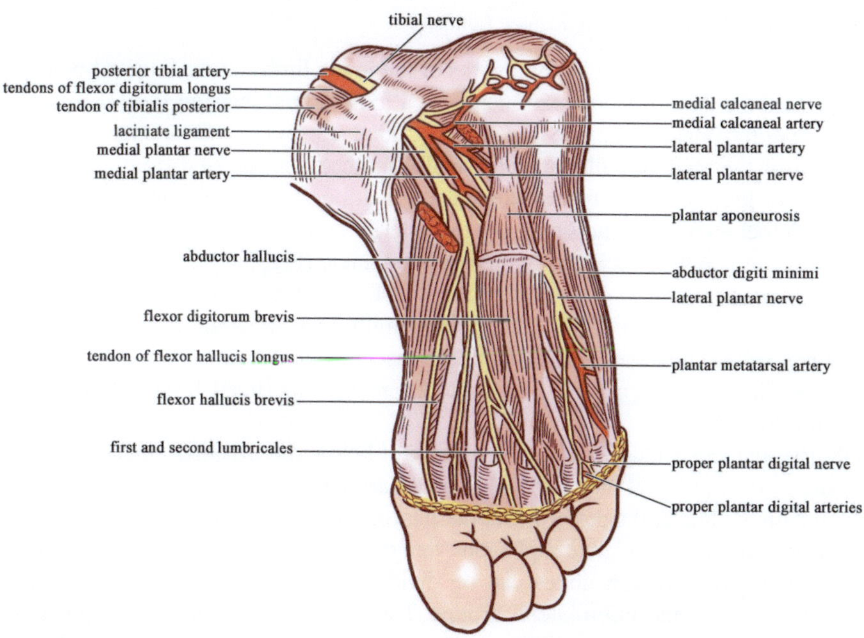

Fig. 5.39 Medial side of the posterior talocrural region and the plantar aspect of the foot

limb bones connections. The lower limb girdle bones connections include the sacroiliac joint, the ligament connections between the hip bone and the spine, the pubic symphysis, the inherent ligaments of the hip bone and the pelvis. The connections of free lower limb bones include those of the hip joint, knee joint, the connections between the tibia and fibula, the joints of foot and arches of the foot.

Anatomy of the Lower Limbs

Objective

1. To observe the morphology, localization, and distribution of superficial veins, cutaneous nerves, and superficial lymph nodes of the lower limbs. To dissect the deep fascia of the lower limbs and to observe the components.
2. To observe the intermuscular septa, localization, contents, and communication of the muscles, blood vessels, and nerve trunks of the lower limbs. To observe the muscles and nerves (orientation, branches, and distribution) of the lower limbs.

Dissection Procedures

Superficial Structures of the Lower Limbs

Step 1. Palpate the important landmarks of the lower limbs on the human bodies.

Step 2. Make the following skin incisions: a longitudinal incision from the medial side of the upper part of the thigh to the medial side of the knee and leg, posterior part of the medial malleolus, and finally the heel; an incision from the medial side of the foot to the medial side of the first toe; incisions on bilateral sides of each toe; an oblique incision from the anterior superior spine to the pubic tuberosity; and circular incisions at the knee and ankle (Fig. 5.40).

Step 3. From inside to outside, remove the skin on the anteromedial side of the lower limbs from the intersection of the longitudinal incisions. Protect the superficial veins, cutaneous nerves, and deep fascia.

Step 4. Remove and observe the contents in the superficial fascia of the anterior thigh.

Observe the superficial inguinal lymph nodes below the inguinal ligament. There are 8–10 superficial inguinal lymph nodes arranged below the inguinal ligament and on the bilateral sides of the upper part of the great saphenous vein. Centered by the site where the great saphenous vein drains into the femoral vein, the superficial inguinal lymph nodes can be divided into superomedial, superolateral, inferomedial, and inferolateral groups. Then, observe the superficial epigastric vein running from the umbilicus to the saphenous hiatus, the external pudendal vein running from the vulva to the saphenous hiatus, and the superficial iliac circumflex vein running inferomedially alongside the lateral part of the inguinal ligament (Fig. 5.24).

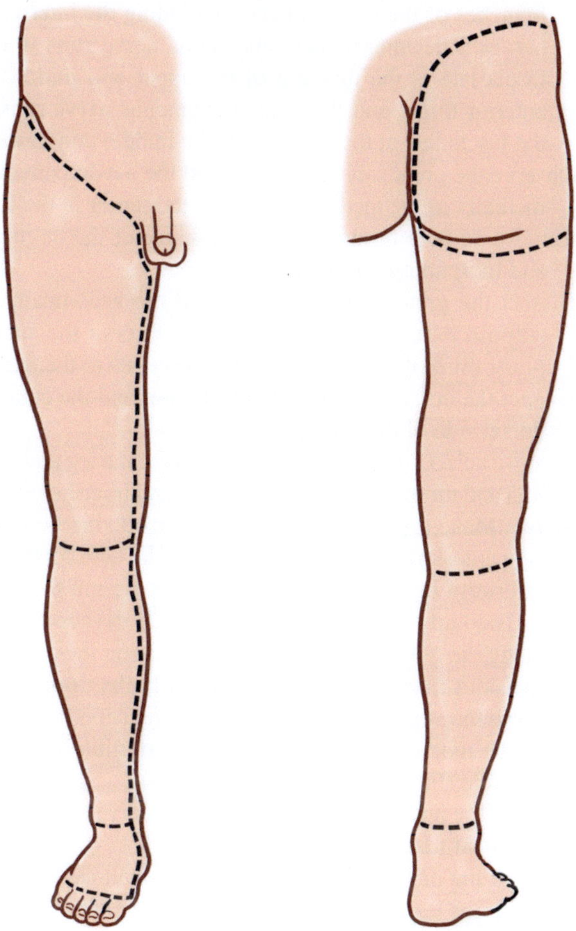

Fig. 5.40 Skin incisions of the lower limbs

Dissect the great saphenous vein and the superficial medial and lateral femoral veins situated within the adipose tissues of the anterior thigh, and free them until the femoral triangle. The great saphenous vein can be observed behind the medial condyle of the femur, and the superficial femoral veins can then be identified above it. Raise up the entire superficial inguinal lymph nodes from the lateral side or remove a part of them. Observe the saphenous hiatus lying 2 cm below the junction of the medial and middle third of the deep layer of the inguinal ligament. Observe the falciform margin of the saphenous hiatus, the morphology of cribriform fascia, and the root of the great saphenous vein that travel through the cribriform fascia. Identify the site of five tributaries draining into the great saphenous vein (Fig. 5.23).

Dissect the cutaneous nerves situated in the adipose tissues of the anterior thigh, including the lateral femoral cutaneous nerve and anterior cutaneous branches of the femoral nerve. The former runs inferiorly after perforating the fascia lata at 8–10 cm below the anterior superior iliac spine. There are 2–3 anterior cutaneous branches of the femoral nerve, including the intermediate and medial cutaneous nerves. The intermediate cutaneous nerve runs inferiorly after perforating the fascia lata at the junction of the upper and middle third of the midline of the anterior thigh, and the medial cutaneous nerve runs inferiorly after perforating the fascia lata at the junction of the middle and lower third of the medial thigh.

Observe the great saphenous vein and the accompanying saphenous nerve posteromedially to the medial condyle of the femur in the lower part of the thigh.

Remove adipose tissues in the lateral side of the thigh and observe the localization and morphology of the iliotibial tract.

Dissect the great saphenous vein and the accompanying saphenous nerve in the adipose tissues of the medial leg. Observe the superficial fibular nerve in the lower third of the lateral leg that descends to the dorsal side of the foot.

Dissect the dorsal venous arch of the foot and the cutaneous nerves running on the dorsal side of the foot.

Remove adipose tissues in the lower part of the leg and the foot. Observe the localization and morphology of the superior and inferior extensor retinaculum (Fig. 5.26).

Step 5. Make the following skin incisions on the body in a prone position: an incision anteriorly from the iliac crest to the anterior superior iliac spine; an incision inferiorly from the middle part of the sacrum to the apex of the coccyx; and an incision inferolaterally from the apex of the coccyx to the lateral side of the thigh along the gluteal fold. Raise up the skin on the thigh, leg, and foot along the skin incisions made on the anterior lower limbs from inside to outside (Fig. 5.40).

Observe the superior cluneal nerves in the superficial fascia of the superior margin of the iliac crest between the lateral portion of the erector spinae and the iliac tubercle (Fig. 5.41).

Observe the posterior femoral cutaneous nerve perforating the deep fascia above the popliteal fossa.

Observe the origin and insertion of the small saphenous vein in the midline of the posterior leg. Observe the accompanying medial-sural cutaneous nerve and the sural nerve formed by the medial-sural cutaneous nerve joining with the lateral sural cutaneous nerve at the junction of the middle and lower third of the leg.

Remove adipose tissues in the sole of the foot. Observe the characteristic and distribution of the plantar aponeurosis. Observe the blood vessels and nerves in the plantar aspect of the bilateral sides of the second toe.

Step 6. Observe the characteristics of the deep fascia of different regions of the lower limbs, including the thickness, tension, site of superficial veins, and cutaneous nerves that perforate.

Step 7. Observe the boundary of the superficial layer of the lower limb muscles through the deep fascia.

Muscles, Nerves, and Blood Vessels in the Anterior Side of the Lower Limbs

Anteromedial Side of the Thigh

Step 1. Separate the great saphenous vein from the deeper layer of tissues and raise it up. Free the five tributaries of the great saphenous vein to the site, where they

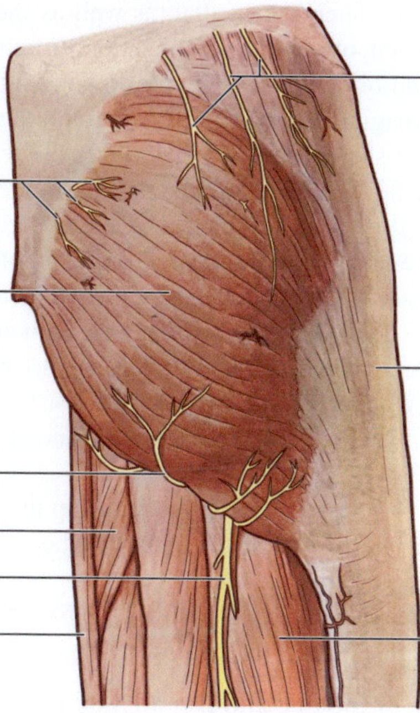

Fig. 5.41 The superficial fascia of the hip

join it, and the cutaneous nerves to the site, where they perforate the deep fascia. Be careful not to cut them off. Cut open the fascia lata, alongside the anterior portion of the iliotibial tract, and the latter is protected and should not be cut off. At 1 cm below the inguinal ligament, cut open the fascia lata to the lateral side of the saphenous hiatus and bypass the incision to the inferior portion. A transverse skin incision is then made until the medial side of the thigh. Be cautious to protect the intact structure of the saphenous hiatus. Raise up the fascia lata to the medial side or remove it. Notably, superficial blood vessels or cutaneous nerves that pierce the fascia lata should be carefully freed to the deep layer and not cut off. At the lateral portion of the sartorius, cut open the fascia sheath of the sartorius that is formed by the enclosed superficial and deep layers of the fascia lata. Remove the superficial layer of the fascia sheath of the sartorius but reserve the deep layer. Separate the fascia lata from the deep tissues in the femoral triangle, and reserve the blood vessels and nerves that pass through the saphenous hiatus. Reserve the superficial inguinal lymph nodes as much as possible. Observe the thicknesses in different regions and the anatomical relationship with the deep tissues during the process of peeling off the fascia lata.

Step 2. Observe the localization of muscles in the superficial layer of the anteromedial side of the thigh and the boundary of the femoral triangle.

Step 3. Remove the contents of the femoral triangle, free the femoral sheath, and observe its morphology and localization. Make a longitudinal incision on the midline of the femoral sheath, and observe the femoral artery, femoral vein, and femoral canal from lateral to medial, as well as the fibrous compartments that separate them. Then, observe the localization, structure, size, and contents of the femoral canal and femoral ring. Gently probe into the femoral canal using forceps without damaging the structure of the femoral ring.

Separate the femoral sheath from the deep-layer tissues, and observe the iliopsoas fascia and pubic fascia situated on the floor of the femoral triangle. Make a longitudinal incision on the iliopsoas fascia, and observe the femoral nerve and the iliopsoas that are situated in the deep layer. Find out the localization, contents, and communications of the lacuna vasorum and lacuna musculorum.

Step 4. Observe the deep femoral artery and its branches of the medial and lateral circumflex femoral arteries and the perforating arteries.

Step 5. Raise up the sartorius in the central part of the thigh, and do not cut it off. Observe the localization, structure, contents, and communications of the adductor canal.

Step 6. Separate and remove the gracilis. Raise up the adductor longus that is situated on the floor of the femoral triangle to the lateral side to expose the adductor brevis in the deep layer. Remove the adductor brevis, and observe the anterior and posterior branches of the obturator nerve passing superficially and deeply to the adductor longus, as well as accompanying obturator vessels.

Anterolateral Side of the Leg and Dorsal Side of the Foot

Step 1. Free but not cut off the superficial veins and cutaneous nerves situated on the anterolateral side of the leg and the dorsal side of the foot. Then, remove the deep fascia, but preserve the superior and inferior extensor retinacula, and protect the main trunk of the superficial veins and cutaneous nerves. Observe the thickness of the deep fascia, its anatomical relationship with the muscles in the deep layer, and the intermuscular septa.

Step 2. Observe the muscles of the anterolateral side of the leg and the tendon sheaths of the dorsal side of the foot.

Step 3. Separate the raphe between the tibialis anterior and the extensor digitorum longus and that between the tibialis anterior and the extensor hallucis longus. Observe the anterior tibial artery and vein and the deep fibular nerve that are situated deeply to the raphe and travel inferiorly at the anterior aspect of the interosseous membrane.

Step 4. Observe the superficial fibular nerve in the space between the fibularis longus and brevis and the tibialis anterior in the central part of the leg.

Step 5. In the posterior portion of the dorsal aspect of the foot, observe the dorsalis pedis artery and vein and the deep fibular nerve situated lateral to the extensor hallucis longus.

Muscles, Nerves, and Blood Vessels in the Posterior Side of the Lower Limbs

The Hip

Step 1. Free the superior cluneal nerves and remove the deep fascia on the surface of the gluteus maximus. Observe the anatomical relationship between the deep fascia and the gluteus maximus.

Step 2. Clean the margin of the gluteus maximus. Observe the gluteus maximus and the superolaterally situated gluteus medius.

Step 3. Remove the connective tissues on the inferomedial side of the gluteus maximus. Find out the inferomedial margin of the gluteus maximus, and raise up its inferomedial portion and separate it from the deep-layer tissues. Gently cut off the origin of the gluteus maximus from bottom to top, and be cautious to protect the sacrotuberous ligament. Then, raise up the gluteus maximus to the inferolateral side, and observe the muscles in the deep layer, suprapiriform and infrapiriform foramen, superior and inferior gluteal blood vessels and nerves, sciatic nerve, internal pudendal vessels, and pudendal nerve. Identify the anatomical relationship between the sciatic nerve and the piriformis and the localization of the sciatic nerve in the hip.

Posterior Side of the Thigh and Popliteal Fossa

Step 1. Make a longitudinal incision in the deep fascia of the posterior thigh along the posterior portion of the iliotibial tract, and remove the deep fascia without damaging the iliotibial tract. Observe the anatomical relationship with the deep-layer tissues and the intermuscular septa.

Step 2. Observe the posterior femoral cutaneous nerve running deep along the midline in the deep fascia of the posterior thigh, muscle groups of the posterior thigh, and the boundary of the popliteal fossa.

Step 3. Separate the posterior compartment between the biceps femoris, the semimembranosus, and the semitendinosus. Observe the sciatic nerve, tibial nerve, common peroneal nerve, and perforating arteries.

Step 4. Remove adipose tissues in the popliteal fossa. Observe the common peroneal nerve inferior to the biceps femoris tendon in the superolateral part of the popliteal fossa. From superficial too deep in the midline, find out the tibial nerve, popliteal vein and artery, and surrounding popliteal lymph nodes. Then, observe the branches of the popliteal vein and artery that travel to the bilateral sides or the deep layer. Finally, observe the components, contents, and communications of the popliteal fossa.

Posterior Side of the Leg

Step 1. Free the small saphenous vein and sural nerve, and carefully remove the deep fascia on the posterior leg. Observe the thickness of the deep fascia, its anatomical relationship with the deep-layer tissues, and intermuscular septa.

Step 2. Observe the muscles in the superficial layer of the posterior leg.

Step 3. Cut off the medial head of the gastrocnemius muscle and raise up the gastrocnemius muscle laterally to expose the soleus. Cut open the partial origin of the soleus and raise it up to the lateral side to expose the posterior compartment of the leg. Remove the deep fascia covering on the surface of the muscles in the deep layer of the posterior leg, and observe the localization of muscle groups in this region. Observe the posterior tibial artery and vein and the tibial nerve in the midline of the posterior leg. Find out the origins of the anterior and posterior tibial arteries and veins in the inferior margin of the popliteus.

Step 4. In the deep layer of the flexor retinaculum posterior to the medial malleolus, observe the posterior tibial tendon, flexor digitorum longus tendon, posterior tibial vessels, tibial nerve, and flexor hallucis longus that course through the medial malleolus to the plantar aspect of the foot.

Plantar Aspect of the Foot

Step 1. Clarify the boundary of the plantar aponeurosis, and cut open the anterior portion of the medial and lateral sides of it. Raise up the plantar aponeurosis from the front, with the distal end attaching on the calcaneal tuberosity. Be careful to protect the deep-layer structures, especially the five bundles of fibrous connective tissues, compartments of the plantar aponeurosis and blood vessels and nerves passing through them. Finally, observe the flexor digitorum brevis situated in the deep layer of the plantar aponeurosis.

Step 2. Observe the medial plantar artery, vein, and nerve between the flexor digitorum brevis and medial plantar muscles of the foot. Raise up the flexor digitorum brevis, and observe the quadratus plantae, flexor digitorum longus tendon, and lateral plantar artery, vein, and nerve that obliquely travel across the superficial layer of the quadratus plantae.

Summary

Similar to the five-layer structure of the upper limbs, the lower limbs are composed of the skin, superficial fascia, deep fascia, intermuscular septa and fascial compartments, and bones and bone connections. The superficial fascia of the lower limbs contains the superficial blood vessels, cutaneous nerves, superficial lymph nodes, and lymphatic vessels. The superficial veins usually accompany the main trunk of the cutaneous nerves. In the lower limbs, important superficial veins mainly include the great saphenous vein and its five tributaries, and the small saphenous vein. The deep fascia of the lower limbs is continuous and thick. The saphenous hiatus is situated on the fascia lata at 3–4 cm inferolateral to the pubic tuberosity, through which the veins and lymphatic pass. The iliotibial tract is the thickening of the fascia lata on the lateral side of the thigh, and the retinacula of the ankle are localized thickening of the crural fascia. Several intermuscular structures and septa of the lower limbs are of great significance, including the lacuna musculorum, lacuna vasorum, femoral sheath, femoral canal, femoral triangle, adductor canal, popliteal fossa, deep gluteal space, suprapiriform, and infrapiriform foramen. Blood vessels and nerves pass through the intermuscular septa of the lower limbs that are composed of loose connective tissues and communicate with each other. As a result, they provide the passageways for inflammation to spread. The femoral canal is an anatomical area of weakness, where femoral hernia occurs. The nerve trunks of the lower limbs that are close to the bones and joints are prone to damage in cases of joint dislocation or fractures.

Clinical Application of Key Anatomical Structures of the Limbs

Application of the Anatomical Structures of the Limbs in Common Surgical Procedures

Application of Key Anatomical Structures of the Upper Limbs

The shoulder joint is a spheroidal joint in the human body, with the greatest range of motion, and composed of the glenoid cavity and the head of the humerus. The rotator cuff tendons, composed of the supraspinatus, infraspinatus, teres minor, and subscapularis tendons, cover the shoulder joint and thus enhance its stability (Fig. 5.42a). The shoulder joint is the most frequently dislocated joint and is unstable due to the specific structures of the large head of the humerus, shallow and small glenoid cavity, and loose joint capsule. Anterior shoulder dislocation usually accompanies with an avulsion fracture of greater tuberosity of humerus, which is caused by the violent contraction of the supraspinatus, infraspinatus, and teres minor that attach on the greater tuberosity (Fig. 5.42d). A dislocated shoulder injury may cause a rotator cuff injury, resulting in recurrent shoulder dislocations. Notably, the dislocated head of the humerus may cause the compression of the brachial plexus, and the potential brachial plexus injury should be assessed prior to shoulder reduction.

The surgical neck of the humerus is situated in the junction between the proximal end of the humerus and the humeral shaft, as the most common site for proximal humerus fractures due to the low bone mineral density. The deltopectoral approach is the most common approach for proximal humerus fractures. Briefly, an incision is made from the palpable coracoid process at the lower portion of the distal clavicle and then extended anterolaterally to the proximal humeral shaft along the deltopectoral groove between the deltoid and pectoralis major. Be careful to protect the cephalic vein and axillary nerve in the deltopectoral groove and the triangular space, respectively. Expose the bony structure of the proximal humerus and rotator cuff after bluntly separating the deltoid and pectoralis major. Reduction of proximal humerus fractures and rotator cuff repair can usually be performed under direct vision. Open reduction and internal fixation of midshaft humeral fractures should be carefully performed to prevent iatrogenic injury of the radial nerve that runs behind the middle portion of the humeral shaft. Surgical exploration of radial nerve, however, is necessary in cases of midshaft humeral fractures presenting the manifestations of radial nerve injuries.

The elbow joint includes the humeroradial joint, humeroulnar joint, and superior radioulnar joint (proximal radioulnar joint) (Fig. 5.43a). The humeroulnar joint is composed of the humeral trochlea and the trochlear notch of the ulna. The humeroradial joint is composed of the capitulum of the humerus and the articular facet of the head of the radius. The superior radioulnar joint is composed of the caudal aspect of the head of radius and the radial notch of the ulna. The triangular

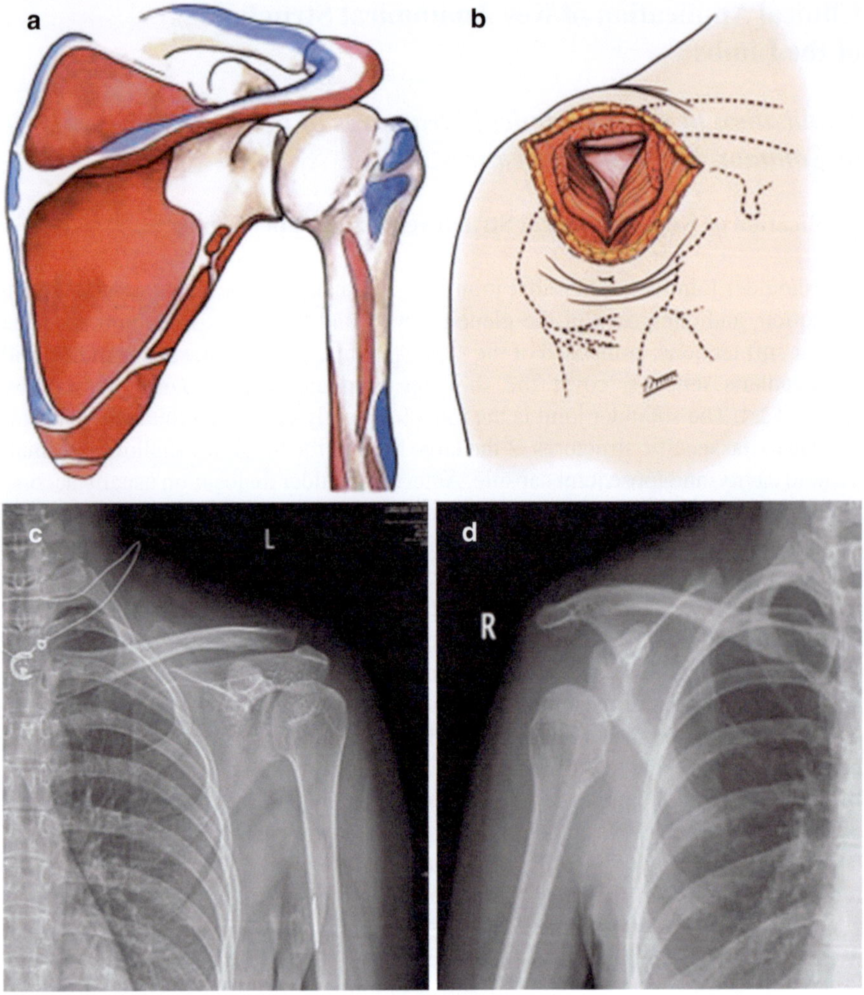

Fig. 5.42 Key anatomical structures of the upper limbs. (**a**) Shoulder joint. (**b**) Deltopectoral approach. c, d. Normal shoulder joint. (**c**) Anterior shoulder dislocation (**d**) On X-ray scans

relationship between the medial and lateral epicondyle of the humerus and the olecranon of the ulna changes in cases of elbow dislocation can be taken as an important sign in identifying elbow dislocation and distal humeral fractures (Fig. 5.43b). Posterior surgical approaches to the elbow are preferred due to the thick anterior muscles of the elbow, medial and lateral collateral ligaments that maintain the stability of the elbow, and loose posterior wall of the joint capsule. Briefly, an incision is made on the midline of the posterior elbow, and the ulnar nerve runs in the superficial fascial on the dorsal side of the medial condyle of the humerus (Fig. 5.43d). During the surgical procedures, the ulnar nerve requires it to be fully exposed and protected. The proximal end of the ulna is exposed after separating the superficial

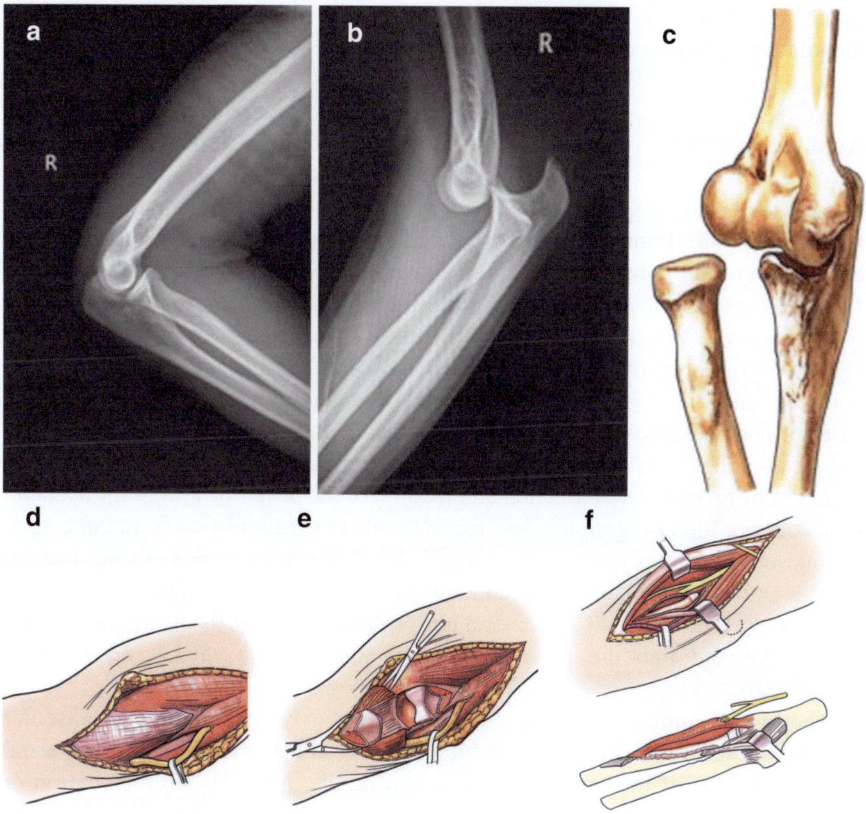

Fig. 5.43 Elbow joint. (**a**, **b**) Normal elbow joint. (**a**) Posterior elbow dislocation. (**b**) On X-ray scans. (**c**) Diagram of the radial head subluxation. (**d**) Posterior approach to the elbow in the midline of the posterior distal humerus and the anatomical position of the ulnar nerve. (**e**) Diagram of a V osteotomy of the olecranon. (**f**) Diagram of the course of the radial nerve through the anterolateral incision of the elbow

fascia, while the distal end cannot be directly exposed due to the obstruction of the olecranon. Therefore, a V osteotomy of the olecranon and the lifting of the bone ends and attached triceps brachii to the proximal end are essential to expose the fractured distal humerus (Fig. 5.43e). Due to the obstruction of lateral ligaments and muscles, posterior surgical approaches are difficult to expose the proximal end of the radius. A curved incision, lateral to the biceps brachii, is usually made on the anterolateral side of the elbow for the surgery of radial head fractures. After the deep fascia is separated through this incision, the radial nerve is exposed between the brachialis and brachioradialis and usually situated anteromedial to the latter muscle (Fig. 5.43f). The annular ligament of the radius encircles the annular articular surface of the proximal radius, both ends of which connect to the ulna. The annular ligament of the radius and radial head are immature in childhood, and therefore, a vigorous stretch of the forearm causes radial head subluxation, in which the radial head slips under the annular ligament or the annular ligament incarcerates in the joint space between the humerus and radius (Fig. 5.43c).

Application of Key Anatomical Structures of the Lower Limbs

The hip joint is the largest spheroidal joint composed of the acetabulum and femoral head (Fig. 5.44a). Protected by the tough joint capsules, ligaments, and strong muscles, the hip joint is highly stable. Hip dislocation is typically caused by a strong force in a specific position, and the posterior hip dislocation is the most common type due to the weakness in the inferior and posterior parts of the joint capsule (Fig. 5.44b). Postoperative hip dislocation may cause sciatic nerve injury due to the compression by the displaced femoral head. Reduction failure is often reported in cases of postoperative hip dislocation combined with the posterior wall fracture of the acetabulum due to the lack of bony obstruction on the posterior side and usually managed by an operative reduction and fixation of the posterior wall of the acetabulum. Anterior hip dislocation is less reported due to the protection from thick anterior muscles. It causes lower limb ischemia due to the compression of anteromedial arteries and veins from the displaced femoral head (Fig. 5.44c). In the central dislocation of the femoral head, the femoral head is forced through the medial wall of the acetabulum and into the pelvis and often succumbs to severe hip fractures (Fig. 5.44d).

The blood supply to the femoral head is primarily provided by the vascular network of the medial and lateral femoral circumflex arteries and the arterial ring at the base of the femoral neck. It can be disrupted by hip dislocation or femoral neck fractures, which eventually results in the avascular necrosis of the femoral head. The femoral artery pierces the thigh below the midpoint of the inguinal ligament, where the femoral head is projected onto the skin. The femoral artery and vein then run along the medial side of the femur in the middle and upper parts of the femur and course to the posterior femur at the distal end. The femoral nerve is situated anterior to the femur and medial to the rectus femoris. A lateral approach to surgical procedures of the femur is therefore recommended. The greater trochanter of the femur is an important surface landmark

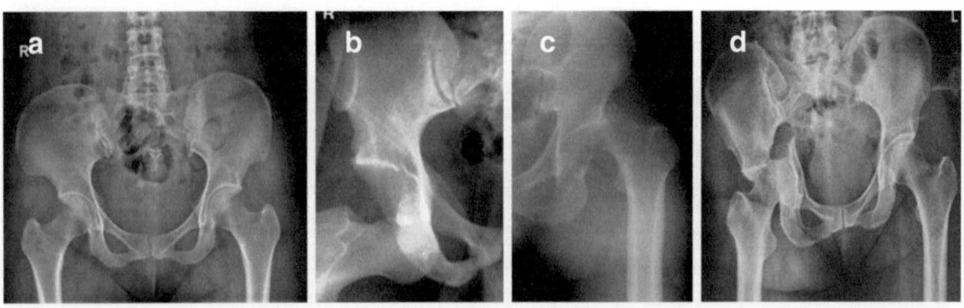

Fig. 5.44 Key anatomical structures of the lower limbs. Normal hip joint (**a**), posterior hip dislocation (**b**), anterior hip dislocation, (**c**) central dislocation of the femoral head (**d**) on X-ray scans

of the proximal femur for skin incisions starting at the proximal or distal end. After making a proximal incision on the lateral femur, the fascia lata and myofascial layer of the vastus lateralis are observed in the superficial and deep layers, respectively. A layer-by-layer suture of incised fascia is required to prevent muscle hernias. The femur is the strongest long bone in the human body, presenting a physiological curvature to the lateral side. In femoral shaft fractures, plate fixation is typically performed on the lateral side (tension side) of the femur to prevent the breakage of the plate.

Application of the Anatomical Structures of the Limbs in Arthroscopic Surgeries

Shoulder Joint

The bony structures of the shoulder joint include the glenoid cavity and the head of the humerus. Important soft tissues inside and outside the shoulder joint capsule include the glenoid labrum, glenohumeral ligaments, supraspinatus, infraspinatus, teres minor, subscapularis, biceps brachii, and deltoid. All of them contribute to the stability and flexibility of the shoulder.

Common shoulder injuries in sports include rotator cuff tears, injuries to the long head of biceps tendon, glenoid cavity tears, acromion impingement, and capsular contracture.

The anatomical characteristics of the shoulder joint under arthroscopic surgeries are described in the following sections.

Position and Approach

After general anesthesia, the affected limb is placed in a 45°of abduction with 5 kg of traction weight in the lateral position. Common surgical approaches for shoulder arthroscopic surgeries include the posterior, anterior, anterosuperior, and lateral approaches. A posterior approach provides the access to the glenoid cavity and subacromial space.

Important Anatomical Structures under the Arthroscope

Glenoid Cavity and Glenoid Labrum

The glenoid labrum attaches to the margin of the glenoid cavity to deepen the glenoid, stabilize the shoulder and limit the excessive movement of the head of the humerus. A Bankart lesion is described as the glenoid labrum tear in patients with the anterior shoulder dislocation, and an osseous Bankart lesion is defined as fractures of the anterior and inferior glenoid (Fig. 5.45a).

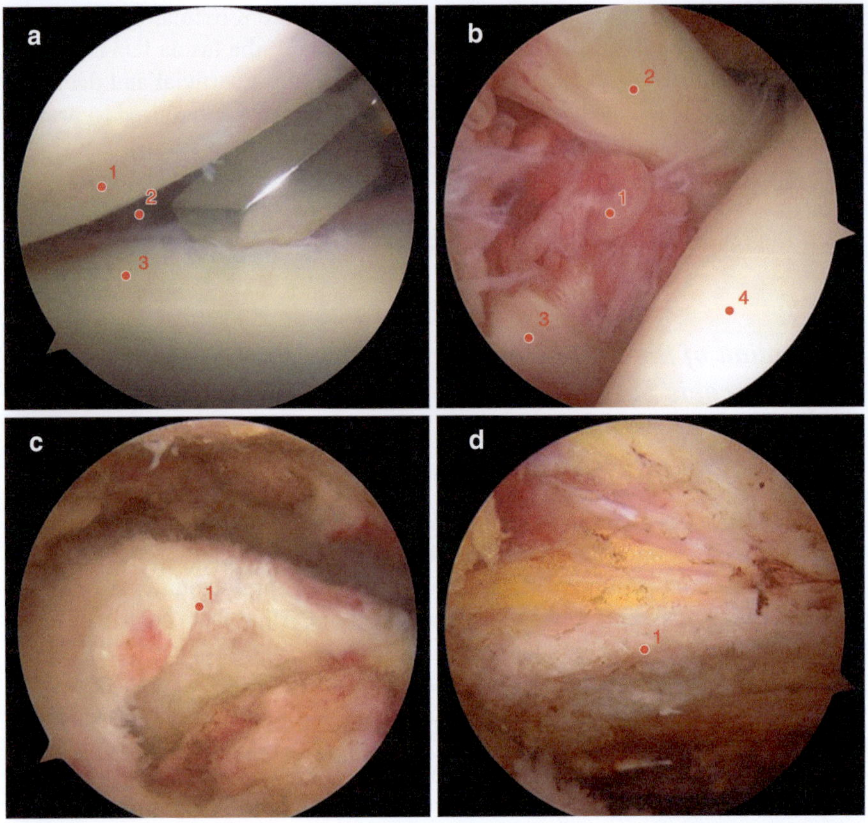

Fig. 5.45 Shoulder joint. (**a**). A Bankart lesion (*1*. head of the humerus; *2*. glenoid labrum tears; *3*. glenoid cavity). (**b**). Dislocated long head of biceps tendon (*1*. rotator cuff space; *2*. long head of biceps tendon; *3*. subscapularis; *4*. head of humerus). (**c**). Ruptured supraspinatus muscle (*1*. ruptured supraspinatus muscle). (**d**). Acromion after decompression (*1*. acromion)

Long Head of Biceps Tendon

The long head of biceps tendon passes through the bicipital groove anterior to the humerus, travels into the shoulder joint by bending by 90°, and inserts into the glenoid labrum at the 12-o'clock position of the glenoid. The long head of biceps tendon degenerates in some manual workers with aging, resulting in pain at the anterior part of the shoulder. Common in overhead throwing athletes, superior labrum anterior and posterior (SLAP) injuries are defined as tear of the long head of biceps tendon and glenoid labrum from anterior to posterior due to the excessive shoulder abduction and internal rotation (Fig. 5.45b).

Rotator Cuff

The rotator cuff is composed of the tendons of the supraspinatus, infraspinatus, teres minor, and subscapularis. It originates from the scapula and inserts into the anterior, superior, and posterior parts of the head of the humerus. The rotator cuff is closely contacted with the joint capsule and responsible for stabilizing the head of the humerus into the glenoid cavity and providing a force couple to achieve the flexible movement of the shoulder. Rotator cuff tears cause pain and weakness in the shoulder joint, especially in the supine position to the affected side. An arthroscopic surgery allows to locate and assess the type and size of the torn rotator cuff, and implant suture anchors through an auxiliary approach for repairing (Fig. 5.45c).

Acromion

The acromion is the flat bony tip on the lateral side of the scapula. Acromial impingement, a common disease among middle-aged and elderly people, was initially described by Neer in 1972. It is caused by the repeated impingements of the greater tubercle and coracoacromial arch when the shoulder joint is flexed and abducted and can result in the pain and limited movement of the shoulder due to subacromial bursa and rotator cuff injuries. Arthroscopic acromion decompression, recommended to patients with acromial impingement and poorly responding to a conservative treatment, can be performed through the resection of the subacromial inflammatory bursa, cleaning of osteophytes on the anterior and inferior acromion, and partial resection of the coracoacromial ligament (Fig. 5.45d).

Knee Joint

The bony structures of the knee joint are composed of the distal end of the femur, the proximal end of the tibia, and the patella. Important tissues outside the knee joint capsule include the quadriceps femoris, biceps femoris, semitendinosus, semimembranosus, and medial and lateral collateral ligaments. All of them contribute to the stability and flexion and extension of the knee joint. Important structures within the knee joint capsule include the medial and lateral menisci and the anterior and posterior cruciate ligaments. The meniscus is a fibrocartilage situated between the femoral condyle and the tibial plateau. Thicker on the outside and thinner on the inside, the meniscus as a cushion prevents knee joint cartilage damage. The anterior cruciate ligament originates from the anteromedial aspect of the tibial intercondylar eminence and inserts into the medial wall of the lateral femoral condyle, maintaining forward and rotational stability of the knee joint. The posterior cruciate ligament originates from the posterior aspect of the tibial intercondylar eminence and inserts into the lateral wall of the medial femoral condyle, maintaining the rotational stability of the knee joint. Meniscal tears and anterior and posterior cruciate ligament tears are common injuries in sports. Injuries to important structures of the knee joint seriously affect the function of the knee joint and limit the range of motion.

The anatomical characteristics of the knee joint under arthroscopic surgeries are described in the following sections.

Position

In a supine position, a pneumatic tourniquet cuffed on the groin of the affected side is usually used in an arthroscopic surgery of the knee, with the pressure of systolic blood pressure set at +150 mmHg and an inflation lasting less than 90 min.

Patella and Trochlea The patellofemoral joint consists of the articular surface of the patella and the trochlea. Instability of the patellofemoral joint and degeneration of articular cartilage lead to pain at the anterior part of the knee joint (Fig. 5.46a).

Menisci

The medial meniscus is a C-shaped cartilage with a narrower anterior portion and wider posterior portion. Its anterior end is attached to the anterior aspect of the tibial insertion of the anterior cruciate ligament, and the posterior end is fixed to the anterior aspect of the tibial insertion of the posterior cruciate ligament. The lateral meniscus is an O-shaped cartilage with narrower anterior and posterior portions and a wider central part. Its anterior end is attached to the posterolateral aspect of the tibial attachment of the anterior cruciate ligament, and the posterior end is fixed to the posterior aspect of the lateral intercondylar eminence and in front of the posterior end of the medial meniscus. The range of motion of the lateral meniscus is greater than that of the medial meniscus (Figs. 5.46b, c).

Cruciate Ligaments

The anterior cruciate ligament originates from the posterior aspect of the lateral side of the intercondylar fossa and descends anteromedially to the anterior aspect of the tibial spine (intercondylar eminence). The posterior cruciate ligament originates from the anterior aspect of the medial side of the intercondylar fossa and descends posterolaterally to the posterior aspect of the tibial spine (Fig. 5.46d).

Ankle Joint

The bony structures of the ankle joint are composed of distal ends of the tibia and fibula and the trochlea of talus. The medial deltoid ligament and the lateral collateral ligament contribute to stabilizing the ankle joint. The anterior talofibular ligament, calcaneofibular ligament, and posterior talofibular ligament make up the lateral collateral ligament of the ankle. The deltoid ligament is divided into superficial and deep layers. The ankle is a type of mortise and tenon joint with a narrow joint space and has been previously considered unsuitable for arthroscopy. Ankle arthroscopy is now extensively performed with the advance in medical technologies. It is applied to treat ankle injuries in sports like chronic ankle instability induced by recurrent ankle sprains, osteochondral lesions of the talus, anterior ankle impingement

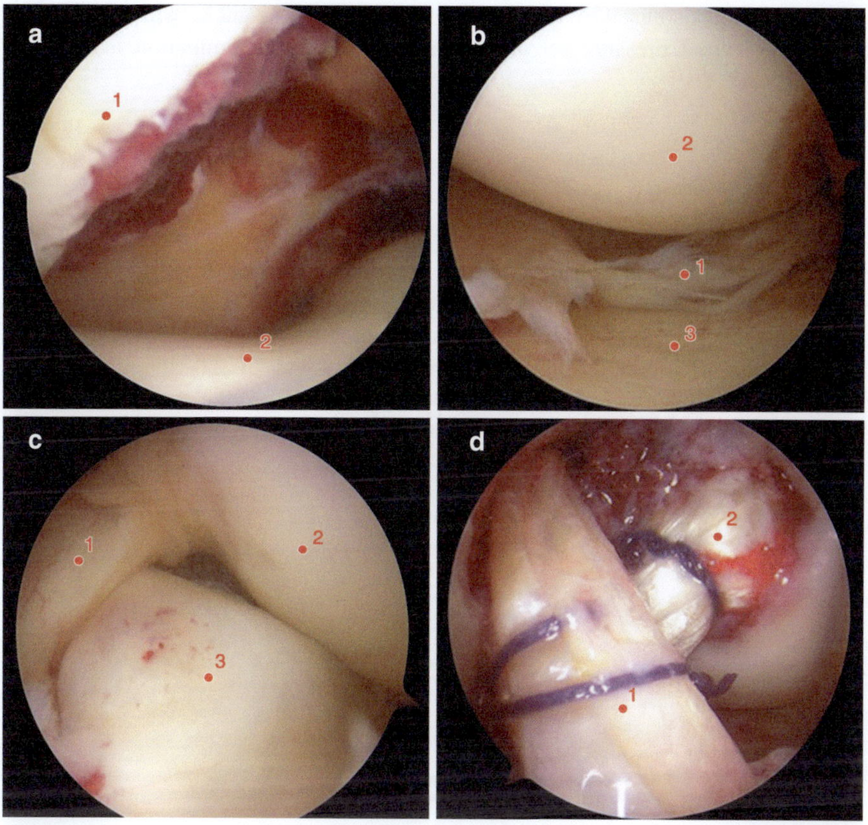

Fig. 5.46 Knee joint. (**a**) Patella and trochlea of a patient with patellar dislocation (*1*. patella, cartilage fracture; *2*. trochlea). (**b**) Torn posterior end of the medial meniscus (*1*. Torn medial meniscus. *2*. Medial femoral condyle. *3*. Medial tibial plateau). (**c**) Ruptured lateral discoid meniscus (*1*. Anterior cruciate ligament. *2*. Lateral femoral condyle. *3*. Lateral discoid meniscus, ruptured). (**d**) Reconstructed cruciate ligaments in a patient with both anterior and posterior cruciate ligament tears (*1*. Reconstructed anterior cruciate ligament. *2*. Reconstructed posterior cruciate ligament)

(footballer's ankle), and posterior ankle impingement induced by fractures of the os trigonum. Ankle arthroscopy is also an option for patients with intraarticular tumors like solitary or diffuse giant cell tumor of the tendon sheath and synovial chondromatosis. The anatomical characteristics of the ankle joint under arthroscopic surgeries are described in the following sections.

Position

Ankle arthroscopy is usually performed with the patient in the supine position, and for anterior and posterior ankle injuries, it is performed with the patient in the supine and prone positions, respectively. A pneumatic tourniquet cuffed on the groin of the affected side is also used in an arthroscopic surgery of the ankle, with the pressure of systolic blood pressure set at+150 mmHg and an inflammation lasting less than 90 min.

Anterior Ankle

The anterior part of the talus is mortised into the anterior ankle, and the middle and posterior parts of the talus can also be observed in the plantar flexed position of the ankle. Osteochondral injuries of the talus typically occur on the anterolateral or posteromedial side of the talus (Fig. 5.47a).

The anterior talofibular ligament, with a thickness of 2.0–2.5 mm, can be observed in the lateral retromalleolar groove. It arises from the anterior margin of

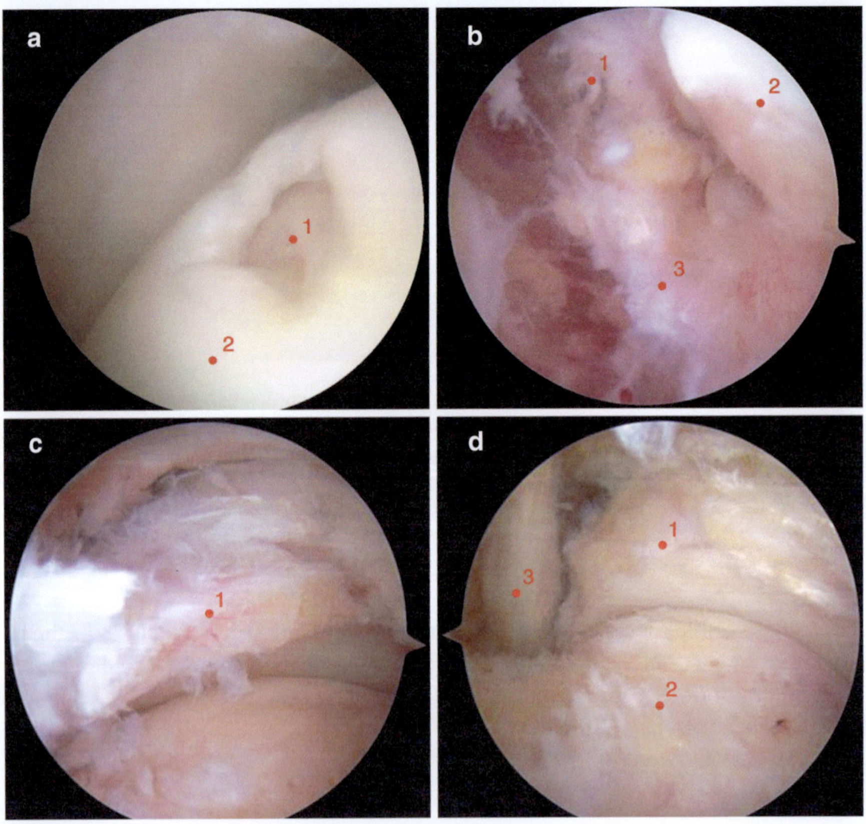

Fig. 5.47 Ankle joint. (**a**) Osteochondral injuries of the talus on the posteromedial side of the talus (*1*. damaged cartilages and subchondral bones; *2*. the talus); (**b**) injuries of the anterior talofibular ligament (*1*. the fibula; *2*. the talus; *3*. the anterior talofibular ligament); (**c**) fractured os trigonum (*1*. the fractured os trigonum); (**d**) released flexor hallucis longus (*1*. the talus; *2*. the calcaneus; *3*. the flexor hallucis longus)

the lateral ankle and descends anteriorly to the lateral side of the talar neck. The anterior talofibular ligament limits the anterior displacement and internal rotation of the talus. Recurrent sprains of the ankle joint result in tears, scarring, and fatty degeneration of the anterior talofibular ligament or even complete absorption in patients with a long course of disease. Injuries of the anterior talofibular ligament cause chronic ankle instability (Fig. 5.47b).

Posterior Ankle

The anatomical scope of the posterior ankle includes the posterior margin of the distal tibia, posterior side of the peroneal groove, posterior tibial tubercle, malleolus groove, and posterior colliculus of medial malleolus. The posterior ankle is a component of the distal tibiofibular syndesmosis that maintains the stability of the posterior part of the ankle and lowers the pressure of the ankle. The posterior ankle joint and subtalar joint can be observed through the posterior approach. Both of the os trigonum and Stieda process are long and large posterolateral processes of the talus, while the former is not fused with the talus. Fractures of the os trigonum or Stieda process occur in some trauma patients, leading to the posterior ankle impingement (Fig. 5.47c). An ankle arthroscopy contributes to alleviating the pain in the posterior ankle by resecting the unstable os trigonum or Stieda process and releasing the flexor hallucis longus. The tarsal tunnel is posteromedial to the flexor hallucis longus in the posterior ankle, and therefore, the medial side of the flexor hallucis longus is the restricted zone for the posterior ankle arthroscopy. Except for the treatment of diffuse giant cell tumors of the tendon sheath, the exposure of the flexor hallucis longus is a hint to stop shaving inward (Fig. 5.47d).

Application of the Anatomical Structures of the Limbs in Vascular Surgeries

The course and communication of muscles, bones, nerves, and blood vessels of the limbs are of great significance in surgical procedures. Clinical applications of key anatomical structures of the lower limbs in the high ligation and stripping of the great saphenous vein are described in the following sections.

Preoperative Marking of Varicose Veins

Bulging varicose veins reduce in the supine position, and therefore, a preoperative marking of varicose veins alongside the courses in the standing position is essential. With the extensive application of ultrasonography in recent years, ultrasound-guided localization of varicose veins, saphenofemoral junction (a connection between the great saphenous vein and femoral vein), and dysfunctional perforating branches is more favorable to the intraoperative localization (Fig. 5.48a).

High Ligation of the Great Saphenous Vein

High ligation of the great saphenous vein is usually performed through an oblique incision in the groin, parallel to or 1 cm above the inguinal groove. The surgical incision for the high ligation of the great saphenous vein aligns with skin tension lines, resulting in a minimal trauma and aesthetic benefit. Generally, the midpoint of the incision lies in the saphenous hiatus at 3–4 cm inferolateral to the pubic tubercle. The incision can also be made on the medial side of the femoral pulse point to accurately expose the root of the great saphenous vein and its tributaries (Fig. 5.48b). Preoperative ultrasound-guided localization of the saphenofemoral junction enhances the accurate location of the skin incision, which further reduces the trauma caused by subcutaneous separation through making a smaller incision. After separating the subcutaneous tissue, the main trunk of the great saphenous vein is exposed along the venous sheath and separated from the proximal end to the saphenofemoral junction. Free and ligate each tributary of the great saphenous vein, and reconfirm the localization of the saphenofemoral junction (Fig. 5.48c). An uncertain localization of the saphenofemoral junction may lead to femoral vein injuries.

The superficial epigastric vein, superficial iliac circumflex vein, external pudendal vein, and superficial medial and lateral femoral veins are five major tributaries at the root of the great saphenous vein. They join the great saphenous vein through various

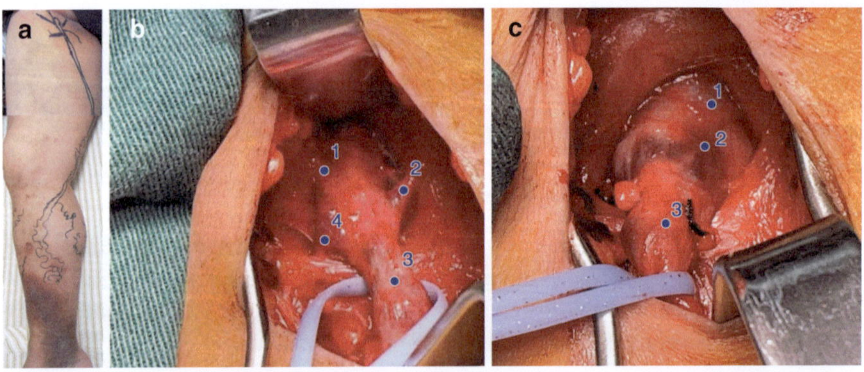

Fig. 5.48 Preoperative marking of varicose veins, the great saphenous vein and its branches. (**a**) The great saphenous vein incompetence on the right side, with cutaneous pigmentation of the leg and local ulcers (healed). The main trunk of the great saphenous vein and its tributaries and varicose veins are preoperatively marked by ultrasound. (**b**) Exposure of the great saphenous vein and its tributaries during the procedures of high ligation (*1*. superficial epigastric vein; *2*. superficial iliac circumflex vein; *3*. great saphenous vein; *4*. external pudendal vein). (**c**) Exposure of the great saphenous vein draining into the saphenofemoral junction after ligating and cutting off the tributaries (*1*. femoral vein; *2*. saphenofemoral junction; *3*. great saphenous vein)

ways, leading to variation in the number and localization of tributaries. Therefore, an intraoperative dissection of the saphenofemoral junction and 2 cm below it ensures the complete ligation of the great saphenous vein tributaries. The distal tributaries of the great saphenous vein are dissected during the procedures of vein stripping. In the procedures of high ligation without stripping, a dissection of 10 cm distal to the main trunk of the great saphenous vein is essential to identify any hidden lower tributaries.

After freeing, the great saphenous vein is ligated at 0.5–1.0 cm away from the saphenofemoral junction. Its proximal end is ligated and sutured to prevent hemorrhage due to the falling of the ligation line. In the procedures of high ligation without stripping, the exposed great saphenous vein should be resected as much as possible for at least 5.0–10.0 cm. The surgical incision is sutured layer by layer.

Stripping of the Great Saphenous Vein

Stripping of the great saphenous vein is an important part in surgical procedures of varicose veins and can greatly lower the postoperative recurrent rate compared with that of a unilateral high ligation without stripping. After the high ligation of proximal end of the great saphenous vein through a skin incision in the groin, a vein stripper is inserted through the distal end of the dissected great saphenous vein, and advanced until the inferior part of the knee. The tip of the stripper is palpable below the knee, where a skin incision is made to cut off the great saphenous vein and take out the tip. After fixing the proximal end of the stripper using a small olive head, and ligating and fixing the vein on the stripper, the main trunk is stripped from top to bottom (Fig. 5.49).

A vein stripper is inserted from the proximal to the distal end and fixed using a small olive head at the proximal end. Ligate and fix the vein on the stripper. Strip the main trunk of the great saphenous vein by slowly removing the stripper from the distal end.

Spot Stripping of Local Varicose Veins

Local varicose veins in the leg are surgically treated with spot stripping. Based on the preoperatively marked sites, a longitudinal incision with 1–3 mm long is made. Subcutaneous tissues are dissociated if necessary, and then varicose veins are removed using vascular hooks or small vascular forceps by clamping and cutting them off. Varicose veins are pulled out from dissected ends for centimeters (Fig. 5.50). A ligation is not necessary after stripping of small veins, and the bleeding can be stopped immediately by applying pressure for a few minutes. Varicose veins should be completely removed. In case of an intraoperative break of the stripped varicose veins, a small skin incision is made at the breaking site for re-stripping. Incompetent perforating veins are ligated and stripped based on the preoperative ultrasound-guided localization. Absorbable sutures are used for skin closure.

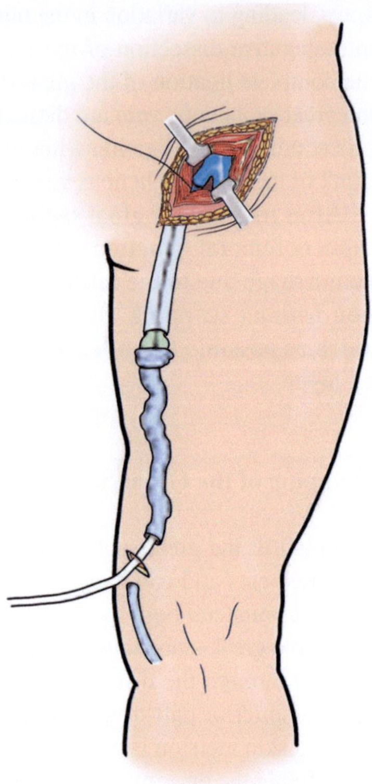

Fig. 5.49 Stripping of the great saphenous vein

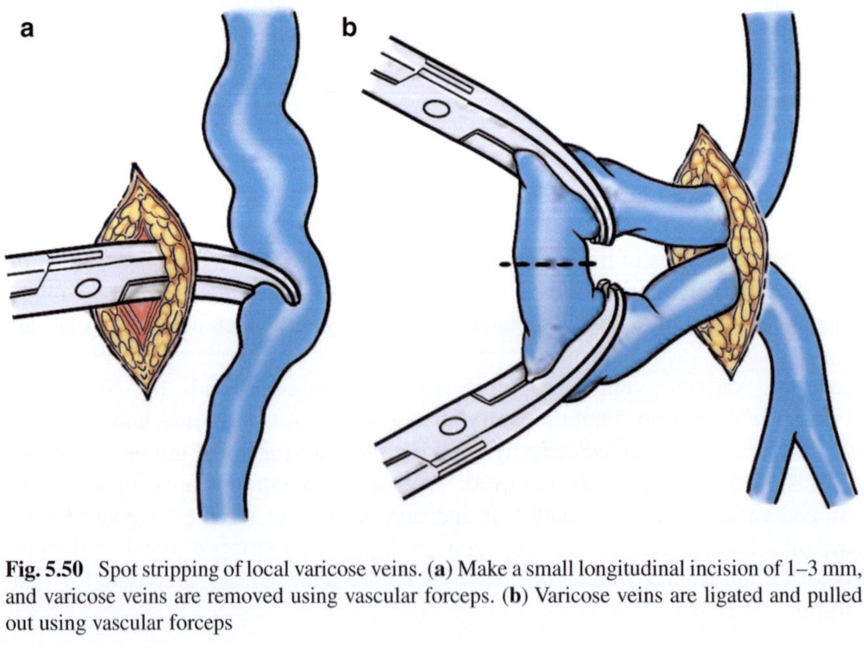

Fig. 5.50 Spot stripping of local varicose veins. (**a**) Make a small longitudinal incision of 1–3 mm, and varicose veins are removed using vascular forceps. (**b**) Varicose veins are ligated and pulled out using vascular forceps

Chapter 6
Regional Anatomy of the Head and Face and Its Clinical Application

Minfeng Tang, Junying Gao, Jian Tang, and Jingping Shi

6.1 Regional Anatomy of the Head and Face

The head rests on the top of the cervical spine and is divided into the cranium (posterior and superior aspects) and the face (anterior and inferior aspects). Their morphologies, structures, and functions vary a lot.

6.1.1 Cranium

The cranium occupies the posterior and superior parts of the head. The intracranial space is known as the cranial cavity that accommodates the brain and its meninges. From the roof to the base, the cranium is divided into extracranial soft tissues, calvarium, intracranial space (three layers of meninges and the gaps between two layers), brain, and cranial base. Only the extracranial soft tissues in the fronto-parieto-occipital region and temporal region are described in the following sections.

6.1.1.1 Boundary

The cranium is delineated by the supraorbital rim, zygomatic arch, external acoustic pore, and mastoid process. It is separated from the face anteriorly and inferiorly.

M. Tang · J. Gao (✉) · J. Tang · J. Shi
Nanjing Medical University, Nanjing, China
e-mail: renjie@njmu.edu.cn; gaojunying@njmu.edu.cn; tangjian@njmu.edu.cn

Q. Ding et al. (eds.), *Clinically Oriented Regional Anatomy*,
https://doi.org/10.1007/978-981-95-9888-5_6

6.1.1.2 Anatomical Landmarks and Surface Projections

Anatomical Landmarks

External Occipital Protuberance
The external occipital protuberance is located at the back of the cranium and is the most prominent protrusion of the occipital bone. The extension of the bone crest on both sides is known as the superior nuchal line, where the sternocleidomastoid muscle and trapezius muscle attach. The confluences of the sinus and transverse sinus are deep to the external occipital protuberance and superior nuchal line, respectively. The occipital emissary veins run inferiorly to the external occipital protuberance. It is essential to protect the above structures during posterior fossa surgery.

Mastoid Process
The mastoid process is situated behind the inferior part of the outer ear. It is a downward projection of the temporal bone. The mastoid process is located behind and below the outer ear and is a downward projection of the temporal bone. The posterior half of the deep aspect of the mastoid process houses the sulcus for the sigmoid sinus, accommodating the sigmoid sinus within this groove. The stylomastoid foramen is situated anteromedially to the mastoid process, through which the facial nerve flows out of the cranium. The above structures should be carefully protected during mastoid surgery.

Parietal Tuber
The parietal tuber is the most prominent projection of the parietal bone. The distal end of the posterior branch of the lateral sulcus is situated 2 cm deep below the parietal tuber. The distance between parietal tubers on both sides represents the maximum transverse diameter of the skull. Caput quadratum describes a "square-headed" appearance in infants and young children with rickets, which is caused by the pathological prominence of the parietal tubers.

Surface Projections

Bregma
Bregma, as the intersection of the coronal suture and the sagittal suture, is situated at the junction of the anterior and middle third of the line connecting the nasion and posterior margin of the foramen magnum. It is 13 cm away from the glabella. The Bregma is often used as the location of palpation to determine changes in intracranial pressure based on its bulge or depression.

Anterior Branch of Middle Meningeal Artery
The anterior branch of the middle meningeal artery runs beneath the pterion. An equilateral triangle is delineated posteriorly and superiorly by the line between the marginal tubercle of the zygomatic bone and the midpoint of the zygomatic arch as the base. The vertical angle is the surface projection of the pterion, where the anterior branch of the middle meningeal artery passes through the deep layer (Fig. 6.1).

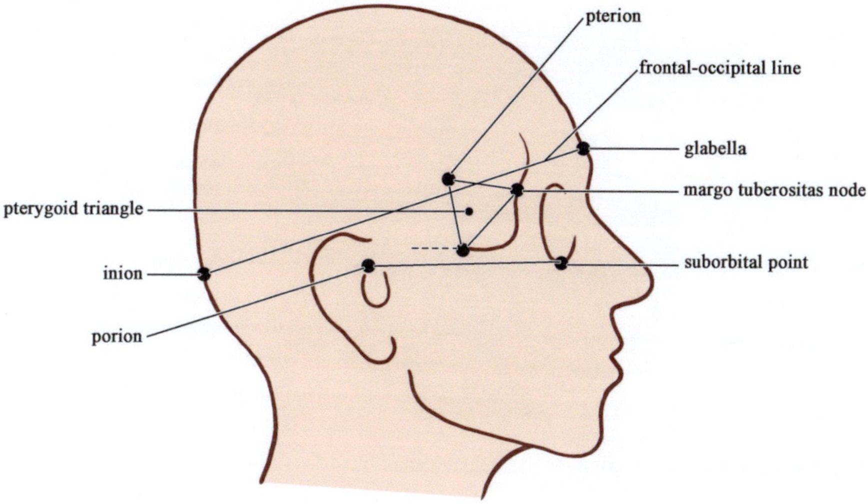

Fig. 6.1 Anatomical landmark of the pterion

Inferior Margin of the Cerebrum
The inferior margin of the cerebrum is projected on the line connecting the point at 1.25 cm above the midpoint of the nasion, the supraorbital margin, the superior margin of the zygomatic arch, the superior margin of the external auditory meatus, and the external occipital protuberance.

6.1.1.3 Layers (Superficial Layer of the Calvaria)

The calvaria is composed of superficial soft tissues and the calvarium. Separated by the superior temporal line, the calvaria is divided into the temporal regions on both sides.

Fronto-Parieto-Occipital Region

The superficial layer of the fronto-parieto-occipital region is composed of five layers (Fig. 6.2).

Skin

The skin on the fronto-parieto-occipital region is dense, thick, and enriched with sweat glands and sebaceous glands. Furuncles and sebaceous cysts often appear in this area. In addition, the fronto-parieto-occipital region contains abundant blood vessels, and significant bleeding may appear after trauma. However, wounds in this region exhibit strong anti-infection properties and heal rapidly.

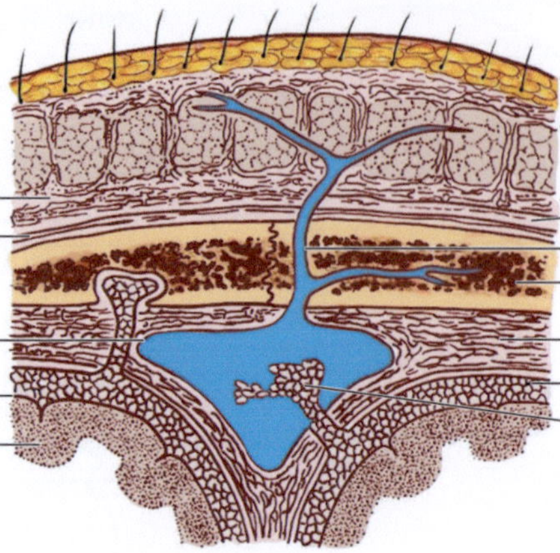

Fig. 6.2 Layers in the calvarium on the frontal plane

Superficial Fascia

Longitudinal fiber bundles are present in the superficial fascia of the fronto-parieto-occipital region, formed by dense connective tissues that connect the skin and the galea in the deep layer. The superficial fascia is separated by many small gaps filled with adipose tissue, where blood vessels and nerves pass through. Infections in this layer are not prone to spreading. Exudate can induce severe pain by compressing nerve endings. The blood vessel walls in these small gaps typically connect with fiber bundles. Traumas in this region may result in significant bleeding due to the poor constriction of blood vessels, requiring suture or compression hemostasis.

The blood vessels and nerves in the superficial fascia of the fronto-parieto-occipital region pass from the base to the roof of the skull. They are divided into anterior, lateral, and posterior groups (Fig. 6.3). The anterior group is situated in the forehead and ascends beyond the supraorbital margin, including the supratrochlear artery, vein, and nerve on the medial side, and the supraorbital artery, vein, and nerve on the lateral side. The lateral group ascends after passing through the anterior and posterior aspects of the ear. The larger ones are situated anterior to the ear, including the auriculotemporal nerve and superficial temporal artery and vein that pierce from the upper edge of the parotid gland. The posterior auricular artery and vein, and the lesser occipital nerve are situated posterior to the ear. The occipital artery and vein and the greater occipital nerve ascend in the occipital region, belonging to the posterior group. The internal and external carotid arteries are major arteries supplying the calvarium. Due to the wide anastomoses on the bilateral sides and those formed by branches, large-scale tears on the scalp generally do not cause ischemic necrosis. Since blood vessels and nerves run from all sides to the calvarium, radial incisions generally should be made in calvarium surgeries to avoid damaging blood vessels and nerves. During craniotomy surgeries, the pedicle of the flap should be positioned below, preserving the blood vessels and nerve trunks within the pedicle to ensure the nutrition of the flap. Although the nerves traveling through the calvarium have

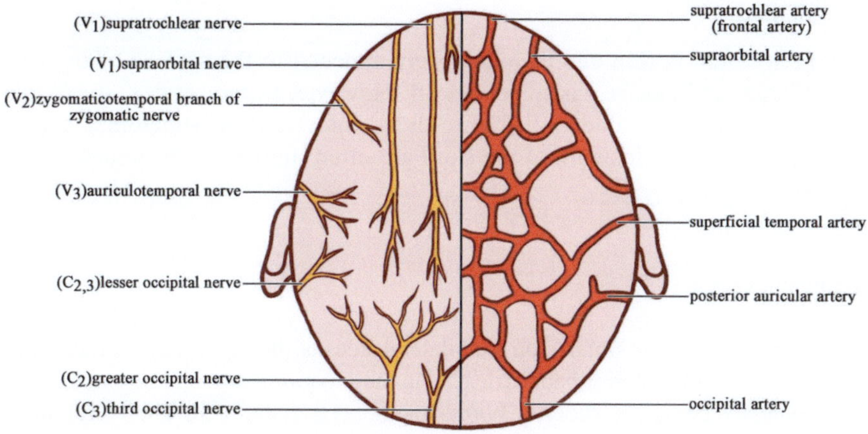

Fig. 6.3 Blood vessels and nerves travel through the calvarium

different origins, they all run within the superficial fascia, and therefore, local block anesthetics should be injected subcutaneously. Due to the thick fiber bundles in the superficial fascia, injections may encounter significant resistance, and the distribution areas of nerves overlap with each other. Therefore, it is necessary to expand the range of block anesthesia to achieve more satisfactory results.

Galea Aponeurotica and Occipitofrontalis Muscle

The galea aponeurotica is connected to the frontal belly of the occipitofrontalis muscle in the front and to the occipital belly of the same muscle in the back. The thinning extensions on both sides communicate with the superficial layer of the temporal fascia. Fibrous bundles of the superficial fascia closely attach to the skin. The skin, superficial fascia, and galea aponeurotica are often collectively termed as the scalp. Wounds involving the galea aponeurotica, especially a transverse one, may split the scalp due to the tension from the frontal and occipital bellies.

Subgaleal Fascia

Subgaleal fascia, also known as the subgalea layer, connects the scalp and pericranium. It covers a wide range of the calvarium, reaching the orbital region in the front and the superior nuchal line in the back. Blood or pus throughout the calvarium within this layer. Scalp tears are prone to avulsion injuries of the deep layer. The veins in the superficial fascia of the calvarium are extensively anastomosed to form a venous network. These veins also communicate with the diploic veins and dural sinus through the emissary blood vessels in this layer. Although this communication can balance the pressure of the intracranial and extracranial veins, it also triggers the infection to spread from the extracranial space to the intracranial cavity. Hence, the subgaleal layer is known as the danger space at the top of the skull.

Pericranium

The periosteum is thin and dense, loosely attached to the surface of the calvarial bone, and can be easily peeled off. However, at the sutures, it extends into the sutures and adheres firmly to them. Infections or hematomas occurring beneath the periosteum of the skull are often limited to the area of a single skull bone.

Temporal Region

The temporal region is situated on the bilateral sides of the calvarium, with its anterior, superior, and posterior boundaries being the superior temporal line and its inferior boundary being the superior border of the zygomatic arch. The hierarchical layers of the temporal region are as follows:

Skin

The skin on the anterior part of the temporal region is thin and mobile, and that on the posterior part is similar to that on the fronto-parieto-occipital region.

Superficial Fascia

The superficial fascia in the temporal region is thin and contains less adipose tissues. In front of the ear, within this layer, are the zygomatic and temporal branches of the facial nerve, the superficial temporal artery, the auriculotemporal nerve, and the superficial temporal vein, which emerge from the upper margin of the parotid gland and travel upward in an anterior to posterior direction (Fig. 6.4). The superficial temporal artery crosses the zygomatic arch in front of the tragus. Its position is superficial and constant, commonly taken as a site for compression hemostasis, retrograde intubation for the interventional treatment of maxillofacial malignancies, and harvesting skin flaps containing the superficial temporal artery and vein and auriculotemporal artery to repair maxillofacial soft tissue defects.

Temporal Fascia

The temporal fascia arises from the superior temporal line and covers the surface of the temporalis muscle. It is divided into a superficial and a deep layer. The superficial layer is thin and is a continuation of the galea aponeurotica; the deep layer is dense and tough, from which some fibers of the temporalis muscle originate. The two layers adhere closely in the superior part of the temporal region and separate 1–2 finger breadths above the zygomatic arch and attach on the lateral and medial sides of the zygomatic arch, respectively.

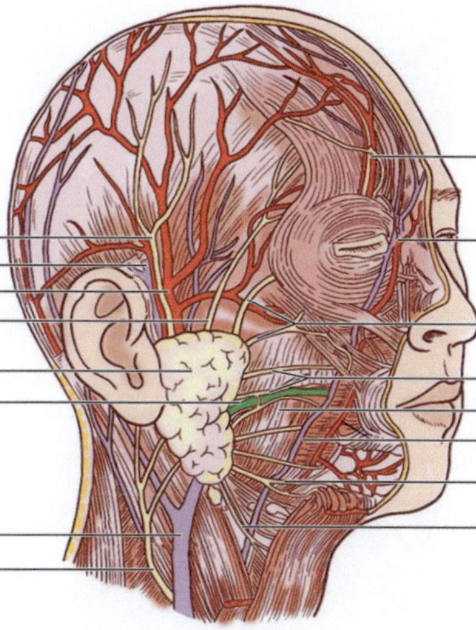

Fig. 6.4 Superficial layers of the face

Temporalis Muscle

The temporalis muscle is a strong, thick, fan-shaped muscle. Two longitudinal blood vessels and nerve bundles travel anteriorly and posteriorly in the deep layer of the temporalis muscle. After piercing into this layer, the blood vessels become the branches of the anterior and posterior deep temporal arteries arising from the maxillary artery, and the nerve becomes a branch of the mandibular nerve.

Pericranium

The pericranium covers the surface of the skull that forms the temporal fossa. The superficial surface of the temporal fossa is a common approach in cranial surgeries, due to the strong protection provided by the temporalis muscle and temporal fascia.

The Temporal Space

The temporal space is a space between the temporal fascia and the periosteum of the temporal fossa and is divided into superficial and deep parts (Fig. 6.5). The superficial temporal space is located superior to the zygomatic arch, between the superficial and deep layers of the temporal fascia. It contains adipose tissues and the middle temporal artery (a branch of the superficial temporal artery). The deep temporal space is situated between the deep layer of the temporal fascia and the periosteum of the temporal fossa and communicates with the buccal space, infratemporal space, and pterygomandibular space of the maxillofacial region. It contains the temporalis muscle along with blood vessels, nerves, and connective tissues in the deep layer.

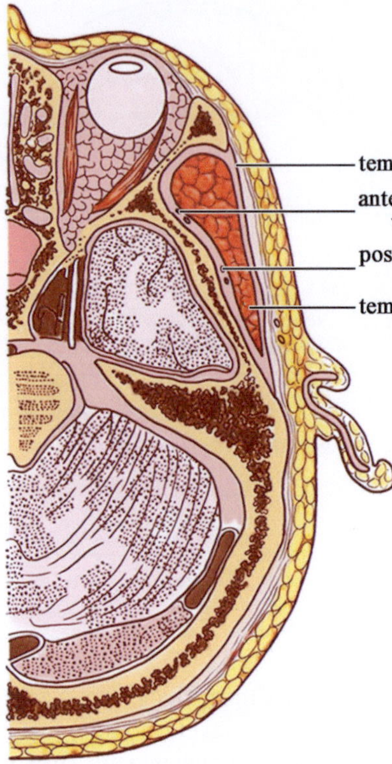

Fig. 6.5 Temporal region and temporal space parallel to the transverse section of the supraorbital rim

6.1.2 Face

6.1.2.1 Boundary

The face is superiorly and posteriorly separated from the cranium by the line connecting the supraorbital rim, zygomatic arch, external acoustic pore, and mastoid process. It is anteriorly and inferiorly separated from the cervical region by the line connecting the lower margin of the body of the mandible, the angle of the mandible, and the top of the mastoid process.

6.1.2.2 Anatomical Landmarks and Surface Projections

Supraorbital Foramen

The supraorbital foramen is situated above the intersection of the medial thirds of the supraorbital margin, through which the supraorbital blood vessels and nerve pass. In some cases, the supraorbital foramen is absent and replaced by the supraorbital notch (Fig. 6.6).

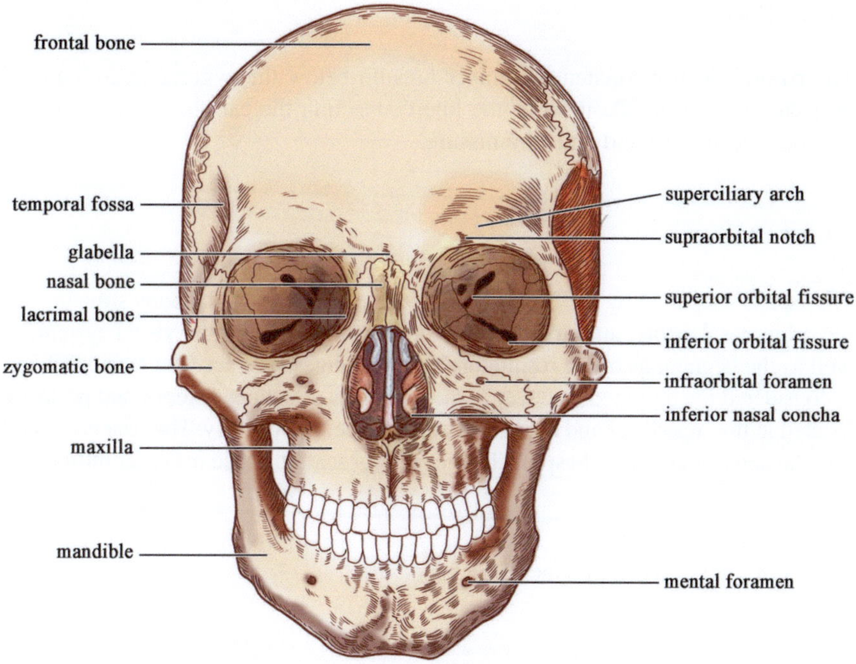

Fig. 6.6 Cranial bones on the anterior aspect

Infraorbital Foramen

The infraorbital foramen is situated 0.5–0.8 cm below the midpoint of the infraorbital rim, serving as the passage for the infraorbital blood vessels and nerve.

Mental Foramen

The mental foramen is situated lateral to the midpoint of the line connecting the superior and inferior margins of the body of the mandible, below the space between the roots of the mandibular first and second premolar, where the mental vessels and nerve pass through. The supraorbital foramen, infraorbital foramen, and mental foramen are usually arranged in a straight line.

Zygomatic Arch

The full length of the zygomatic arch, which is approximately 3 finger breadths long, can be palpable. It is located at the level anterior to the external auditory meatus.

Parotid Duct

The parotid duct is situated one finger breadth below the zygomatic arch and is projected on the middle third of the line connecting the earlobe to the midpoint between the ala nasi and oral commissure.

6.1.2.3 Layers

The face is supported by the facial skeleton and participates in the bony structures of the orbit, nasal cavity, and oral cavity. It houses the organs of the visual system, as well as the beginnings of the respiratory tract and digestive tract. The facial skeleton is considered the intermediate layer of the face, with structures anterior and posterior located in the superficial and deep layers of the face, respectively. The face is divided into the anterior and lateral aspects by the anterior margin of the masseter muscle.

Layers of the Superficial Layer of the Face

Skin

The skin on the face is thin, soft, and greatly mobile. Blood supply to the face is rich, resulting in a large volume of bleeding after trauma. Its strong anti-infection property favors wound healing. The skin, containing abundant sebaceous glands, sweat glands, and hair follicles, is a common site for sebaceous cysts and furuncles. Visceral motor nerves are widely distributed in the face, and the skin color is easily changed by emotions. The dermal layer of the skin is attached to the fibers of the superficial fascia and the muscles of facial expression, forming complex skin tension lines (Fig. 6.7). A facial incision aligned with skin tension lines can minimize postoperative scars.

Superficial Fascia and Muscles of Facial Expression

The face contains minimal subcutaneous tissues with adipose tissues arranged in small granules, notably less in the frontal, palpebral, and nasal regions. The buccal region contains abundant adipose tissues, known as the buccal fat pad. Subcutaneous tissues in the palpebral region are loose, making them prone to exhibiting early signs of edema due to heart and kidney diseases. The muscles of facial expression, also known as mimetic muscles, are situated in the superficial fascia of the face. Most of these muscles originate from the facial skeleton and insert into the skin. Contraction of these muscles pulls on the skin to make various facial expressions. The muscles of facial expression are arranged in circular or radial patterns around the palpebral fissure, oral fissure, and nostrils, allowing for functions such as opening and closing (Fig. 6.4).

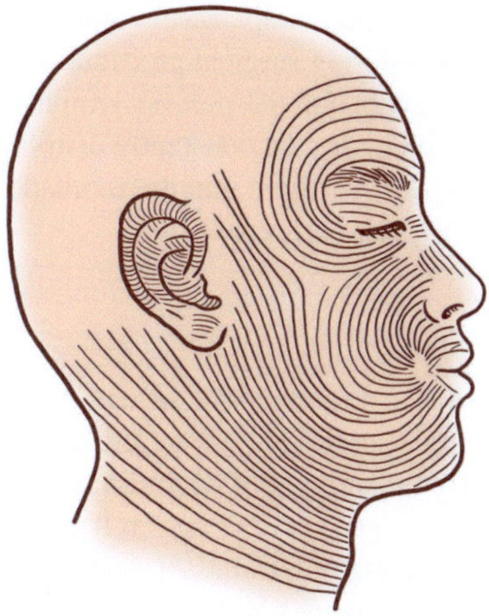

Fig. 6.7 Skin tension lines of the face

Blood vessels are abundant in the superficial fascia of the face. The facial artery and vein travel laterally to the mouth and nose and medially to the palpebral fissure. The facial vein lies behind the facial artery. It communicates with the superior ophthalmic vein through the angular vein and drains into the pterygoid venous plexus in the infratemporal fossa through the deep facial vein. The superior ophthalmic vein and pterygoid venous plexus communicate with the cavernous sinus. Due to the absence of valves in the facial vein above the oral commissure, a retrograde infection from the triangle area (the danger triangle of the face), bounded by the bilateral corners of the mouth to the bridge of the nose, can spread to the cavernous sinus through the above-mentioned communications. The superficial temporal artery and vein pass through the superior margin of the parotid gland and travel along the superior part of the tragus. Terminal branches of deep arteries, such as the supraorbital artery, infraorbital artery, and mental artery, pierce into the superficial layer of the face.

The sensory terminal branches of the trigeminal nerve and the motor terminal branches of the facial nerve are distributed in the superficial layer of the face. The supraorbital nerve (terminal branch of the ophthalmic nerve), infraorbital nerve (terminal branch of the maxillary nerve), and mental nerve (terminal branch of the inferior alveolar nerve) exit the supraorbital foramen, infraorbital foramen, and mental foramen to the superficial fascia, respectively, and provide sensory innervation to the skin of the superior aspect of the face. Trigeminal neuralgia causes tenderness in the three foramina. The auriculotemporal nerve accompanies the superficial temporal artery and vein on the lateral side of the face. The temporal branch (pass through the superior margin of the parotid gland), zygomatic branch (pass through the anterosuperior margin of the parotid gland), buccal branch (pass through the anterior margin of the parotid gland), marginal mandibular branch (pass through the anteroinferior margin of the parotid gland), and cervical branch of the facial nerve (pass through the inferior margin of the parotid gland) innervate the facial expression muscles and platysma muscle. Terminal branches of the facial nerve superficially travel within the superficial fascia of the face and should be protected during surgical procedures of the face to prevent facial paralysis.

Except for the parotid lymph nodes superficial to the parotid gland, no other lymph nodes are constantly distributed in the fascia. The superficial lymphatic vessels directly drain into the submandibular lymph nodes and submental lymph nodes in the cervical region.

Deep Fascia

The deep fascia of the face is generally thin and weak. However, the parotideomasseteric fascia that covers the surface of the masseter muscle and parotid gland is a prominent layer of deep fascia, being the upward extension of the superficial layer of the deep cervical fascia. It attaches superiorly to the zygomatic arch. Its anterior part, lying on the masseter muscle, is called the masseteric fascia. The posterior part splits into two layers that enclose the parotid gland to form the capsule of the parotid gland.

Layers of the Lateral Aspect of the Face

The lateral side of the face is posterior to the anterior margin of the masseter muscle, inferior to the zygomatic arch; superior to the line connecting the inferior margin of the mandible, angle of the mandible, and top of the mastoid process; and anterior to the mastoid process and anterior margin of the sternocleidomastoid muscle. The parotideomasseteric region and deep layer of the lateral aspect of the face are of great anatomical significance.

Parotideomasseteric Region
The parotideomasseteric region is situated in the superficial layer of the lateral aspect of the face. It contains the parotid gland, masseter muscle, ramus of the mandible, facial nerve, external carotid artery, maxillary artery, and retromandibular vein. From superficial to deep, the parotideomasseteric region is divided into five layers, including the following: (1) skin; (2) superficial fascia containing the platysma muscle and greater auricular nerve; (3) parotideomasseteric fascia; (4) masseter muscle (anterior part) and superficial part of the parotid gland (posterior part, including blood vessels and nerves that pass through the parotid gland); (5) submasseteric space and ramus of the mandible (anterior half) and deep layer of the parotid gland (posterior half); and (6) bottom of the posterior mandibular fossa (Fig. 6.8).

Localization of the Parotid Gland
The parotid gland is situated anteroinferior to the external auditory canal, superior to the zygomatic arch, inferior to the angle of the mandible, and posterior to the anterior margin of the mastoid process. A part of the parotid gland extends anteriorly to cover the surface of the masseter muscle, and a major part of the gland fills the posterior mandibular fossa. The deep layer of the parotid gland is adjacent to the stylohyoid muscle and accompanying blood vessels and nerves, including the

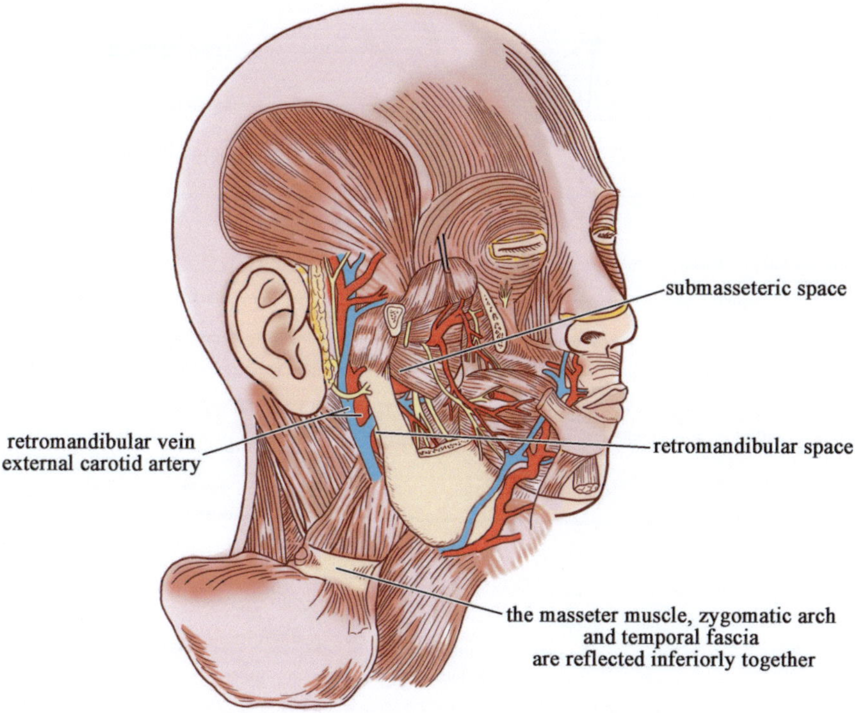

Fig. 6.8 Deep structure of the parotideomasseteric region

internal carotid artery and vein, glossopharyngeal nerve, vagus nerve, accessory nerve, and hypoglossal nerve. These structures that surround the parotid gland form the parotid bed.

Morphology of the Parotid Gland

The parotid gland is irregular and wedge-shaped, with the base facing outward and the tip protruding anteromedially toward the side wall of the pharynx. The outline of the parotid gland surface is an irregular quadrilateral with four extensions, including the anterior extension to the facial process, superior extension to the articular process, posterior extension to the auricle, and inferior extension to the cervical process (Fig. 6.9). The general outline of the parotid gland is an upside-down pyramid (indistinct superior extension to the temporomandibular joint), an inverted "L" shape (pronounced anterior extension to the facial process), or oval (indistinct four extensions). The process of the pharynx, situated in the deep space of the parotid gland, extends to the side wall of the pharynx. Tumors at this site manifest obvious pharyngeal symptoms that are difficult to diagnose in the early phase.

Capsule of the Parotid Gland

The capsule of the parotid gland is formed by the two layers of the parotideomasseteric fascia that enclose the superficial and deep aspects of the parotid gland, respectively. The superficial layer of the capsule is dense, closely attached to the

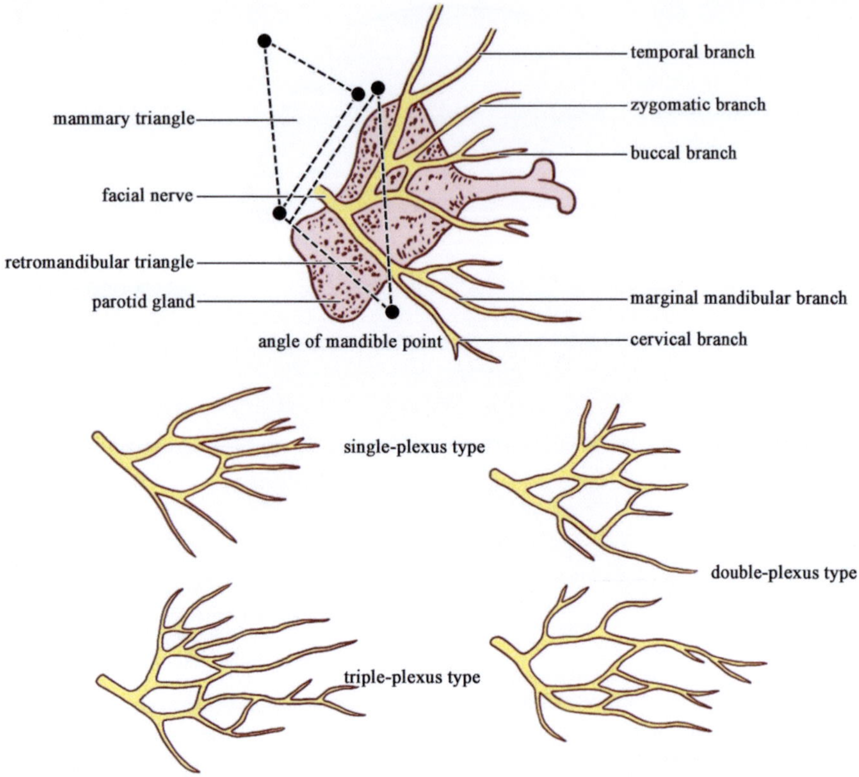

Fig. 6.9 The morphology of the parotid gland and classifications of facial nerves

parotid gland, and deeply invested in the lobules of the parotid gland. Therefore, when the parotid gland is inflamed, swelling is restricted, and pain is severe. The deep layer of the capsule is weak, and abscesses usually affect the deep structures rather than the superficial layer, leading to a parapharyngeal abscess or protrusions to the neck.

Parotid Duct

The parotid duct arises from the deep layer of the anterior margin of the parotid gland, coursing anteriorly at one finger's breadth below the inferior margin of the zygomatic arch (Fig. 6.10). After running across the surface and the anterior margin of the masseter muscle, the parotid duct takes a right-angle turn and travels inward to pass through the buccal fat pad and buccinator muscle. It finally opens into the buccal mucosa of the second maxillary molar tooth. The elevation at the opening of the parotid duct is known as the papilla of the parotid duct, where a tube is often inserted to perform parotid sialography. The buccal branch of the facial nerve, the transverse facial artery, and vein accompany the parotid duct, and sometimes, an accessory parotid gland is found superior to the main parotid gland with an isolated relation.

Blood vessels and nerves pass through the parotid gland.

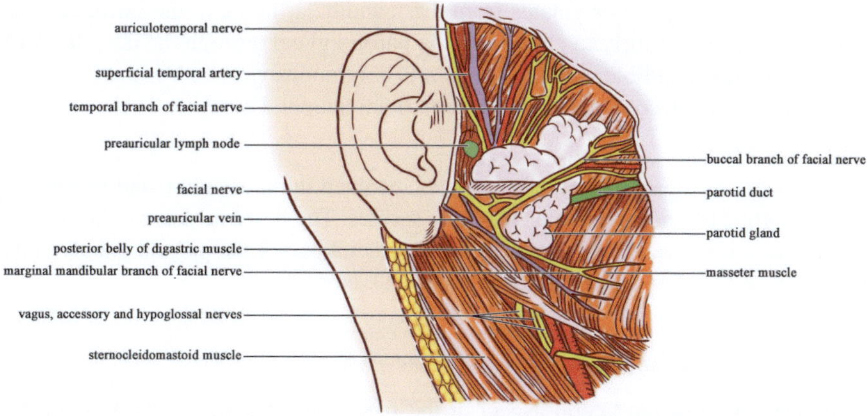

Fig. 6.10 The parotid gland, blood vessels, and nerves passing through the parotid gland

The facial nerve and the parotid plexus transversely course through the parotid gland. The external carotid artery and its terminal branches, retromandibular vein and its branches, and the auriculotemporal nerve longitudinally course through the parotid gland (Fig. 6.10).

The main trunk of the facial nerve exits the skull at the stylomastoid foramen, passes anteriorly through the superficial surface of the base of the styloid process, and travels about 1 cm to pierce into the parotid gland, where it splits into the superior and inferior trunks. Branches are bifurcated from the two trunks of the facial nerve to form the parotid plexus, which further divides into five terminal branches (temporal, zygomatic, buccal, marginal mandibular, and cervical) to exit the parotid gland. The extracranial branches of the facial nerve can be divided into three segments based on their relationship with the parotid gland. The first is the segment where the facial nerve trunk passes through the stylomastoid foramen and pierces into the parotid gland. The second is the inner segment within the parotid gland, and the third is the segment of the facial nerve leaving the parotid gland. The trunk and plexus of the facial nerve divide the parotid gland into superficial and deep parts, which are closely related to the parotid gland. Inflammations or tumors of the parotid gland cause facial paralysis by compressing the facial nerve. The facial nerve and its branches should be carefully protected during parotidectomy.

Blood vessels and nerves that longitudinally course through the parotid gland are generally situated in the deep aspect of the facial nerve. The external carotid artery passes through the deep layer of the posterior belly of the digastric muscle and enters the parotid gland in the posterior mandibular fossa. Behind the neck of the mandible, it divides into two terminal branches: the superficial temporal artery and the maxillary artery. The former ascends and pierces the superior margin of the parotid gland, giving off the transverse facial artery within the parotid gland. The latter travels anteriorly to the infratemporal fossa. The retromandibular vein runs behind the external carotid artery and descends after being formed within the parotid gland by the confluence of the maxillary vein and superficial temporal vein. The auriculotemporal nerve originates from the mandibular nerve in the infratemporal fossa, courses posteriorly to pierce into the parotid gland through the deep layer of the neck of the mandible, and then curves to continuously ascend. It travels out of the parotid gland accompanied by the superficial temporal artery and vein.

Masseter Muscle
The masseter is a pair of powerful muscles involved in mastication, and its quadrilateral outline can be palpable on the body surface. The posterior superficial surface of the masseter muscle is covered by the superficial part of the parotid gland, while the anterior part is covered by the parotideomasseteric fascia.

Deep Space of the Lateral Aspect of the Face

The deep space of the lateral aspect of the face is situated below the base of the skull, deep to the ramus of the mandible, posterolateral to the oral cavity, and lateral to the pharynx. Above it are the infratemporal fossa and infratemporal space, while below it is the pterygomandibular space. The retropharyngeal and parapharyngeal spaces are located within its deep space.

6.1.2.4 Fascial Spaces of the Face

Fascial spaces are potential gaps between two layers of fasciae, or those between fascia and periosteum. Under normal circumstances, fascial spaces serve as passageways for blood vessels and nerves, and are filled with adipose and connective tissues. The spatial structure of fascial space becomes clear when connective tissues are infiltrated by inflammation. Anesthetic agents for nerve blocks of the face and mouth are usually injected around nerves within a fascial space. In cases of purulent infections, exudates generally spread along the weak structures, like fascial spaces and passageways for blood vessels and nerves. Therefore, fascial spaces are of great significance in the anatomy of the maxillofacial region. It is important to learn the localization, contents, and communications of fascial spaces of the face, in order to accomplish accurate procedures of local block anesthesia and drainage of maxillofacial infections.

Bounded by the maxilla and mandible, the fascial spaces of the face are classified into the superficial and deep fascial spaces. The superficial fascial space includes the infraorbital space, buccal space, submasseteric space, temporal space, and retromandibular space. The deep fascial space comprises the infratemporal space, pterygomandibular space, pterygopharyngeal space, extraorbital space, and the space of the floor of the mouth.

Infraorbital Space

The infraorbital space is an inverted triangular space situated below the orbit, between the deep surface of the musculus quadratus labii superioris (which includes the zygomaticus minor muscle, levator labii superioris, and levator labii superioris alaeque nasi) and the anterior part of the maxilla (Figs. 6.11 and 6.12). Its superior, medial, and inferolateral boundaries refer to the infraorbital rim, lateral portion of the nose, and zygomaticus major muscle and zygomatic bone, respectively. The bottom of the infraorbital space is situated anterior to the body of the maxilla, and the infraorbital foramen is situated in the central part of the bottom. The canine fossa and levator anguli oris are located inferolateral to the infraorbital foramen, with the latter running obliquely forward and downward to the corner of the mouth. The infraorbital space is filled with adipose and connective tissues, blood vessels, and

Fig. 6.11 Infraorbital space

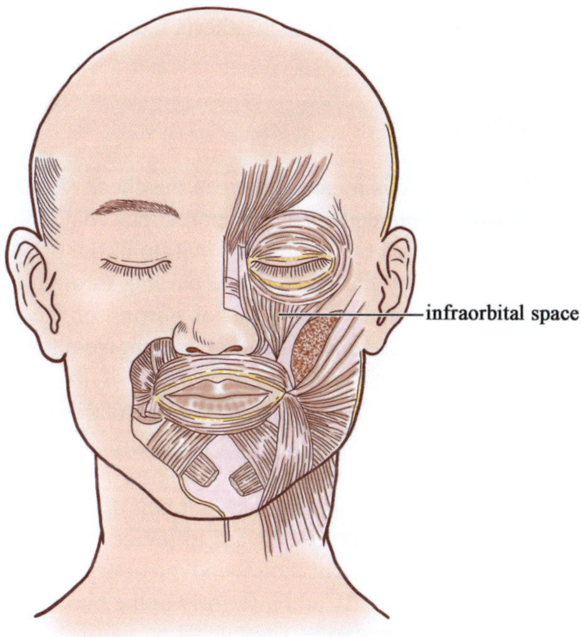

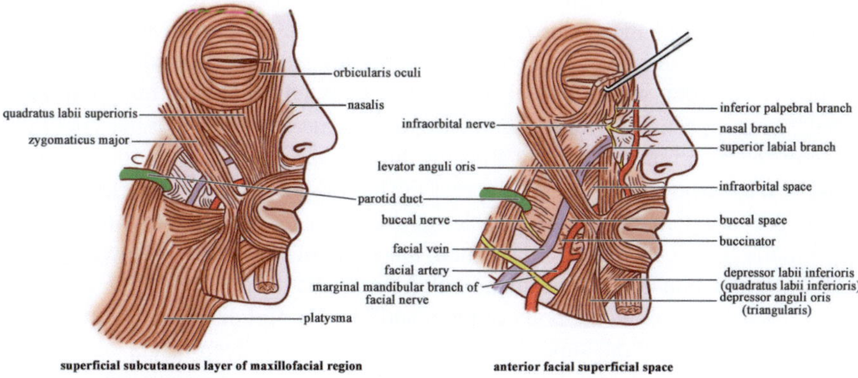

Fig. 6.12 Infraorbital and buccal spaces

nerves. The infraorbital nerve and artery pass out of the infraorbital foramen and split into branches to reach the lower eyelid, external nose, and upper lip. The facial artery ascends within the medial side of the infraorbital foramen, where it becomes the angular vein. The facial vein descends behind the facial artery. The transverse facial artery and the terminal zygomatic branch of the facial nerve travel along the superior part of the zygomaticus major muscle on the deep side.

The infraorbital space communicates with the buccal space through the deep surface of the zygomatic major muscle. Infections in the infraorbital space mostly spread from odontogenic infections of the maxillary canines and premolars. The infraorbital nerve, as well as the anterior and middle superior alveolar nerves, can be blocked through regional anesthesia within the infraorbital canal.

Buccal Space

The buccal space is located between the cheek skin and the buccinator muscle. It is superiorly bounded by the zygomaticus major muscle and zygomatic bone, inferiorly bounded by the inferior margin of the body of the mandible, anteromedially bounded by the vertical line passing through the corner of the mouth, and posteriorly bounded by the anterior portion of the masseter muscle (superficial space) and the pterygomandibular ligament from the medial pterygoid plate to the posterior aspect of the alveolar process of the mandibular third molar (deep space). The anterior half of the buccal space is shallow and becomes deeper in the posterior half. The buccal fat pad fills the posterior part of the buccal space and extends to other deep spaces, providing a passageway for infections. The parotid duct runs transversely in the posterior half of the buccal space, passes through the buccal fat pad, and travels inward to pierce into the buccinator muscle, opening into the buccal mucosa of the second maxillary molar tooth. The buccal artery and nerve course superiorly and inferiorly to the buccinator muscle, where the parotid duct pierces, respectively. The buccal nerve further travels to the superficial part of the buccal space to innervate the buccal skin and mucosa. The facial artery and vein run in the anterior half of the buccal space. The buccal and marginal mandibular branches of the facial nerve travel from back to front in the superficial fascia of the buccal space. The buccal branches are situated superior and inferior to the parotid duct, with the thicker branch usually adjacent. The marginal mandibular branch, usually with 1–2 branches, travels along the inferior margin of the body of the mandible or slightly above it through the deep layer of the platysma muscle. It then curves and ascends across the blood vessels in the superficial space of the face and pierces into the muscles of the lower lip. Damage to the marginal mandibular branch can lead to movement disorders of the ipsilateral lower lip due to fewer anastomoses. During mandibular surgeries, a skin incision is typically made 1.0–1.5 cm below the body of the mandible. Careful dissection between the platysma muscle and the superficial layer of the cervical deep fascia, along with low ligation of facial blood vessels, can help protect the marginal mandibular branch of the facial nerve (Fig. 6.12).

The buccal space communicates superiorly with the infraorbital space; posteriorly and superiorly with the pterygomandibular space, infratemporal space, and extraorbital space; and posterolaterally with the submasseteric space. Infections in the buccal space often spread from adjacent spaces or the oral cavity.

Submasseteric Space

The submasseteric space is a narrow, flat space located between the deep layer of the masseter muscle and the superior half of the mandibular ramus.

Anteriorly, it is bounded by the anterior margin of the masseter muscle and the buccal space; posteriorly by the posterior portion of the mandibular ramus; superiorly, by the inferior portion of the zygomatic arch; and inferiorly, by the attachment of the masseter muscle to the mandibular ramus (Fig. 6.13). This space contains a small amount of connective tissues. The masseteric artery and nerve emerge from the infratemporal space superior to the mandibular notch and anterior to the neck of the mandible, and then pierce into the deep layer of the masseter muscle through the superior part of the submasseteric space. Anesthetic agents are typically injected from a site superior and posterior to the midpoint of the mandibular notch for masseteric nerve block.

The superior part of the submasseteric space communicates with the deeply located infratemporal space and pterygomandibular space via the mandibular notch, and with the temporal space via the deep side of the zygomatic arch. It communicates anterior-superiorly with the extraorbital space, anteriorly with the buccal space, and posteriorly with the retromandibular space. Infections in the submasseteric space mostly derive from pericoronitis of the mandibular wisdom tooth, mandibular osteomyelitis, or the spread of infections from the parotid gland and adjacent spaces.

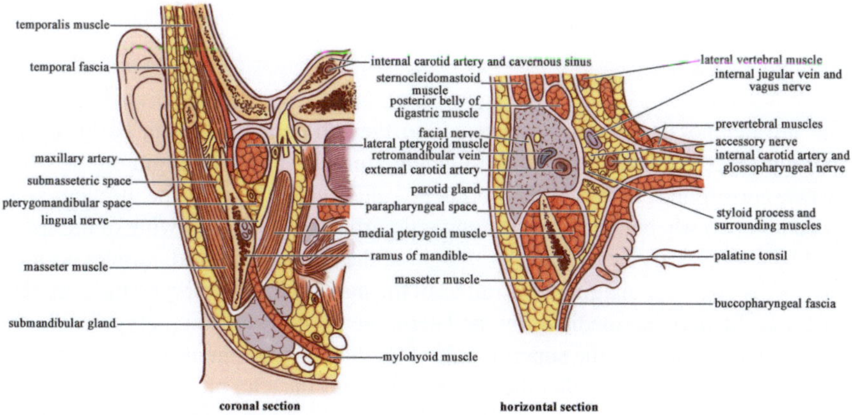

Fig. 6.13 Spaces within the lateral side of the face (right side)

Retromandibular Space

The retromandibular space is situated within the posterior mandibular fossa, located between the ramus of the mandible and the mastoid process. It is superiorly bounded by the external auditory canal, inferiorly bounded by a line connecting the angle of the mandible and the apex of the mastoid process, anteriorly bounded by the mandibular ramus and the masseter (superficial layer) and medial pterygoid muscles (deep layer), and posteriorly bounded by the mastoid process and the anterior border of the sternocleidomastoid muscle. The floor of the space, from top to bottom, includes the styloid process, muscles attached to the styloid process, the transverse process of the atlas, and the posterior belly of the digastric muscle. The retromandibular space lies between the superficial layer of the parotid capsule and the floor of the posterior mandibular fossa, containing the parotid gland and structures passing through it (Fig. 6.10). Along the floor of the space and deep to the digastric muscle, structures are arranged from posterior to anterior as follows: the accessory nerve, internal jugular vein, hypoglossal nerve, internal carotid artery, and external carotid artery. Anteriorly, the retromandibular space communicates with the infratemporal space, pterygomandibular space, pterygopharyngeal space, and the submandibular space in the neck.

Temporal Space

As previously mentioned, the temporal space is situated between the temporal fascia and the periosteum of the temporal fossa. Although the temporal space is located on the lateral side of the cranium, it contains the temporalis muscle, which is critical for chewing function. Inferiorly, the temporal space communicates with the buccal space, infratemporal space, and pterygomandibular space. We therefore describe the temporal space in the section on the fascial spaces of the face (Fig. 6.5).

Infratemporal Space

The infratemporal space is situated within the infratemporal fossa, covering the lateral pterygoid muscle and its surrounding area. Its superior margin on the body surface corresponds to the superior border of the zygomatic arch. The infratemporal space is superiorly bounded by the temporal portion of the greater wing of the sphenoid bone; inferiorly by the inferior margin of the lateral pterygoid muscle; posteriorly by the posterior margin of the ramus of the mandible; anteriorly by the posterior aspect of the maxilla; medially by the lateral pterygoid plate and pterygomaxillary fissure; and laterally by the superior half of the mandibular ramus and the temporalis muscle tendon. It contains the lateral pterygoid muscle, blood vessels, nerves, and adipose and connective tissue. The infratemporal space is divided by the lateral pterygoid muscle into three layers: the superficial layer on the superficial side of the lateral pterygoid muscle, the intermediate layer where the lateral pterygoid muscle is located, and the deep layer on the deep side of the lateral pterygoid muscle (Fig. 6.14).

The superficial part of the infratemporal space, which serves as the passageway for the maxillary blood vessels, contains the maxillary artery and its branches, as well as the pterygoid plexus. In a small percentage of cases (about 10.0%), the maxillary artery may course deep to the lateral pterygoid muscle. The maxillary artery gives rise to the middle meningeal artery and the posterior deep temporal artery on the posterior and inferior aspects of the lateral pterygoid muscle, which travel upward. The inferior alveolar artery runs downward. Before entering the pterygopalatine fossa, the maxillary artery gives off the anterior deep temporal artery, which travels upward, and the buccal artery and posterior superior alveolar artery, which run downward. The pterygoid plexus accompanies the maxillary artery. It is formed by venous anastomoses and is distributed around the superficial surface of the lateral pterygoid muscle on its deep side. Posteriorly, the pterygoid plexus converges to form the maxillary vein, which drains into the retromandibular vein. Anteriorly, the deep facial vein communicates with the facial vein after passing through the superficial layer of the buccinator muscle. On the deep side, the pterygoid plexus communicates with the cavernous sinus through the small venous foramina, the foramen ovale, and the foramen lacerum of the sphenoid bone. These channels form a buffer device for venous return and also serve as pathways for extracranial infections to spread into the intracranial area.

The middle part of the infratemporal space is occupied by the lateral pterygoid muscle. The buccal nerve exits between the upper and lower heads of the lateral pterygoid muscle. The lingual nerve and inferior alveolar nerve exit between the lateral and medial pterygoid muscles.

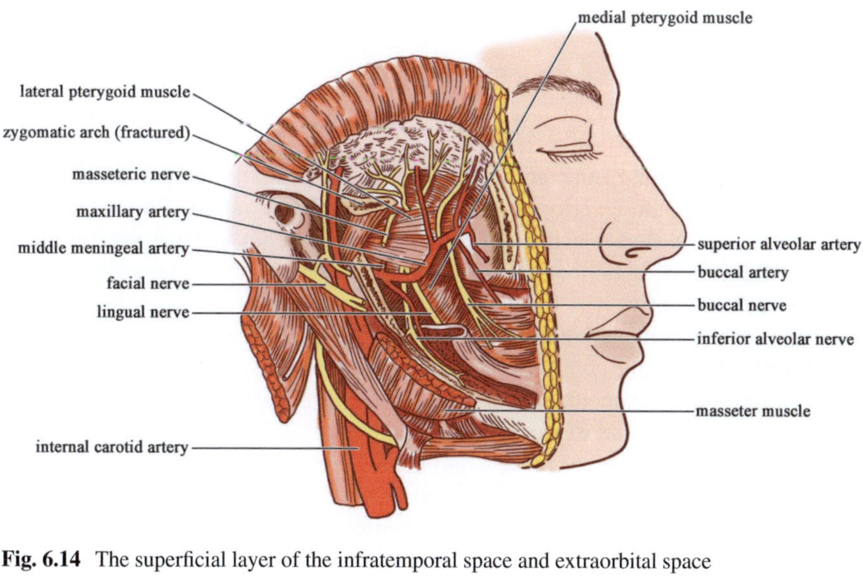

Fig. 6.14 The superficial layer of the infratemporal space and extraorbital space

The deep part of the infratemporal space can be exposed after removing the lateral pterygoid muscle. The anterior and posterior temporal nerves run upward along the superior wall of the infratemporal fossa. In the posterior part of the deep infratemporal space, deep to the temporomandibular joint, lies the upper end of the sphenomandibular ligament. The auriculotemporal nerve runs horizontally upward and outward. The middle meningeal artery passes through the two roots of the auriculotemporal nerve and ascends into the cranium through the foramen spinosum. Deep to the middle meningeal artery, the chorda tympani emerges from the sutures at the base of the skull, then runs obliquely forward and downward to join the lingual nerve. The above structures must be carefully protected during temporomandibular joint surgeries. In the middle part of the deep infratemporal space, there are the foramen ovale, the mandibular nerve, and its branches (the masseteric nerve, buccal nerve, lingual nerve, inferior alveolar nerve, and auriculotemporal nerve). The foramen ovale is projected onto the mid-point of the line connecting the mid-point of the lower margin of the zygomatic arch and the mid-point of the mandibular notch, at a depth of about 4.0 cm. in the anterior part of the deep infratemporal space are the lateral pterygoid plate and the upper end of the medial pterygoid muscle. Deep to the medial pterygoid muscle are the. Superior border of the superior pharyngeal constrictor muscle, the tensor veli palatini muscle, the cartilaginous part of the pharyngotympanic tube (Eustachian tube), and the levator veli palatini muscle.

The infratemporal space communicates with the temporal space superiorly, with the cranium through the cranial foramen at the base of the skull, with the extraorbital space anteroinferiorly, with the pterygomandibular space inferolaterally, with the submasseteric space by crossing the mandibular notch laterally, with the retromandibular space posteriorly through the maxillary blood vessels, and with the pterygopalatine fossa medially through the pterygomaxillary fissure.

Pterygomandibular Space

The pterygomandibular space is situated between the medial side of the mandibular ramus and the lateral surface of the medial pterygoid muscle. It is anteriorly bounded by the anterior margin of the temporalis muscle, the posterior margin of the buccinator muscle, and the anterior margin of the mandibular ramus. Posteriorly, it is bounded by the posterior margin of the mandibular ramus and the parotid gland capsule. Superiorly, it is bounded by the inferior margin of the lateral pterygoid muscle, and inferiorly, it is bounded by the attachment of the medial pterygoid muscle to the mandibular ramus. The pterygomandibular space contains a small amount of adipose and connective tissues, two ligaments, and three nerves. The pterygomandibular ligament, also known as the buccopharyngeal raphe, is situated at the anterior—most part of the pterygomandibular space. It serves as the common origin of both the buccinator muscle and the superior pharyngeal constrictor muscle. Once covered with mucosa in the oral cavity, it forms the pterygomandibular fold, which is an important marker for the inferior alveolar nerve block and the intra-oral incision in the pterygomandibular space. Approximately 0.6 cm posterior and slightly deeper to the buccal nerve, the lingual nerve descends. Passing through the deep side of the mucosa behind the third mandibular molar to the submandibular space, about 1.5 cm posterior to the lingual nerve, at the middle of the lateral surface of the medial pterygoid muscle, the inferior alveolar nerve and its accompanying blood vessels descend and enter the mandibular foramen. The sphenomandibular ligament is situated at the posterior—most part of the pterygomandibular space and descends to attach to the lingula of the mandible (Figs. 6.13, 6.15 and 6.16).

The pterygomandibular space communicates with the temporal space and the infratemporal space superiorly, with the infraorbital space superomedially, with the buccal space anteriorly, with the retromandibular space posteriorly, and with the submandibular space inferiorly, along with the lingual nerve. The pterygomandibular space is situated centrally, and inflammation here can spread widely to the surrounding spaces. Anesthetic agents are injected into the pterygomandibular space for an inferior alveolar nerve block. Generally, the needle is inserted slightly outside the mid-point of the pterygomandibular fold inside the mouth and enters the pterygomandibular space through the buccal mucosa and the buccinator muscle. After reaching the superior part of the mandibular foramen, the inferior alveolar nerve can be blocked. The lingual nerve and the buccal nerve can be blocked successively during the process of withdrawing the needle. As a result, three ligaments are blocked spontaneously, achieving the anesthesia of the ipsilateral mandibular alveolar and gingivae (Fig. 6.15).

Extraorbital Space

The extraorbital space is situated posterolateral to the lateral orbital wall. From anterior to posterior, the medial wall of the extraorbital space is composed of the maxillary tuberosity, pterygomaxillary fissure, and the anterior end of the lateral

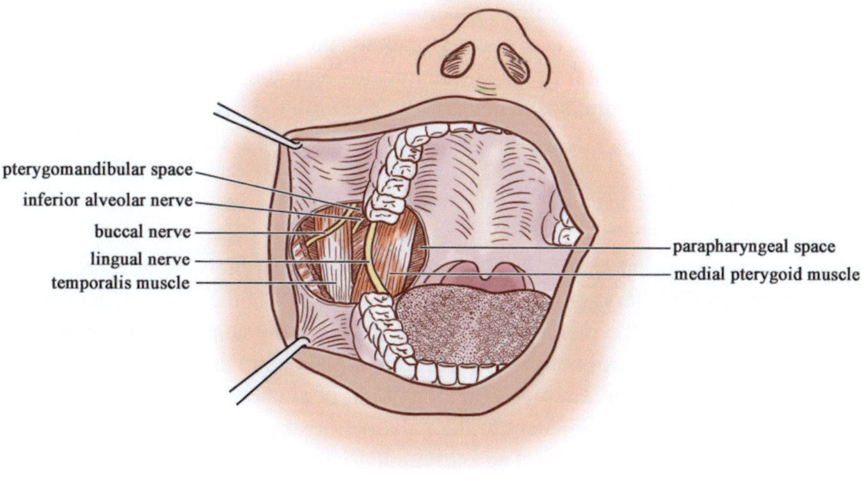

Fig. 6.15 Pterygomandibular space and pterygopharyngeal space (intraoral view)

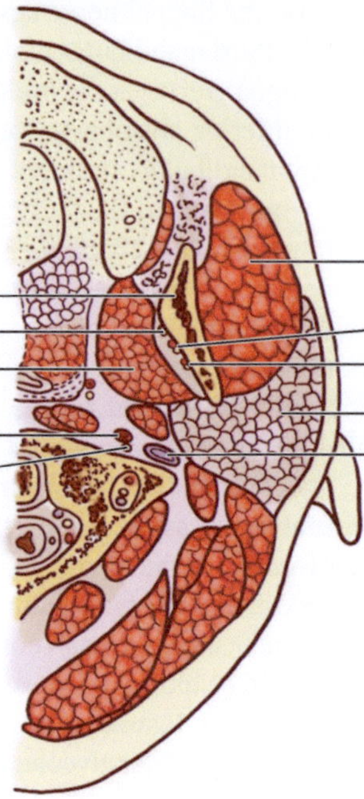

Fig. 6.16 Pterygomandibular space (transverse section parallel to the ramus of the mandible)

pterygoid muscle. The anterior wall and the lateral wall of the extraorbital space are formed by the zygomatic bone and the anterior end of the zygomatic arch, respectively. The anterior edge of the lower part of the temporalis muscle and the coronoid process of the mandible form the posterior wall of the extraorbital space. This space is filled with adipose tissues. The posterior superior alveolar artery and nerve, which are closely attached to the maxillary tuberosity, descend into the alveolar foramina. Anesthetic agents can be injected here to block the posterior superior alveolar nerve (Fig. 6.14). The extraorbital space communicates with the temporal space superiorly, with the infratemporal space posteriorly, and with the buccal space inferiorly.

Pterygopharyngeal Space

The pterygopharyngeal space, also known as the parapharyngeal space, is situated between the medial pterygoid muscle and the lateral wall of the pharynx. Its anterosuperior boundary is the pterygomandibular ligament; the anteroinferior boundary reaches the superior margin of the submandibular gland; and the posterior boundary is the prevertebral fascia. There is a small amount of connective tissue in the pterygopharyngeal space. It is adjacent to the palatine tonsils, separated by the superior pharyngeal constrictor muscle. The pterygopharyngeal space communicates with the retropharyngeal space posteriorly, with the infratemporal space and pterygomandibular space through the space between the medial and lateral pterygoid muscles, with the buccal space and extraorbital space anteriorly, and with the submandibular space inferiorly (Figs. 6.16 and 6.17).

Space of Mouth Floor

The space of the mouth floor, also known as the sublingual space, is in the "∩"-shaped configuration encircling the root of the tongue. Its anterolateral side is bounded by the body of the mandible; the inferior side is bounded by the diaphragma oris (mylohyoid muscle and geniohyoid muscle); the superior side is bounded by the oral floor mucosa; and the medial side is bounded by the hyoglossus muscle and the roof of the tongue. The anterior end of the space of mouth floor communicates with each other deep to the sublingual caruncle. The lingual artery and hypoglossal nerve are housed in the posterior space of the mouth floor, and the sublingual gland and submandibular duct (Wharton's duct) in the anterior space. The lingual nerve first runs anteroinferiorly on the superolateral side of the submandibular duct, winds around from the lateral side of the duct to its inferior disc, and then turns to the superomedial side of the duct and ascends, with branches entering the anterior two-thirds of the tongue. When ligating the submandibular duct during submandibular gland

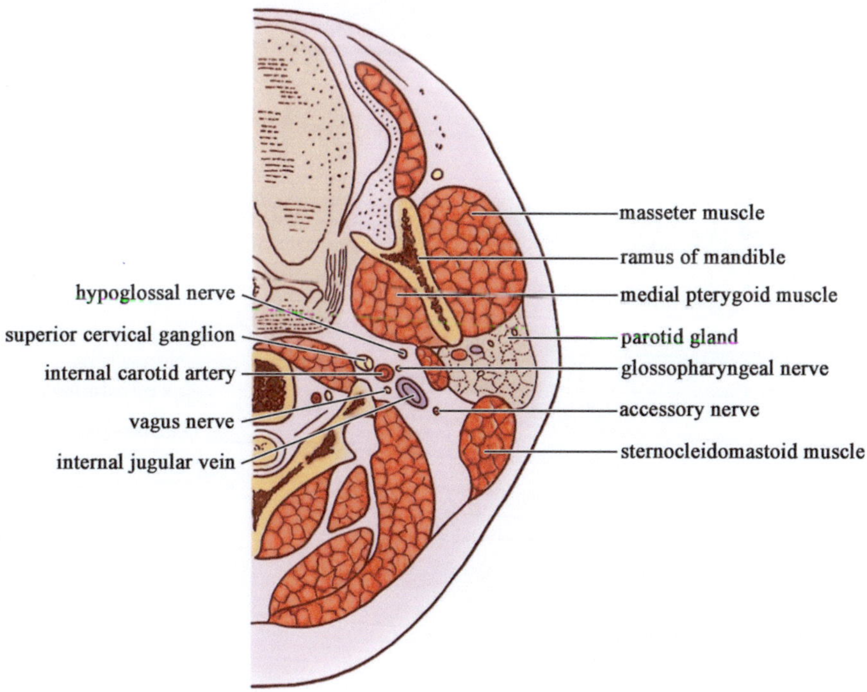

Fig. 6.17 Pterygopharyngeal space(transverse section parallel to the second cervical vertebra)

surgery, attention should be paid to the semi-spiral crossing relationship between the lingual nerve and the duct. The hypoglossal nerve runs obliquely anterosuperiorly in the middle and lower part of the hyoglossus muscle and enters the middle part of the inferior surface of the tongue.

The space of the floor of the mouth communicates with the submandibular space, pterygomandibular space, and pterygopharyngeal space through the posterior portion of the mylohyoid muscle.

The anatomical locations of the deep spaces in the maxillofacial region are illustrated in Fig. 6.18.

6.1.2.5 Anatomy of the Head

Objective

1. Master the structural characteristics of the superficial layers of the cranium.
2. Master the structural characteristics of the superficial layers of the face.
3. Students majoring in stomatology are also required to master the structural characteristics of the facial spaces.

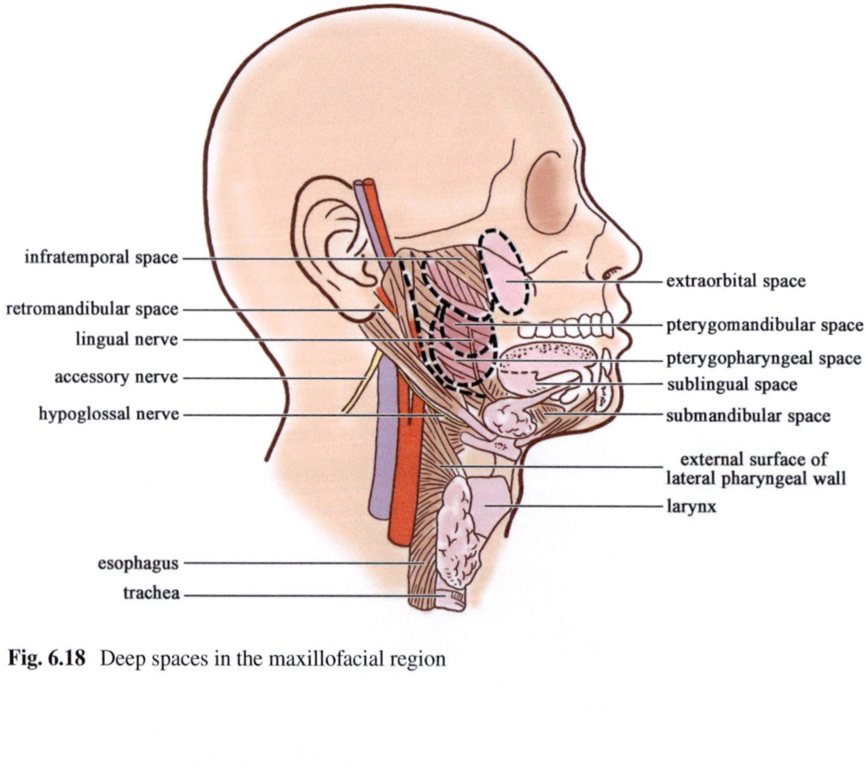

Fig. 6.18 Deep spaces in the maxillofacial region

Anatomical Position

Place the subject in a supine position, and place a wooden pillow under the shoulder.

Dissection Procedures

Dissection of the Calvaria and Superficial Layers of the Face

Step 1. Make a 5 cm × 8 cm incision on the calvaria, 2.5 cm away from the midline. After dissecting the skin, successively make incisions layer by layer, reducing the size by 0.5 cm × 0.5 cm for each layer until reaching the skull. Observe each layer as it is dissected. Pay special attention to observing the thick fibrous bundles in the superficial fascia, the composition of the scalp, the loose environment beneath the galea aponeurotica, and the attachment condition between the pericranium and the skull.

Step 2. Incise the facial skin. The incisions are made as shown in Fig. 6.19. Start from the midpoint of the hairline and make a midline incision downward until

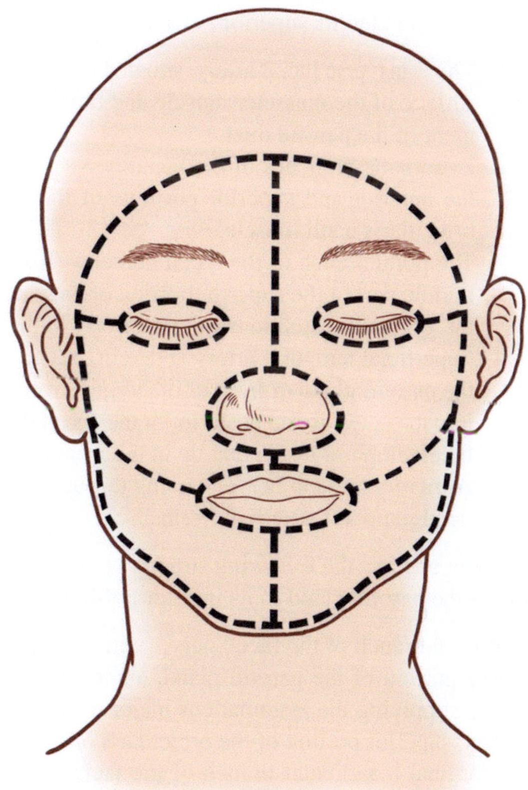

Fig. 6.19 Skin incisions on the head

reaching the neck. When passing the alar of the nose and the oral fissure, make circular incisions. Ensure that the incisions are not too deep. Along the midline incision, make a transverse cut starting from the corner of the mouth and extending outward to the root of the external ear. When dealing with the palpebral fissure, make circular incisions along the lower margin of the upper eyelid and the upper margin of the lower eyelid.

Step 3. Carefully raise the facial skin from the midline incision to both sides. Due to the thin facial skin and its attachment to the facial muscles, subcutaneous structures beneath the facial skin should be protected during dissection.

Step 4. Remove adipose tissues in the superficial fascia to expose the outline of the facial muscles.

Step 5. Remove the capsule of the parotid gland anterior to the ear and the parotideomasseteric fascia to expose the parotid gland, parotid duct, and masseter muscle. Observe the presence of the parotid lymph nodes within the capsule of the parotid gland.

Step 6. Starting from the parotid duct that is situated one finger's breadth below the zygomatic arch, dissect the structures that pass through the parotid gland sequentially.

Observe the following structures from the superior part of the anterior portion of the parotid gland to its superior portion.

1. The transverse facial artery, situated inferior to the zygomatic arch and on the surface of the masseter muscle and travelling anteriorly with the accompaniment of the parotid duct.
2. Zygomatic branches of the facial nerve, with 2–3 branches, passing through the anterior and superior portions of the parotid gland, and supplying the orbicularis oculi muscle.
3. Temporal branch of the facial nerve, with 1–2 branches, passing through the middle part of the superior portion of the parotid gland, and coursing through the zygomatic arch to travel superiorly to the epicranius muscle.
4. Superficial temporal artery and vein, passing through the superior portion of the parotid gland in front of the tragus, over the zygomatic arch, and splitting into the anterior and posterior branches on the superficial surface of the superficial temporal fascia that lie in the frontal and parietal regions, respectively.
5. Auriculotemporal nerve, passing through the parotid gland behind the superficial temporal artery and vein.

Then, observe the following structures from the inferior part of the anterior portion of the parotid gland to its inferior portion.

1. Buccal branch of the facial nerve, with 3–4 branches, passing through the anterior portion of the parotid gland, anteriorly above and below the parotid duct, and supplying the zygomaticus major muscle, musculus quadratus labii superioris, superior portion of the orbicularis oris muscle, and buccinator muscle.
2. Marginal mandibular branch of the facial nerve, with 1–2 branches, travelling anteriorly above and below the inferior portion of the body of the mandible,

coursing through the superficial side of the facial artery and vein, and supplying the inferior portion of the orbicularis oris muscle, depressor anguli oris muscle, depressor labii inferioris muscle, and mentalis muscle.

3. Cervical branch of the facial nerve, usually with 1 branch, passing through the inferior portion of the parotid gland, and descending into the deep layer of the platysma muscle.

Step 7. Dissect the parotid gland and retromandibular space. Following the buccal branch or marginal mandibular branch of the facial nerve into the parenchyma of the parotid gland, isolate the parotid plexus of the facial nerve, and carefully dissect the superficial part of the parotid gland on the superficial side of the plexus. Raise up the superficial part of the parotid gland and parotid duct anteriorly to expose the upper, lower, and main trunks of the facial nerve. Remove the deep part of the parotid gland on the deep side of the facial nerve. Observe the contents in the retromandibular fossa and space. Isolate the external carotid artery and its terminal branches and the retromandibular vein and its branches on the deep side of the facial nerve.

Dissection of the Superficial Fascial Spaces and Intermediate Layer of the Face

Step 1. Cut the orbicularis oculi muscle between it and the frontal belly, and turn it downward. Dissect the supraorbital blood vessels and nerves, and supratrochlear blood vessels and nerves on the medial side that pass through the supraorbital foramen or notch.

Step 2. Dissect the buccal space, facial arteries, and veins. Outline and preserve the zygomaticus major muscle. It is the anatomical landmark for distinguishing the infraorbital space and buccal space. Observe the range of the buccal space between the inferior part of the zygomaticus major muscle and the anterior part of the masseter muscle. In the posterior half of the buccal space, the parotid duct, and the buccal and marginal mandibular branches of the facial nerve travel transversely. Take out the buccal fat pad from the deep side of the parotid duct, and observe the morphology and depth. From the anteroinferior margin of the masseter muscle to its attachment to the inferior body of the mandible, identify the facial artery and superior and inferior labial arteries situated below the muscular layer of the corner of the mouth from the lateral side. The facial vein lies behind the accompanying artery. The deep facial vein lies in the middle part of the buccal space. Below the corner of the mouth, raise up the depressor anguli oris muscle and depressor labii inferioris muscle (musculus quadratus labii inferioris) to expose the mental foramen. Observe the location of the mental foramen inferior to the second mandibular premolar, at 2.0–3.0 cm from the midline, its posterior opening, and the mental artery and nerve pass through it.

Step 3. Dissect the infraorbital space. Cut off the musculus quadratus labii superioris from its inferior end, and raise it up to expose the infraorbital space. Remove the contents from the infraorbital space. Observe the location of the infraorbital foramen, and the infraorbital blood vessels and nerves passing through it. Trace the facial artery already identified upwards to its terminal branch - the angular artery. The facial vein originates from the angular vein and descends behind the facial artery.

Step 4. Dissect the submasseteric space and temporal space. Cut off the end of the terminal branches of the facial nerve, and turn up all the terminal branches, parotid plexus, and main trunk of the facial nerve towards the stylomastoid foramen. Cut open the superficial layer of the temporal fascia above the zygomatic arch transversely to expose the superficial part of the temporal space. Remove the adipose tissues, explore the range of the superficial part using the handle of the forceps, and observe the middle temporal artery and the deep layer of the temporal fascia. Subsequently, cut open the temporal fascia along the anterior, superior, and posterior portions, and turn it downward to the superior margin of the zygomatic arch to expose the deep temporal space and temporalis muscle. Insert a probe into the deep surface of the zygomatic arch from top to bottom, identify the anterior and posterior ends, and cut them off. Turn the temporal fascia, zygomatic arch, and masseter muscle downward to the attachment to the ramus of the mandible, and observe the masseteric blood vessels and nerves that travel from the deep layer of the superior mandibular notch to the masseter muscle. Observe the location and communication of the submasseteric space.

Step 5. Dissect the pterygomandibular space and the superficial part of the infratemporal space. Saw or bite off about 2.0 cm of the compact bone in the middle and lower part of the ramus of the mandible, and scrape off the cancellous bone to expose the mandibular canal formed by the compact bone in the mandible. Then, scrape the compact bone out of the mandibular canal upward to expose the inferior alveolar blood vessels and nerves and protect them. Saw the compact bone deep to the ramus of the mandible that is situated on the deep side of the inferior alveolar blood vessels and nerves, and dissect the ramus of the mandible until reaching the mandibular foramen. Dissect and cut open the capsule of the temporomandibular joint, and leave the articular disc within. Free the head of the mandible, and raise up the dissected ramus of the mandible and the inferior half of the temporalis muscle to expose the pterygomandibular space on the deep side of the ramus of the mandible, the superficial part of the infratemporal space above the pterygomandibular space, and the deep part of the temporal space on the deep side of the temporalis muscle. Protect the buccal nerve that passes through the anteroinferior part of the temporalis muscle.

From anterior to posterior, dissect the buccal nerve, lingual nerve, and inferior alveolar nerve and blood vessels situated on the surface of the medial pterygoid muscle in the pterygomandibular space, and measure their intervals.

On the deep surface of the temporalis muscle, dissect the anterior and posterior deep temporal blood vessels and nerves that attach to the surface of the temporal fossa.

In the superficial part of the infratemporal space, dissect the maxillary artery and its branches, and observe the location and development of the pterygoid plexus. Observe the site of the buccal nerve, lingual nerve, and inferior alveolar nerve that perforate the infratemporal space.

Step 6. Dissect the extra-orbital space and the deep part of the infratemporal space. Remove the adipose tissues in the extra-orbital space on the deep surface of the zygomatic arch, behind the body of the maxilla. Observe the posterior alveolar blood vessels and nerves and their branches that descend into the alveolar foramina, closely attaching to the posterior body of the maxilla. Dissect the origins of the superior and inferior heads of the lateral pterygoid muscle, and separate the remaining capsule of the mandibular joint and its inner articular disc around the mandibular fossa. Pull out the lateral pterygoid muscle situated on the deep surface of the maxillary artery, as well as the capsule and articular disc of the mandibular joint, backward to expose the deep part of the infratemporal space. Dissect the mandibular nerve and its branches that pass through the foramen ovale. Observe the relationship between the middle meningeal artery and auriculotemporal nerve, and that between the chorda tympani exiting from the base of the skull and lingual nerve.

Step 7. Dissect the pterygopharyngeal space. Cut off the origin of the medial pterygoid muscle in the pterygoid fossa. Completely remove the medial pterygoid muscle to expose the pterygopharyngeal space, and clean the bottom of the space and the blood vessels on the wall of the pharynx. Dissect the tensor veli palatini muscle, levator veli palatini muscle, and cartilage of the Eustachian tube on the deep side of the anterior infratemporal space. Observe the properties of the pterygomandibular ligament between the superior pharyngeal constrictor muscle and buccinator muscle.

Step 8. Dissect the space of the mouth floor. Saw or bite off the body of the mandible below the mandibular canal to the front of the mental foramen. Cut off the origin of the mylohyoid muscle on the medial side of the mandible, turn it downward, and expose the space of the mouth floor. Identify the hypoglossal nerve, lingual nerve, submandibular duct, and sublingual gland, and observe the cross-relationship between the lingual nerve and submandibular duct.

All the dissected and raised structures are reset for future review.

6.1.2.6 Summary

The scalp is tightly composed of the skin, superficial fascia, and galea aponeurosis on the calvaria, and therefore, a violent traction by trauma causes a large - scale scalp avulsion injury. The connective tissue under the galea is loose, and bleeding in the subgaleal layer easily spreads to cause a calvarial hematoma. Subperiosteal hematoma is bleeding limited to one bone, because the periosteum heals tightly at the skull sutures.

The superficial fascia of the face is characterized by a complex structure, rich blood vessels, and the component of expressive muscles. In addition to the sensory terminal branches of the trigeminal nerve, motor terminal branches of the facial nerve lie in the superficial fascia that supply expressive muscles. The parotid duct also runs in the superficial fascia of the face. Be careful to protect the branches of the facial nerve and parotid duct during facial surgeries.

Abundant fascial compartments exist in the face. These compartments provide buffer spaces for the functions and activities of facial organs. They also serve as passageways for blood vessels and nerves, and become the routes for the spread of inflammation when infected. It is of great clinical significance to be familiar with the locations, contents, and communications of these compartments. Specifically, there are five superficial fascial spaces, namely the infraorbital space, buccal space, temporal space, submasseteric space, and retromandibular space; and there are also five deep fascial spaces in the face, namely the infratemporal space, extraorbital space, pterygomandibular space, pterygopharyngeal space, and sublingual space.

6.2 Clinical Application of Key Anatomical Structures of the Head and Face

From superficial to deep, the head is divided into the skin, superficial fascia, epicranius muscle, and galea aponeurosis, subgalea tissues, and pericranium. The soft tissue of the head has a rich blood supply. These are the supratrochlear artery, the supraorbital artery, the superficial temporal artery, the postauricular artery, and the occipital artery from anterior to posterior, and there are many arterial anastomoses. The frontotemporal flap, retroauricular flap, temporo-occipital flap, supraorbital flap, and temporoparietal flap are frequently used in skin flaps of the head. Because the blood vessels in the scalp are surrounded and fixed by fibrous tissues and the blood vessel lumen is not easy to close, ischemia rarely occurs in the skin flaps.

The sensory innervation to the face comes from the trigeminal nerve. The branches of the trigeminal nerve provide nervous supply to the skin, mucosa, and soft tissues of the face. Consistent with the three embryonic divisions of the face, namely the frontonasal, maxillary, and mandibular processes, is the distribution of the trigeminal nerve. Sensations in the posterior scalp, inferior border of the mandible, and neck are innervated by the cervical nerve branches and plexus. Most of the skin and subcutaneous tissues on the face are supplied by branches of the external carotid artery. After the external carotid artery branches off from the common carotid artery in the neck, it gives off a series of branches, including the superior thyroid artery, lingual artery, facial artery, ascending pharyngeal artery, postauricular artery, occipital artery, maxillary artery, and superficial temporal artery.

Clinical application of common skin flaps on the head and face based on their characteristics is described as follows (Fig. 6.20).

1. Forehead Flap

   The forehead flap is a skin flap with a pedicle based on the frontal branch of the superficial temporal artery. According to the range of excision, the flap can

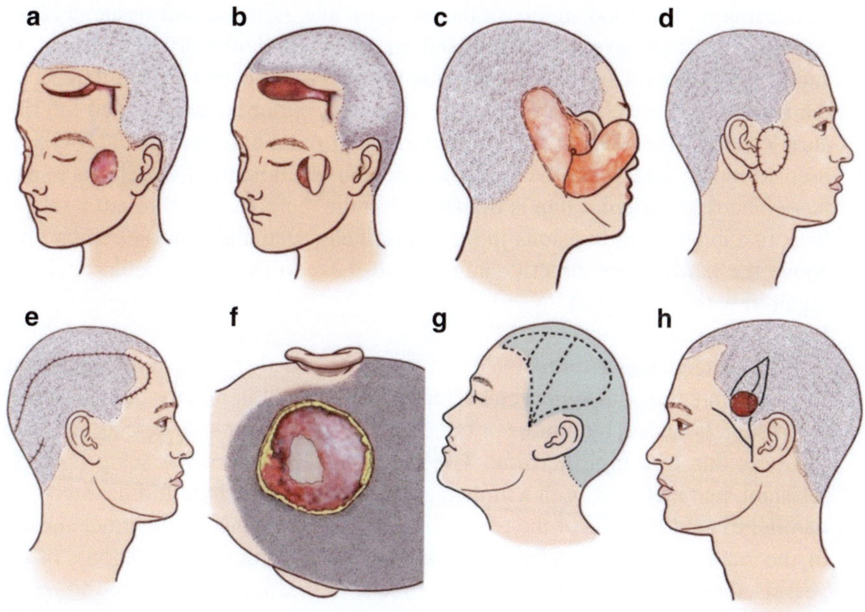

Fig. 6.20 Common skin flaps on the head and face. (**a**) Design of a forehead flap; (**b**) Repair of facial defect using a frontotemporal flap. (**c**) Design of a postauricular flap. (**d**) Repair of facial defect using a postauricular flap. (**e**) Design of a parietal rotation flap. (**f**) Repair of scalp defects after tumor resection using a parietal rotation flap. (**g**) Design of a temporoparietal flap. (**h**) Repair of skin defects in the temporal region of the face using a temporoparietal flap

be divided into a unilateral forehead flap and a full-forehead flap based on the repair of facial skin and intraoral mucosa. The forehead flap is mainly used to repair defects on the upper lip, nasal tip, and cheek perforations. The forehead mainly receives blood supply from the frontal branch of the superficial temporal artery, followed by the supraorbital artery and supratrochlear artery. It is important to determine the running direction of the superficial temporal artery trunk before surgery. The width and length of the flap pedicle should be appropriate to ensure that the flap can cover the wound surface without tension after transfer. When harvesting the flap, first cut open the skin of the pedicle, only cut to the dermis layer, and preserve the main blood vessels underneath and the capillary network in the surrounding subcutaneous tissue. Adequate intraoperative hemostasis should be carried out to prevent the compression of the pedicle vessels by postoperative hematomas. The forehead flap needs to be transferred to the site where the defect needs to be repaired through the subcutaneous tunnel, so the subcutaneous tunnel should be made large enough to allow the flap to pass easily.

2. Retroauricular Flap

   The retroauricular flap, also known as the retroauricular mastoid flap, is prepared from the skin and soft tissues on the posterior auricle and mastoid area.

According to the blood supply to the postauricular skin and soft tissue, a retroauricular flap can have a pedicle based on the postauricular artery and vein, or superficial temporal artery and vein. The former type is used to repair defects on the anterior ear, cheek under the zygomatic arch, earlobes, helixes, and inferior auricles, and a free flap graft is applied to repair nasal defects. The latter type is used to repair defects on the zygomatic region, eyelids, intraorbital space, and nose. The retroauricular flap is transferred to the recipient site through a subcutaneous tunnel. Skin incisions in the preauricular area and supra-auricular area above the hairline are directly sutured, and those in the postauricular area are repaired with a skin graft.

3. Parietal Flap

   The parietal flap is prepared from the region with blood supply from the parietal branch of the superficial temporal artery and is mainly used to repair scalp defects caused by tumors or trauma and preauricular skin defects and treat baldness due to a high hairline. The galea aponeurosis of the scalp is thick, resistant, and inelastic, with a limited extension. Multiple longitudinal incisions parallel to the long axis of the parietal flap need to be made on the inner surface of the scalp, aiming to increase the flap width; during these incisions, blood vessels should be carefully protected. Free skin grafting is performed to repair large scalp defects. The defect should be completely covered to avoid excessive tension.

4. Temporoparietal Fascia Flap

   The temporoparietal fascial flap is prepared from the temporoparietal fascia, serving as the pedicled graft to repair soft tissue defects on the head and face and reconstruct ears and noses, or a free graft to achieve vascular anastomosis and soft tissue reconstruction of the hands or feet. It is supplied by the parietal branch of the superficial temporal artery, which features many vascular anastomoses, a rich blood supply, and a thick arterial branch with a diameter of 1.8–3.3 mm. Therefore, the success rate of anastomosis and patency rate remain high in the repair using the temporoparietal fascial flap. The dissection plane of the temporoparietal fascial flap is a key factor for postoperative survival. As a difficult and time-consuming procedure, the dissection of the superficial layer of the temporoparietal fascial flap that closely attaches to the skin is performed beneath the hair follicles. If accurately located, the deep layer in the loose tissue under the galea aponeurosis can be easily dissected.

5. Cheek Flap

   The cheek flap is a skin flap with the pedicles supplied by the branches of the facial artery and is often used to repair small-scale tissue defects on the superficial cervicofacial skin and fascia and small-scale defects in the adjacent organs of the nasolabial region (Fig. 6.21). The cervicofacial region is covered by the skin outside and the mucous membrane inside, where nerves, blood vessels, and the parotid duct pass through. This flap is filled with muscles and loose adipose tissues, forming a dynamically functional morphology of the cheek. Therefore, cervicofacial tissues should not be used to repair less critical cheek defects. Adjacent or distant skin flaps are usually used to repair large defects on the skin

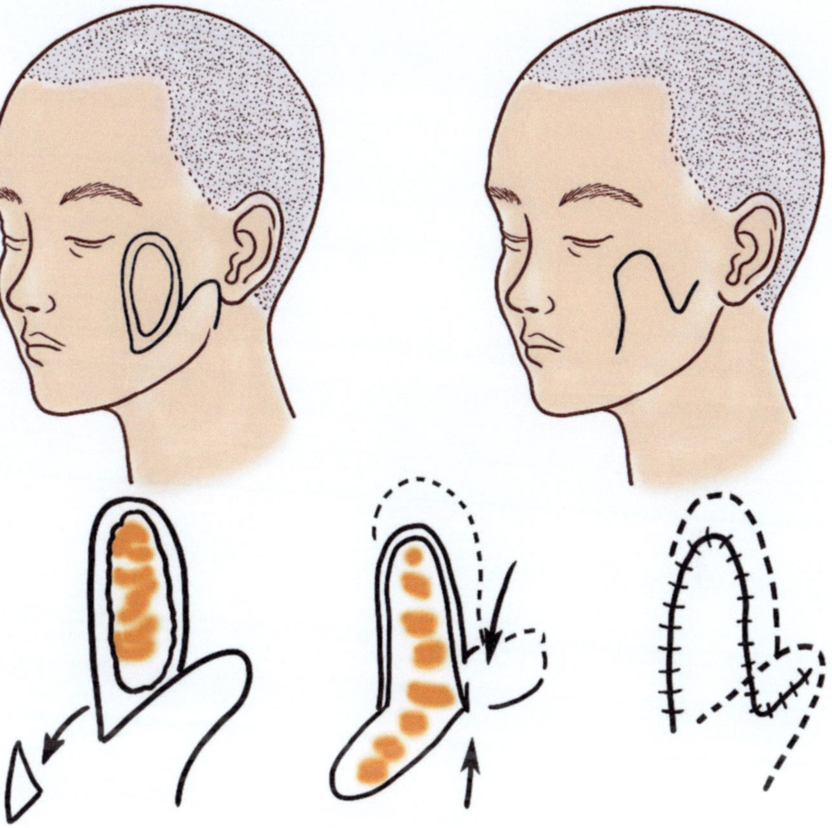

Fig. 6.21 Design of a cervicofacial sliding rotation flap

and mucosa or full-thickness perforation defects in the cervicofacial region. Moreover, cosmetic effects should be considered during the cervicofacial flap repair for the reconstruction of large cheek defects. Tissue flaps in the cervicofacial region or adjacent to the cheek and neck are adopted to repair medium-sized and small cheek defects to maintain a similar skin texture, thickness, and color, thus preventing facial disfigurement from skin-color mismatch.

Chapter 7
Regional Anatomy of the Neck and Its Clinical Application

Zhanchi Zhang, Junying Gao, Ming Xiao, and Yan Si

7.1 Regional Anatomy of the Neck

The neck connects the head, trunk, and upper limbs. Posteriorly, it is supported by the cervical spine of the neck. In the anterior midline, there are organs such as the thyroid gland, parathyroid glands, larynx, trachea, pharynx, and esophagus. Their positions can change with the movements of the neck. The blood vessels and nerves in the neck are generally distributed in an "L" shape. The longitudinally running ones are located on both sides of the viscera including the common carotid artery, internal and external carotid arteries, internal jugular vein, vagus nerve, sympathetic trunks, etc., connecting the head, thorax, and other parts. The transversely arranged ones are located at the root of the neck, including the subclavian artery and vein, and the brachial plexus, etc., connecting the thorax and the upper limbs. The lymphatic return of the whole body also occurs in the neck, where the thoracic duct and the right lymphatic duct respectively empty into the left and right venous angles. There are fascial spaces among various structures in the neck, which facilitate the movement of the viscera and serve as passages for blood vessels and nerves.

Z. Zhang
Hebei Medical University, Shijiazhuang, China

J. Gao (✉) · M. Xiao · Y. Si
Nanjing Medical University, Nanjing, China
e-mail: gaojunying@njmu.edu.cn; mingx@njmu.edu.cn

Q. Ding et al. (eds.), *Clinically Oriented Regional Anatomy*,
https://doi.org/10.1007/978-981-95-9888-5_7

7.2 Boundary and Regions

7.2.1 *Boundary*

The neck is superiorly bounded by a line connecting the inferior margin of the mandible, angle of the mandible, tip of the mastoid process, superior nuchal line, and external occipital protuberance; this line distinguishes the neck from the head. The neck is inferiorly bounded by a line connecting the sternal jugular notch, sternoclavicular joint, clavicle, acromion, and spinous process of the seventh cervical vertebra (C7) to distinguish the neck from the chest wall and upper limbs.

7.2.2 *Regions*

The neck is divided into the cervical region and nuchal region by the anterior portion of the bilateral trapezius muscles. The cervical region, located between the anterior portion of the bilateral trapezius muscles, is thoroughly described in the following section, while the nuchal region is situated posterior to the anterior portion of the bilateral trapezius muscles, as described in Chap. 2.

Bounded by the sternocleidomastoid muscle, the neck is divided into the anterior area, sternocleidomastoid muscle area, and lateral area (Fig. 7.1). The anterior area of the neck is an inverted triangle anterior to the sternocleidomastoid muscle, between the midline of the neck and inferior margin of the mandible. It is further divided into the submandibular triangle, submental triangle, carotid triangle, and muscular triangle by the anterior and posterior bellies of the digastric muscle and the superior belly of the omohyoid muscle. The area of the sternocleidomastoid muscle is a narrow and oblique space between the anterior and posterior portions of

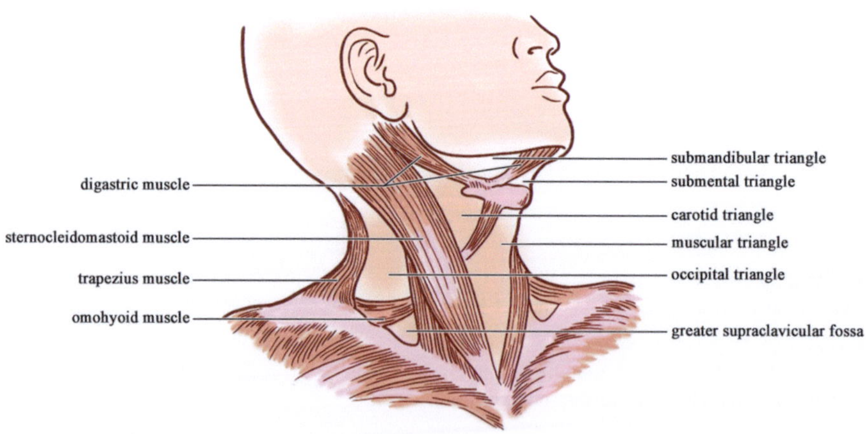

Fig. 7.1 Regions of the neck

the sternocleidomastoid muscle. The lateral area of the neck is delimited by the posterior margin of the sternocleidomastoid muscle, the anterior margin of the trapezius muscle, and the superior margin of the clavicle. It is further divided into the occipital triangle and the greater supraclavicular fossa by the inferior belly of the omohyoid muscle.

7.3 Surface Anatomy

7.3.1 Anatomical Landmarks

Numerous anatomical landmarks of the neck are visible and palpable. From superior to inferior, anatomical landmarks of the central part of the neck include the base of the mandible, hyoid bone and greater horn, thyroid cartilage and laryngeal prominence, cricoid cartilage, cervical trachea, suprasternal fossa, and jugular notch. Those on the lateral side of the neck include the sternocleidomastoid muscle, external jugular vein, greater supraclavicular fossa, clavicle, acromion, and scalenus anterior tendon (Fig. 7.2). Important anatomical landmarks of the neck are described as follows.

7.3.1.1 Cricoid Cartilage

The cricoid cartilage is located at the level of the sixth cervical vertebra (C6) and serves as the junction between the larynx and trachea. It is an anatomical landmark used for counting tracheal rings. The cervical ganglia of the sympathetic trunk and carotid tubercle of C6 are situated at the level of the cricoid cartilage. The carotid tubercle is a common site for compression hemostasis of the neck.

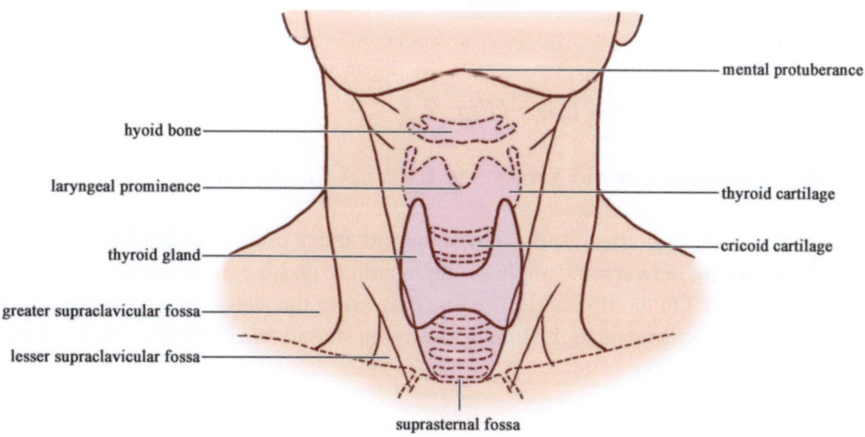

Fig. 7.2 Landmarks of the neck

7.3.1.2 Hyoid Bone

Viewed from the front horizontally, the body of the hyoid bone is situated parallel to the inferior margin of the mental protuberance and, posteriorly, parallel to the third cervical vertebra (C3). The greater horn of the hyoid bone can be palpated from each side of the hyoid bone backward.

7.3.1.3 Thyroid Cartilage

The thyroid cartilage is located inferior to the hyoid bone and parallels the fourth cervical vertebra (C4) superiorly. The superior end of the anterior horn of the thyroid cartilage is the laryngeal prominence, situated in the midline of the neck.

7.3.1.4 Sternocleidomastoid Muscle

The sternocleidomastoid muscle is a significant muscle landmark in the neck, and both its anterior and posterior portions are visible. The midpoint of its posterior edge is where the cutaneous branches of the cervical plexus emerge. Inferior to the muscle, the sternal head, clavicular head, and superior margin of the clavicle form the lesser supraclavicular fossa.

7.3.1.5 Scalenus Anterior Muscle

The scalenus anterior muscle is located deep, inferolateral to the sternocleidomastoid muscle. The scalenus anterior tendon and the first rib to which it attaches can be palpable in the deep area along the posterior side of the clavicle, serving as landmarks of the supraclavicular brachial plexus block.

7.3.2 Surface Projections (Fig. 7.3)

7.3.2.1 Common Carotid Artery and External Carotid Artery

The common carotid artery and external carotid artery project on the line connecting the midpoint between the angle of the mandible and the tip of the mastoid process downward. On the right side, the line extends to the sternoclavicular joint, and on the left side, it extends to the line between the sternal and clavicular heads of the

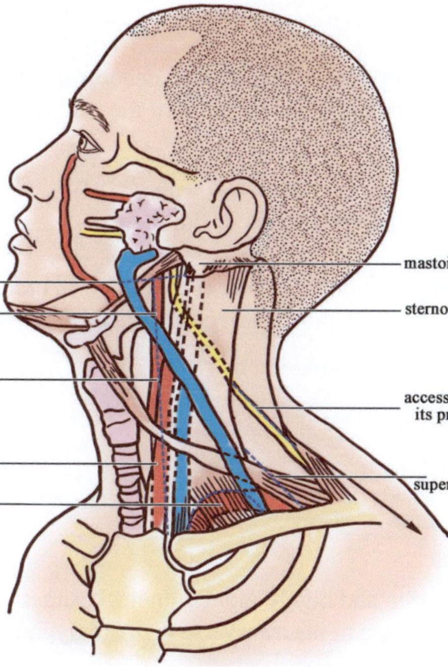

Fig. 7.3 Surface projections of the neck

sternocleidomastoid muscle. The superior margin of the thyroid cartilage serves as the boundary between the two arteries.

7.3.2.2 Brachial Plexus

At the level of the cricoid cartilage, the superior portion of the brachial plexus is projected on the line connecting the lower third of the posterior margin of the sternocleidomastoid muscle and the lateral third of the clavicle. The inferior portion of the brachial plexus is projected along the line connecting the lateral side of the anterior scalenus tendon and the midpoint of the clavicle.

7.3.2.3 Subclavian Artery

The subclavian artery is projected upward along the arc between the sternoclavicular joint and the midpoint of the clavicle, reaching its highest point at 2.0 cm above the clavicle.

7.3.2.4 Accessory Nerve

The accessory nerve is projected along the line connecting the upper third of the sternocleidomastoid muscle and the lower third of the anterior margin of the trapezius muscle.

7.3.2.5 Apex of the Lung and Cupula of the Pleura

The apex of the lung and cupula of the pleura are projected onto the skin above the medial third of the clavicle, with the highest point located approximately 2.5–3.0 cm above the clavicle.

7.4 Layers

7.4.1 Skin

The skin of the neck is thin and highly mobile. In neck surgeries, a transverse skin incision is typically made due to the transverse dermatoglyphic pattern.

7.4.2 Superficial Fascia

The superficial fascia of the neck contains minimal adipose tissues, and its anterolateral part has the broad, thin, cutaneous platysma muscle. The following structures are situated in the deep layer of the platysma muscle (Fig. 7.4).

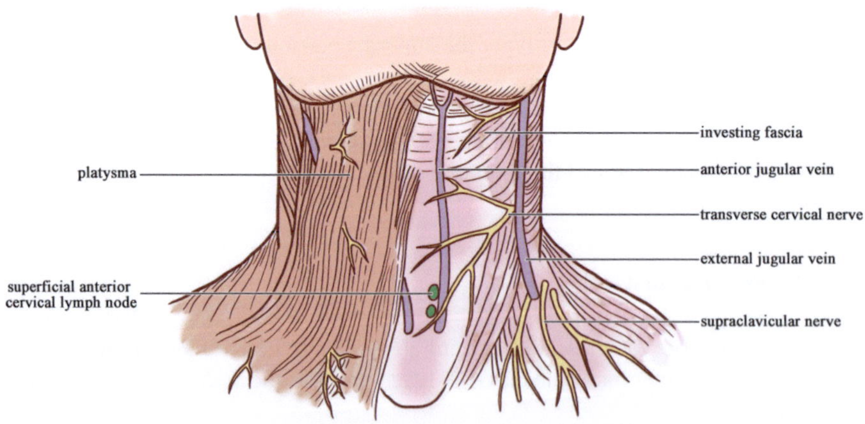

Fig. 7.4 Structures in the superficial layer of the platysma muscle in the neck

7.4.2.1 Cervical Branch of the Facial Nerve

The cervical branch of the facial nerve perforates the platysma muscle approximately 1.0 cm below the angle of the mandible, with the submental artery (a branch of the facial artery) lying anteriorly. The platysma myocutaneous flap is commonly employed for repairing oral and maxillofacial tissue defects. It is crucial to protect the mentioned nerves and blood vessels during platysma myocutaneous flap reconstruction.

7.4.2.2 Cutaneous Branches of the Cervical Plexus

The lesser occipital, great auricular, transverse cervical nerves, and the supraclavicular nerves are cutaneous branches of the cervical plexus. The former two travel superiorly, while the latter two travel anteriorly and inferiorly, respectively. They all penetrate the deep fascia at the midpoint of the posterior portion of the sternocleidomastoid muscle and supply the skin of corresponding areas. Therefore, cervical plexus block for neck surgeries can be achieved by administrating analgesic agents at the midpoint of the posterior portion of the sternocleidomastoid muscle.

7.4.2.3 Superficial Veins of the Neck

The external jugular vein runs down along the surface of the sternocleidomastoid muscle, pierces the deep fascia, and ultimately drains into the subclavian vein or venous angle. In cases where necessary, an intravenous catheter can be inserted into the external jugular vein. Obstruction of the superior vena cava vein to the heart, typically seen in right-sided heart failure, can cause distention of the external jugular vein. The anterior jugular vein is a small vein situated bilaterally along the midline of the neck, descending to laterally drain into the external jugular vein. The two anterior jugular veins are connected by a transverse trunk, known as the venous jugular arch.

7.4.2.4 Superficial Lymph Nodes of the Neck

The superficial lateral cervical lymph nodes are distributed along the external jugular vein, collecting lymph from the retroauricular and occipital regions before draining into the deep lateral cervical lymph nodes. There are superficial anterior cervical lymph nodes near the anterior jugular vein.

7.4.3 Muscles and Deep Fascia of the Neck

7.4.3.1 Muscles of the Neck

Muscles of the neck are categorized into three layers: superficial, intermediate, and deep. The superficial layer includes the platysma and sternocleidomastoid muscle, the intermediate layer contains the suprahyoid and infrahyoid muscles, while the deep layer consists of the scalenus anterior, medius, and posterior muscles, as well as the anterior vertebral muscles.

7.4.3.2 Deep Fascia

The deep fascia is located beneath the superficial fascia and platysma muscle in the neck. It surrounds the muscles, organs, and blood vessels in the neck and is segmented into superficial, intermediate, and deep layers, as well as a pair of carotid sheaths (Fig. 7.5).

Superficial Layer

The superficial layer of the deep fascia of the neck, also known as the investing fascia, is the general fascial sheath that envelops the entire neck structure. It is attached posteriorly to the nuchal ligament and, wrapping around the sternocleidomastoid and trapezius muscle, forms the sheaths for these two muscles. Anteriorly, at the midline, it intertwines with the corresponding fascia on the opposite side to form the linea alba of the neck. Superiorly, it attaches to the superior nuchal line and mastoid process; extends forward to enclose the parotid gland, forming the parotid sheath; and then continues as the parotideomasseteric fascia. Below the mandible, it wraps around the submandibular gland, forming the submandibular gland sheath, and attaches superiorly to the mandibular base. Inferiorly, it attaches to the acromion and clavicle, splitting into two layers above the manubrium of the sternum, and extending to the anterior and posterior edges of the jugular notch, forming the suprasternal space that contains the jugular venous arch.

Intermediate Layer

The intermediate layer of the deep fascia of the neck, also known as the pretracheal fascia or visceral fascia, is situated in the deep layer of the infrahyoid muscles. It envelops various structures in the neck, such as the pharynx, cervical esophageal, larynx, cervical trachea, and thyroid gland, forming structures like the thyroid pseudocyst, esophageal fascia, and tracheal fascia. The anteroinferior part of the

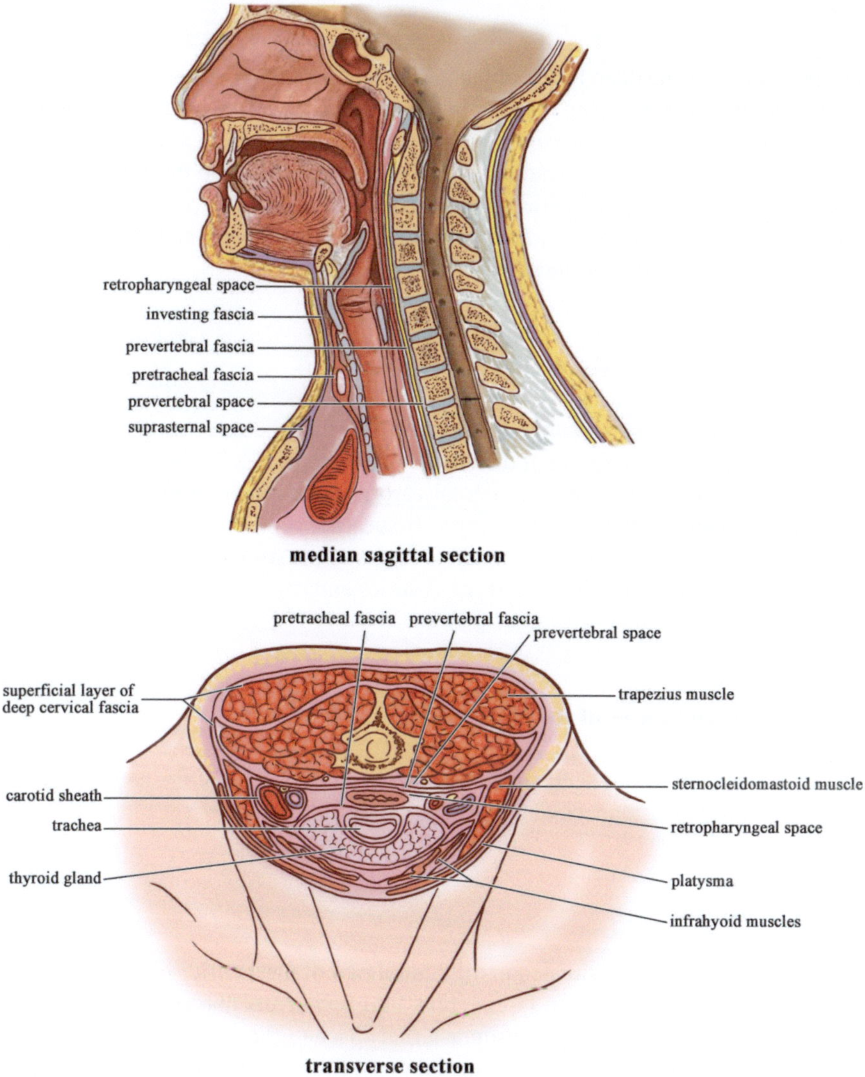

Fig. 7.5 Fasciae of the neck

intermediate layer covers the trachea, known as the pretracheal fascia, while the posterosuperior part covers the buccinator muscle and pharyngeal constrictor muscle, known as the buccopharyngeal fascia. The pretracheal fascia attaches superiorly to the arch of cricoid cartilage arch, oblique line of thyroid cartilage, and hyoid bone; it descends along and the front and sides of the trachea into the thoracic cavity, ultimately attaching to the fibrous pericardium.

Deep Layer

The deep layer of the deep fascia of the neck, also known as the prevertebral fascia, covers the surface of the deep muscles in the neck. It attaches to the base of the skull above and enters the thoracic cavity with the longus colli muscle of the neck below, attaching to the anterior longitudinal ligament at the level of the third thoracic vertebra (T3). In the interval between the scalene muscles, the prevertebral fascia encloses the brachial plexus and the subclavian artery and vein and extends to the axilla, forming the axillary sheath.

Carotid Sheath

The carotid sheath, also known as the cervical vascular sheath or cervical sheath, is a thickening of the deep fascia of the neck that envelops large blood vessels. It contains the common carotid artery, internal carotid artery, internal jugular vein, and vagus nerve. Through the loose connective tissues, the carotid sheath anteriorly connects with the superficial and intermediate layers of the deep fascia of the neck and posteriorly connects with the deep layer. Arteries and veins in the carotid sheath are separated by longitudinal fibers.

7.4.3.3 Fascial Spaces of the Neck

The fascial spaces of the neck are located between the layers of the cervical fascia and filled with loose connective tissues (Fig. 7.5).

Suprasternal Space

The suprasternal space is situated in the central part of the anterior neck, superior to the manubrium. The investing fascia splits into two layers above the manubrium, with the inferior part forming the suprasternal space (3.0 cm in height) along with the manubrium. This space contains the jugular venous arch and a small number of adipose tissues.

Pretracheal Space

The pretracheal space is located between the pretracheal fascia and the trachea and contains the thyroid isthmus, adipose and connective tissues, and inferior thyroid veins. The thyroid ima artery, upper end of the thymus, left brachiocephalic vein, and brachiocephalic trunk are occasionally observed in the inferior half of the pretracheal space. These structures should be protected during tracheotomy. The pretracheal space communicates inferiorly with the superior mediastinum.

Retropharyngeal Space

The retropharyngeal space is located between the posterior pharynx and prevertebral fascia and divided into left and right halves by connective tissues. It extends superiorly to the base of the skull and connects inferiorly with the posterior mediastinum through the retroesophageal space. The parapharyngeal space is situated on the lateral side of the pharyngeal wall.

Prevertebral Space

The prevertebral space is located between the prevertebral fascia and the cervical spine. In cases of cervical tuberculosis with abscess formation, the purulent exudate often accumulates in this space. It can spread inferiorly to the posterior mediastinum, laterally to the lateral regions of the neck, and further along the axillary sheath to the axilla. It may also penetrate through the prevertebral fascia into the retropharyngeal space.

7.5 Main Structures in the Three Areas of the Neck

7.5.1 Anterior Area of the Neck

The anterior area of the neck is medially bounded by the midline of the neck, laterally by the anterior portion of the sternocleidomastoid muscle, and superiorly by the base of the mandible. This area is further divided into the submandibular triangle, carotid triangle, muscular triangle, and submental triangle.

7.5.1.1 Submandibular Triangle

Boundary

The submandibular triangle is located between the base of the mandible and anterior and posterior bellies of the digastric muscle. The base (deep surface) of the submandibular triangle is composed of the mylohyoid muscle and hyoglossus muscle. Its surface is covered by the skin, superficial fascia, platysma muscle, and investing fascia.

Contents

The submandibular triangle mainly contains the submandibular gland and its surrounding blood vessels, nerves, and lymph nodes (Fig. 7.6).

The submandibular gland occupies most of the submandibular triangle, the surface of which is enclosed by the capsule of the submandibular gland formed by the investing fascia. The submandibular gland is divided into a superficial lobe and a deep lobe. The superficial lobe is larger and situated on the superficial part of the mylohyoid muscle, while the deep lobe is smaller and arises from the posterior portion of the mylohyoid muscle, extending to the anteromedial portion.

The submandibular duct starts from the anterior portion of the submandibular gland, ascends anteriorly between the mylohyoid muscle and hyoglossus muscle to the mouth floor, and opens at the sublingual caruncle on the oral mucosa of the floor of the mouth. The submandibular lymph nodes are distributed around the submandibular gland. Arising from the external carotid artery, the facial artery enters the submandibular triangle through the deep layer of the posterior belly of the digastric muscle, passes through the deep surface of the posterior submandibular gland, and courses through the inferior mandible to the face. The facial vein lies behind the facial artery and descends posteriorly to the submandibular gland. The lingual artery lies deep within the submandibular triangle and ascends anteriorly on the deep surface of the hyoglossus muscle. Between the deep aspect of the submandibular gland and the superficial aspect of the hyoglossus muscle, the lingual nerve is located in the upper one-third and the hypoglossal nerve in the lower one-third, both running transversely forward. The lingual nerve inferiorly connects with the submandibular ganglion.

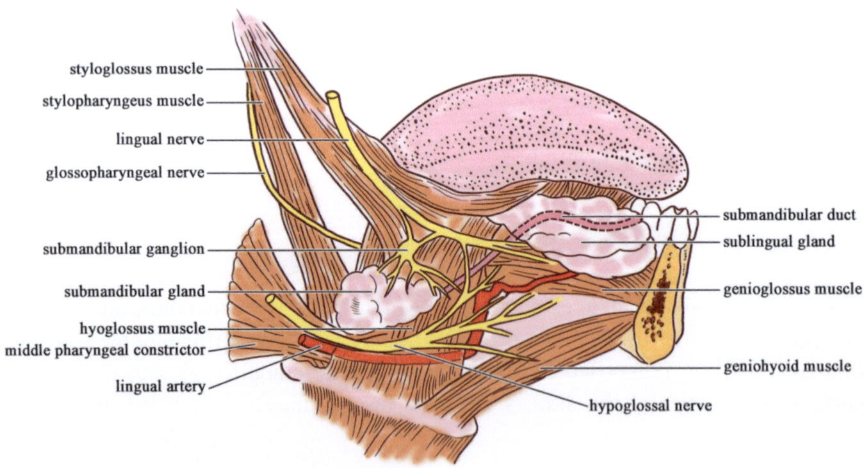

Fig. 7.6 Contents in the submandibular triangle

The investing fascia and the base of the submandibular triangle together form the submandibular space, which communicates with the space of mouth floor anteriorly and the pterygomandibular space posteriorly.

7.5.1.2 Submental Triangle

The submental triangle is situated between the anterior belly of the digastric muscle and the hyoid bone and contains the submental lymph nodes.

7.5.1.3 Carotid Triangle

Boundary

The carotid triangle is situated anterior to the sternocleidomastoid muscle, inferior to the posterior belly of the digastric muscle, and superior to the superior belly of the omohyoid muscle. Its floor is formed by the prevertebral fascia, and the superficial layer contains the skin, superficial fascia, platysma muscle, and investing fascia.

Contents

The carotid triangle contains the greater horn of the hyoid bone, common carotid artery and its branches (internal and external carotid arteries), internal jugular vein and its tributaries, hypoglossal nerve and its descending branch, and vagus nerve and its branches (superior laryngeal nerve, etc.) (Fig. 7.7).

The greater horn of the hyoid bone is a landmark within the carotid triangle. The common carotid artery is divided into the internal and external carotid arteries posterior to the greater horn of the hyoid bone and parallel to the superior margin of the thyroid cartilage. The carotid bifurcation contains the carotid body and carotid sinus, serving as the chemoreceptors and baroreceptors, respectively. Within the carotid triangle, the common carotid artery and its bifurcation are superficially located. Carotid sinus massage is a therapeutic strategy for supraventricular tachycardias, and carotid sinus stimulation may reflexively cause cardiac arrest. Arising from the common carotid artery, the external carotid artery travels anteromedially to the internal carotid artery and then ascends on its lateral side. Below the greater horn of the hyoid bone, the external carotid artery gives off the superior thyroid artery, which descends anteriorly. Above the greater horn, it branches into the lingual artery and facial artery anteriorly in sequence and the occipital artery posteriorly. In addition to the difference in the anatomical position, the external carotid artery has branches, but the internal carotid artery does not in the neck.

Above the greater horn of the hyoid bone, the hypoglossal nerve travels in an arched shape across the surfaces of the internal and external carotid arteries from posterior to anterior and then gives off its descending branch, the superior root of

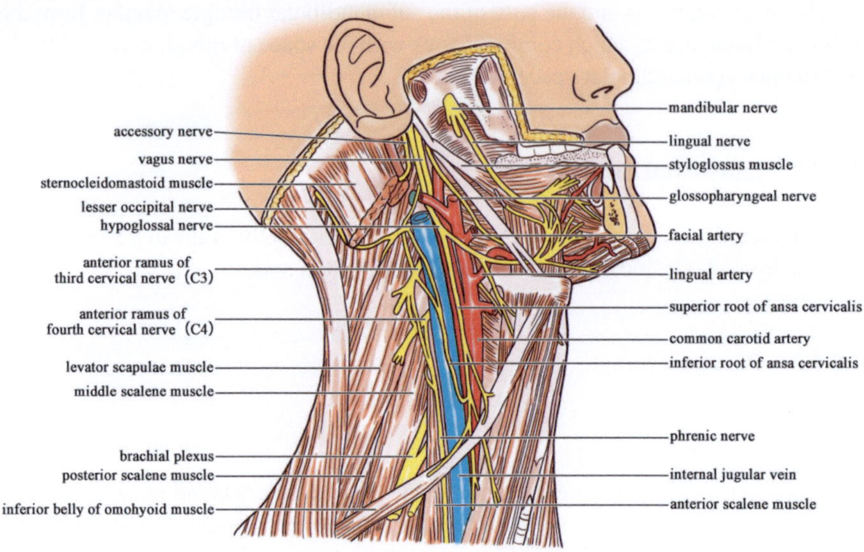

Fig. 7.7 Contents in the carotid triangle

the ansa cervicalis. The superior root of the ansa cervicalis enters the submandibular triangle through the deep surface of the posterior belly of the digastric muscle.

Below the greater horn of the hyoid bone, the branches of the vagus nerve (the internal and external branches of the superior laryngeal nerve) pass through the deep surfaces of the internal and external carotid arteries, respectively. The larger internal branch pierces the thyrohyoid membrane to enter the larynx, while the smaller external branch descends to the cricothyroid muscle. The superior laryngeal artery originating from the superior thyroid artery accompanies the internal branch of the superior laryngeal nerve.

7.5.1.4 Muscular Triangle

The muscular triangle, also known as the omotracheal triangle, is delineated by the midline of the neck, anterior portion of the sternocleidomastoid muscle, and the superior belly of the omohyoid muscle. The superficial layer of the muscular triangle comprises the skin, superficial fascia, investing fascia, infrahyoid muscles, and pretracheal fascia, while its deep layer consists of the prevertebral fascia. Within the muscular triangle are the thyroid gland, parathyroid glands, larynx, trachea, esophagus, as well as the blood vessels and nerves that supply these structures (Fig. 7.8).

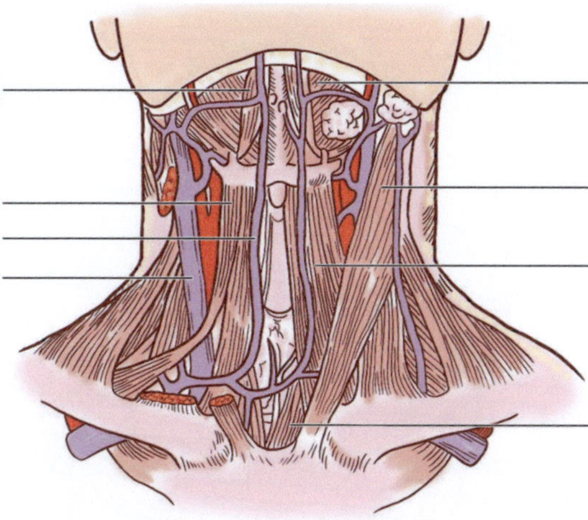

Fig. 7.8 Anterior area of the neck

7.5.2 Sternocleidomastoid Muscle Area of the Neck

The sternocleidomastoid area is the space located between the anterior and posterior portions of the sternocleidomastoid muscle. Deep within this area, it encompasses the carotid sheath, ansa cervicalis, deep cervical lateral lymph nodes, cervical sympathetic trunk, and cervical plexus and its branches.

7.5.2.1 Carotid Sheath

The carotid sheath is formed by the deep fascia of the neck. Within the carotid sheath, the internal jugular vein is situated on the lateral side, while the common carotid artery and internal carotid artery are positioned on the medial side. The vagus nerve is located on the posterior aspect, situated between the arteries and veins within the carotid sheath. The wall of the internal jugular vein is closely attached to the carotid sheath and not easy to collapse, so injury to the internal jugular vein could lead to air embolism.

7.5.2.2 Ansa Cervicalis

The ansa cervicalis is formed by the fusion of the superior and inferior roots at the level of the cricoid cartilage (Fig. 7.9). The anterior ramus of the first cervical nerve (C1) initially travels with the hypoglossal nerve and then separates below the posterior belly of the digastric muscle to form the superior root of the ansa cervicalis

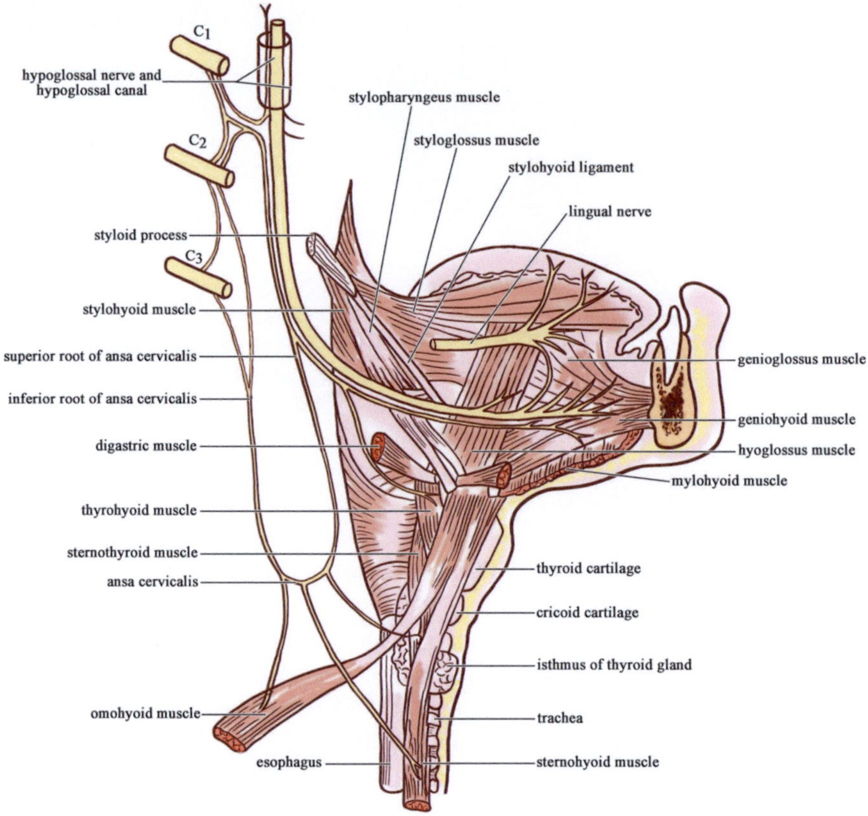

Fig. 7.9 Ansa cervicalis and the muscles it innervates

(known as descendens hypoglossi). The inferior root of the ansa cervicalis is formed by the anterior rami of the second and third cervical nerves (C2, C3). After departing from the cervical plexus, the anterior rami of C2 and C3 collectively descend along the surface of the internal jugular vein and unite with the superior root on the anterolateral aspect of the carotid sheath, thus constituting the ansa cervicalis. Branches of the ansa cervicalis innervate most of the infrahyoid muscles. During thyroid surgeries, cutting the infrahyoid muscles group below the cricoid cartilage can avoid injury to the ansa cervicalis. In clinical practice, the infrahyoid muscle group myocutaneous flap can be taken to reconstruct the tongue, and when harvesting the flap, the branches of the ansa cervicalis should be protected.

7.5.2.3 Deep Lateral Cervical Lymph Nodes

Deep lateral cervical lymph nodes are arranged along the internal jugular vein, expanding from the base of the skull to the root of the neck. The efferent vessels of the lowermost deep cervical lymph nodes form the jugular trunk.

Among them, the lymph nodes positioned between the posterior belly of the digastric muscle and the internal jugular vein are known as the jugulodigastric lymph nodes, and those between the superior belly of the omohyoid muscle and the internal jugular vein are termed the juguloomohyoid lymph nodes. Tumors in the oral and maxillofacial region often involve these lymph nodes. Additionally, a small number of lymph nodes are arranged posteriorly along the accessory nerve.

7.5.2.4 Cervical Plexus

The cervical plexus is located between the deep side of the sternocleidomastoid muscle and the superficial layer of the scalenus medius and levator scapulae muscles. The cervical plexus gives off superficial and deep branches. The superficial branch is a cutaneous branch that superficially emerges through the deep fascia at the midpoint of the posterior portion of the sternocleidomastoid muscle. The deep branch extends into the deep muscles of the neck and gives rise to the phrenic nerve.

7.5.2.5 Cervical Sympathetic Trunk

The cervical sympathetic trunk is located on both sides of the cervical vertebrae, deep to the prevertebral fascia. It consists of three interconnected ganglia: superior, middle, and inferior cervical ganglia. The superior cervical ganglia is the largest and spindle shaped, positioned anterior to the transverse processes of the second to third cervical vertebrae (C2, C3). The middle cervical ganglia are the smallest and located at the level of the carotid tubercle. The inferior cervical ganglia commonly fuse with the first thoracic segmental sympathetic ganglia to form the cervicothoracic (stellate) ganglion. These ganglia give rise to the cervical cardiac nerves, contributing to the formation of the cardiac plexus.

7.5.3 Lateral Cervical Region

The lateral cervical region is delineated anteriorly by the posterior margin of the sternocleidomastoid muscle, inferiorly by the superior margin of the clavicle, and posteriorly by the anterior margin of the trapezius muscle. This region is further partitioned into the occipital triangle and the supraclavicular fossa by the inferior belly of the omohyoid muscle.

7.5.3.1 Occipital Triangle

The occipital triangle, also known as the trigonum omotrapezium, is enclosed by the inferior belly of the omohyoid muscle, the anterior margin of the trapezius muscle, and the posterior margin of the sternocleidomastoid muscle. The deep surface of the triangle consists of the prevertebral fascia and the underlying deep muscles of the neck, while the superficial surface is covered by the investing layer of deep cervical fascia. The triangle contains loose connective tissues and is traversed by the accessory nerve. The accessory nerve enters deep to the sternocleidomastoid muscle from its upper anterior margin, gives off branches to innervate this muscle, and then emerges at the intersection of the upper and middle thirds of the posterior margin of the muscle. It enters the occipital triangle, descends, and penetrates deep to the trapezius muscle at the intersection of the middle and lower thirds of its anterior margin (Fig. 7.10). Around the accessory nerve, lymph nodes are arrayed, with muscular branches from the cervical plexus descending to the trapezius. During lymphadenectomy within the occipital triangle, care must be taken to protect the accessory nerve.

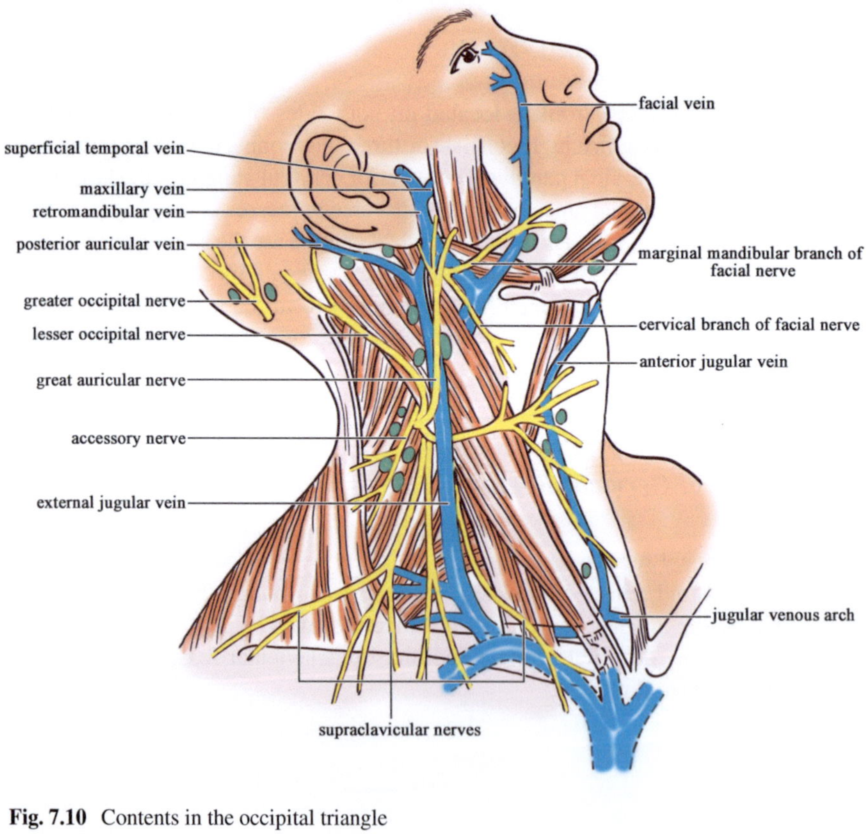

Fig. 7.10 Contents in the occipital triangle

7.5.3.2 Greater Supraclavicular Fossa and Root of the Neck

Boundary

The greater supraclavicular fossa, also known as the omoclavicular triangle, is formed by the posterior margin of the sternocleidomastoid muscle, the inferior belly of the omohyoid muscle, and the clavicle. The root of the neck is situated within two fingers' breadth above the clavicle and serves as a transitional area between the neck, thoracic inlet, and axilla.

Contents

Taking the scalenus anterior muscle as the central landmark, the structures within the root of the neck and the greater supraclavicular fossa are arranged as follows: Medially to the anterior scalene muscle are the longitudinal structures between the neck and chest as well as the apex of the pleura. These longitudinal structures include the internal jugular vein and the brachiocephalic vein, the common carotid artery and the brachiocephalic trunk, the vagus nerve, the sympathetic trunk, and the phrenic nerve. Anterior, posterior, and lateral to the anterior scalene muscle are the transverse structures between the thorax, neck, and upper limb, which include the subclavian vein and its tributaries, the subclavian artery and its branches, and the brachial plexus (Fig. 7.11). Among these, the following are notable.

Cupula of the Pleura and Apex of the Lung
The cupula of the pleura and apex of the lung are situated deep within the root of the neck, approximately 2.0–3.0 cm above the medial one-third of the clavicle. Anterior to the cupula of the pleura is the subclavian artery, and anterolateral lie the anterior scalenus muscle, the phrenic nerve, the subclavian vein, and the vagus nerve, with the thoracic duct additionally on the left side. Posterior to the cupula of the pleura are the cervical sympathetic trunk and cervicothoracic ganglion, while laterally is the middle scalenus muscle. Surgical interventions at the root of the neck demand cautious protection of the pleural apex to avert injury that could precipitate pneumothorax.

Thoracic Duct
The thoracic duct ascends along the left margin of the esophagus. It turns laterally at the level of the seventh cervical vertebra (C7) to form the arch of the thoracic duct. It then crosses over the left cupula of the pleura and drains into the left venous angle in an outward and downward direction. In the neck region, the carotid sheath is in front of the thoracic duct, and behind it are the cupula of the pleura, the subclavian artery, and its branches. Injury to the thoracic duct in the neck can lead to chylous leakage.

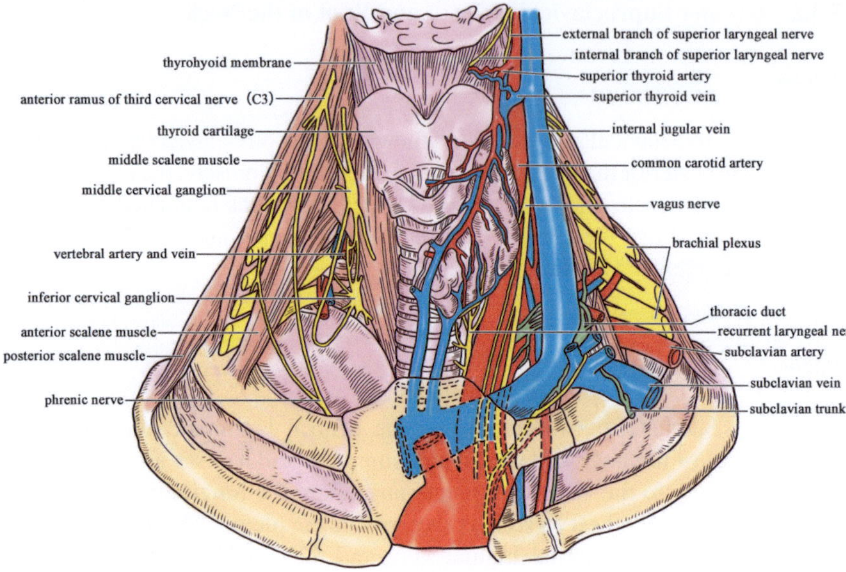

Fig. 7.11 Root of the neck

Subclavian Vein

The subclavian vein courses superficially to the anterior scalenus muscle at the root of the neck, proceeding medially anterior to the cupula of the pleura to join with the internal jugular vein, thus forming the brachiocephalic vein. Inferior and anterior to the subclavian vein are the clavicle and the subclavian muscles; posterior are the anterior scalenus muscle, the subclavian artery, and the cupula of the pleura; and inferior is the first rib. The subclavian vein is intimately associated with adjacent structures, occupying a relatively fixed position, and its walls are resistant to collapse. Consequently, it is frequently utilized for venipuncture and catheterization, prolonged intravenous infusions, and conducting cardiac catheterization and central venous pressure monitoring.

Subclavian Artery and Brachial Plexus

The subclavian artery and brachial plexus course laterally toward the axilla after passing through the interscalene space, which lies between the scalenus anterior and medius muscles and the first rib. Within the scalenus interspace, the brachial plexus occupies the upper three-fourths and the subclavian artery occupies the lower one-fourth. The superior, middle, and inferior trunks of the brachial plexus are concentrated superior to the midpoint of the clavicle, which is a common site for supraclavicular approach for brachial plexus block anesthesia.

Phrenic Nerve

The phrenic nerve is positioned deep to the prevertebral fascia and travels inferomedially over the surface of the anterior scalene muscle. It traverses the interval between the subclavian artery and vein before entering the thoracic cavity.

Supraclavicular Lymph Node
The supraclavicular lymph nodes are the lowermost group of deep lateral cervical lymph nodes, also known as the deep cervical inferior lymph nodes. They are situated deep to the inferior aspect of the sternocleidomastoid muscle, posterolateral to the internal jugular vein. Their efferent vessels form the jugular trunk. Tumor cells from the thoracic and abdominal organs may ascend through the thoracic duct to the left supraclavicular lymph node, causing lymphadenopathy. Clinically, the left supraclavicular lymph node is referred to as Virchow's node.

Triangle of the Vertebral Artery
The triangle of the vertebral artery is defined by the lateral anterior scalenus muscle, the medial longus colli muscle, and the inferior subclavian artery. Superficial to the triangle are the thyrocervical trunk, the vagus nerve, the sympathetic trunk, and the cervicothoracic ganglia. In the deeper layer, one can find the vertebral artery and vein, with the vertebral vein commonly positioned anterolateral to the vertebral artery.

7.6 Organs at the Neck

7.6.1 Thyroid Gland and Parathyroid Gland

7.6.1.1 Thyroid Gland

Localization and Morphology

The thyroid gland typically exhibits an "H" shape, composed of left and right lobes along with an isthmus, but variations in thyroid morphology are common (Fig. 7.12). The left and right lobes of the thyroid gland are situated anterolateral to the larynx and trachea, with the superior poles at the midpoint of the thyroid cartilage and the inferior poles extending to the level of the sixth tracheal ring. The isthmus lies anterior to the second to fourth tracheal rings. Approximately 50% of individuals possess a pyramidal lobe, which is often connected to the upper margin of the isthmus or at the junction where the isthmus meets the lateral lobes.

Thyroid Capsule

The thyroid gland is enveloped by a capsule composed of two layers. The thyroid capsule has an inner and an outer layer (false capsule or sheath of the thyroid gland). The inner layer, closely adherent to the thyroid parenchyma and extending between the lobes, is referred to as the true capsule or fibrous capsule. The outer layer, derived from the pretracheal fascia, is termed as the false capsule or the thyroid sheath. The false capsule is connected to the cricoid cartilage and the annular

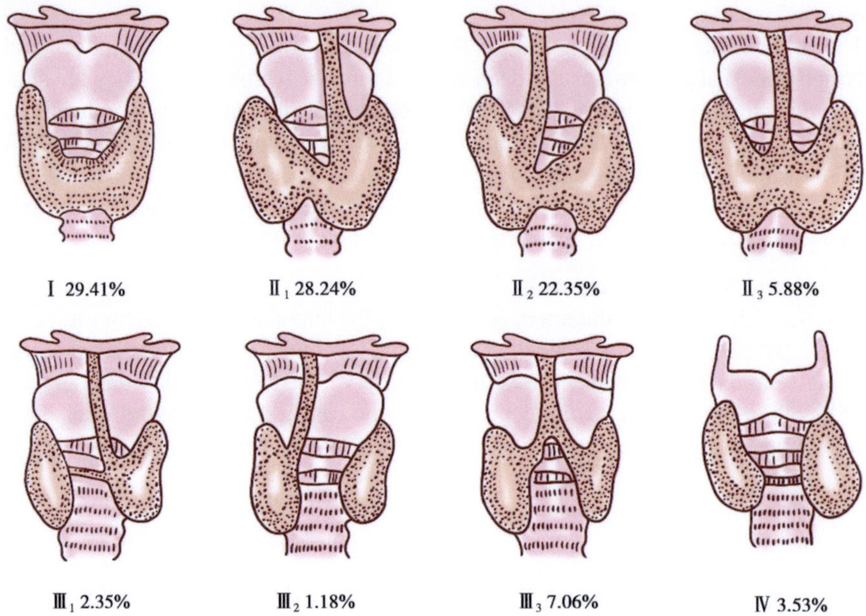

Fig. 7.12 Morphology of the thyroid gland

ligament of the tracheal cartilages, forming the suspensory ligament of the thyroid. Therefore, the thyroid gland can move superiorly and inferiorly with the larynx during swallowing. Situated between the true and false capsules are blood vessels, nerves, and the parathyroid glands.

Blood Vessels of the Thyroid Gland and Nerves of the Larynx (Fig. 7.13)

The thyroid gland is supplied by the superior and inferior thyroid arteries. The superior thyroid artery originates from the external carotid artery and descends alongside the external branch of the superior laryngeal nerve. Approximately 1.0 cm above the superior pole of the thyroid gland, the artery enters the gland at the superior pole of its lateral lobe, whereas the external branch of the superior laryngeal nerve diverges from the artery and courses anteromedially to the cricothyroid muscle. During thyroidectomy, ligation of the superior thyroid artery close to the superior pole can prevent inadvertent injury to the external branch of the superior laryngeal nerve. The inferior thyroid artery arises from the thyrocervical trunk of the subclavian artery and passes medially and inferiorly behind the carotid sheath to the posterior aspect of the lower pole of the thyroid gland, where it crosses posteriorly to the recurrent laryngeal nerve before entering the gland. The left recurrent laryngeal nerve, originating from the thoracic portion of the left vagus nerve, hooks around the aortic arch and ascends vertically in the laryngotracheal groove, typically crossing posteriorly to the inferior thyroid artery. The right recurrent laryngeal

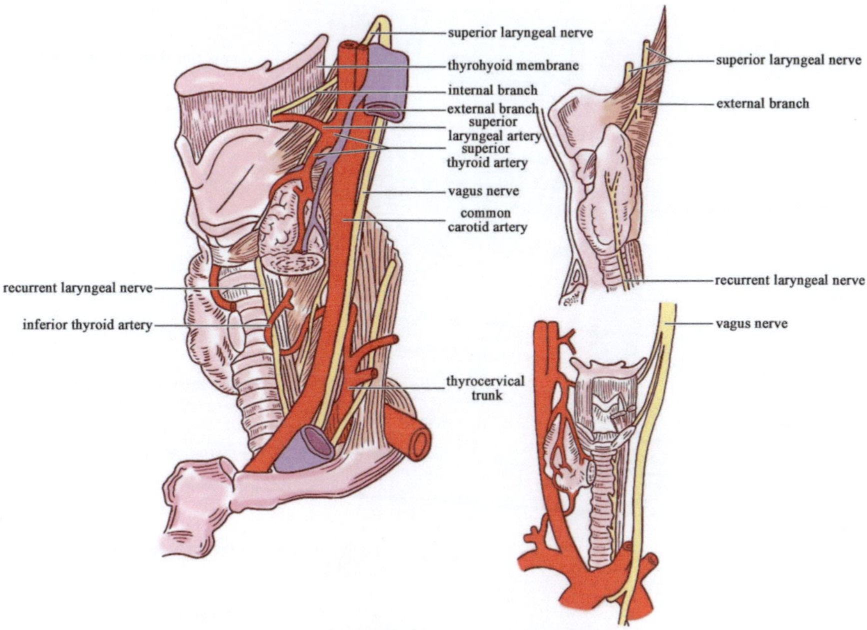

Fig. 7.13 Blood vessels of the thyroid gland and nerves of the larynx

nerve, emanating from the right vagus nerve, hooks around the right subclavian artery and ascends obliquely to the superior and medial part in the laryngotracheal groove, crossing anteriorly to the inferior thyroid artery. Studies in China on the relationship between the recurrent laryngeal nerves and the inferior thyroid artery indicate that the nerve passes posteriorly to the artery in 38.2% of cases, anteriorly to the artery in 13.7%, and between the branches of the artery in 45.2% and has no direct relationship with the artery in 2.9%. During surgery, the intricate relationship between the blood vessels and nerves should be considered, and care should be taken to avoid damage to the recurrent laryngeal nerve when ligating the inferior thyroid artery, which otherwise could result in severe complications, such as vocal cord paralysis. Additionally, approximately 10% of individuals may have an artery known as the lowest thyroid artery, which originates from the brachiocephalic trunk or aortic arch and ascends anteriorly to the trachea to reach the thyroid isthmus. This vessel requires attention during low tracheotomy procedures.

The thyroid gland is drained by three pairs of veins: superior, middle, and inferior thyroid veins (Fig. 7.14). The superior thyroid vein accompanies the superior thyroid artery and drains into the internal jugular vein. The middle thyroid vein originates from the lateral middle portion of the lobe, is short and thick, and empties into the internal jugular vein. The inferior thyroid vein arises from the inferior pole of the lateral lobe and descends to drain into the brachiocephalic vein. The left and right inferior thyroid veins anastomose anteriorly to the trachea to form the thyroid

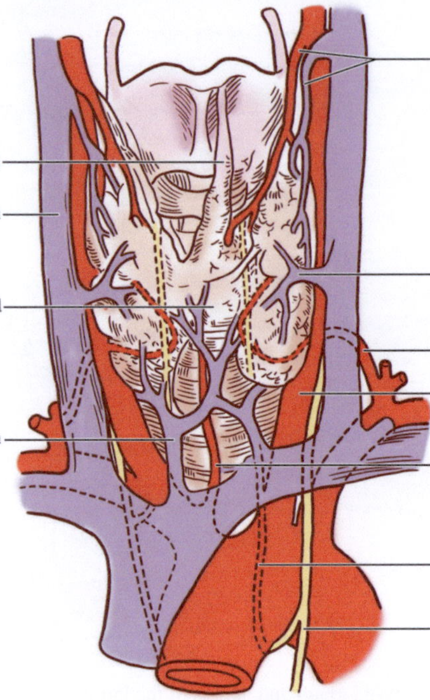

Fig. 7.14 Veins of the thyroid gland

plexus (azygos vein). Hemostasis should be carefully maintained during tracheotomy procedures to manage these venous structures.

Adjacent Structures of the Thyroid Gland

Anterior to the thyroid gland and from superficial to deep are the skin, superficial fascia, investing fascia, infrahyoid muscles, and pretracheal fascia. The posteromedial aspects of the left and right lobes of the thyroid are adjacent to the larynx and trachea, pharynx and esophagus, and the recurrent laryngeal nerve, while the posterolateral aspects are adjacent to the carotid sheath and the cervical sympathetic trunk. An enlarged thyroid gland can posteriorly compress the larynx, trachea, pharynx, esophagus, and recurrent laryngeal nerve, potentially leading to symptoms such as dyspnea, dysphagia, and hoarseness. If the enlargement extends posterolaterally and compresses the cervical sympathetic trunk, it may cause the Horner syndrome, characterized by ipsilateral constricted pupil (miosis), ptosis, and enophthalmos.

7.6.1.2 Parathyroid Glands

The parathyroid glands are typically in two pairs (superior and inferior), situated posterior to the thyroid gland nestled between the true and false capsules (Fig. 7.15). The number of parathyroid glands and their anatomical position vary greatly. Their numbers and positions show considerable variations; approximately 44% of individuals have four glands, 54% have fewer than four, and about 2% possess five. The superior parathyroid glands are more consistently located and numbered, positioned above the midpoint of the posterior portion of lateral lobes at the level of cricoid cartilage. In contrast, the numbers and positions of the inferior parathyroid glands show greater variability, with the majority (around 60%) situated near the lower third of the posterior portion of lateral lobes.

7.6.2 Larynx and Trachea

The larynx is situated in the anterior midline of the neck, at the level of the fifth or sixth cervical vertebra (C5–C6). It shows significant age-related variability: In children, the superior border of the larynx may reach the level of the third cervical

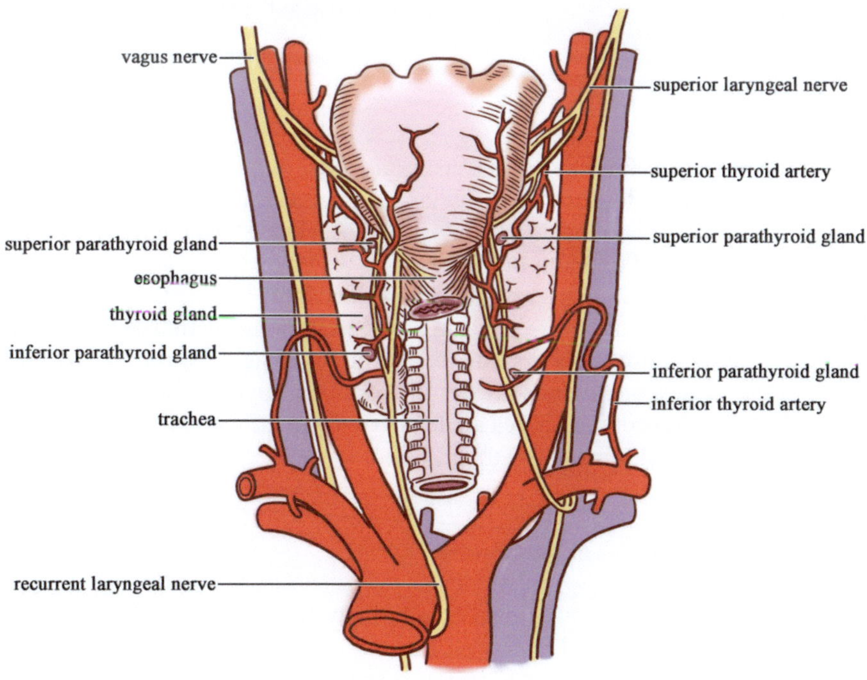

Fig. 7.15 Anatomical positions of the superior and inferior parathyroid glands

vertebra (C3), while in the elderly, it may descend to the upper border of the sixth cervical vertebra (C6). The larynx can move vertically during deglutition. The larynx is supplied by the blood derived from branches of the superior thyroid artery, known as the superior laryngeal artery, and branches of the inferior thyroid artery, referred to as the inferior laryngeal artery. Innervation of the larynx is provided by branches of the vagus nerve, namely, the superior laryngeal nerve and the recurrent laryngeal nerve.

7.6.2.1 Trachea

The cervical trachea is composed of six to eight tracheal rings, situated in the anterior midline of the neck, and connected with the larynx. The upper part of the cervical trachea is relatively superficial, while the lower part is deeper and can be palpated in the suprasternal notch. The position of the trachea can change with movements of the head and neck; it elongates and becomes shallower when the head extends backward and shortens and deepens when the head is lowered. The trachea can move approximately up or down by 1.5 cm during extension or flexion of the head. When the head is turned to one side, the trachea deviates toward the same side while the esophagus behind it shifts to the opposite side. Therefore, during tracheotomy procedures, it is essential to keep the head in the midline position and tilt it back as much as possible to ensure that the trachea is centrally located and close to the body surface.

Surrounding Structures of the Trachea

The structures adjacent to the trachea anteriorly, from superficial to deep, include the skin, superficial fascia, investing fascia, the suprasternal space with the jugular venous arch within it, infrahyoid muscles, pretracheal fascia, and pretracheal space. Anterior to the second to fourth tracheal rings is the thyroid isthmus, below which lie the inferior thyroid vein, the azygos thyroid plexus, and occasionally the thyroid ima artery. The trachea is bordered by the lateral lobes of the thyroid gland on both sides, and its posterior aspect is adjacent to the esophagus. Within the groove between the trachea and esophagus lies the recurrent laryngeal nerve, while the posterolateral aspects of the trachea are in proximity to the carotid sheath, its contents, and the cervical sympathetic trunk.

Blood Vessels and Nerves of the Cervical Trachea

The cervical trachea receives arterial blood supply from branches of the inferior thyroid artery. Venous blood is drained into the inferior thyroid vein. Lymphatic vessels drain into the deep lateral cervical lymph nodes. Sympathetic innervation originates from the middle cervical ganglion, while parasympathetic nerves innervation comes from branches of the recurrent laryngeal nerve.

7.6.3 Pharynx and Esophagus

7.6.3.1 Pharynx

The pharynx extends superiorly to the base of the skull with a blind end; anteriorly connects with the nasal, oral, and laryngeal cavities; laterally communicates with the tympanic cavity; and inferiorly continues with the esophagus at the level of the sixth cervical vertebra (C6). It is surrounded by loose spaces, namely, the parapharyngeal space and retropharyngeal space.

7.6.3.2 Esophagus

The cervical esophagus is located posterior to the trachea on the left side, making the left side a more common approach for cervical esophagus surgeries. It is posterolateral to the sympathetic trunk, lateral to the carotid sheath and lateral lobes of the thyroid gland, and posterior to the prevertebral fascia, longus colli muscle, and spine on its deep side. The esophagus is separated from these structures by the loose retroesophageal space.

The cervical esophagus is supplied with blood from the branches of the inferior thyroid artery. The venous blood drains into the inferior thyroid vein. It is innervated by the small branches of the vagus nerve and sympathetic nerves, forming the esophageal plexus.

7.7 Anatomy of the Neck

7.7.1 Objective

Understand the landmarks of the neck and surface projections of major structures

Identify the boundary and contents of the muscular triangle of the neck through layer-by-layer dissection as well as the distribution of fascial spaces

Recognize the distribution of blood vessels and nerves in the neck.

Understand the anatomical position, morphology, blood vessels, nerves, and surrounding structures of major neck structures

7.7.2 Position

With the body in a supine position, elevate the shoulders with a wooden pillow underneath to achieve a head-tilt/chin-lift posture.

7.7.3 Dissection Procedures

7.7.3.1 Landmarks of the Neck

Observe the bony landmarks of the neck, such as the base and angle of the mandible, mastoid process, hyoid bone and its greater horn, thyroid cartilage and laryngeal prominence, cricoid cartilage, jugular notch, clavicle, and acromion.

Palpate and observe the landmarks of the neck, including the suprasternal fossa, greater supraclavicular fossa, common carotid artery, external jugular vein, and sternocleidomastoid muscle.

7.7.3.2 Skin Incisions and Peeling

Make a skin incision along the midline of the neck, the base of the mandible, and the superior border of the clavicle. Skin incisions in the neck should not be too deep, considering that the thin skin is closely connected to the platysma muscle. Carefully peel the skin from the midline incision to both sides, till the anterior portion of the trapezius muscle. Ensure to protect the platysma muscle on the deep side during the peeling.

7.7.3.3 Dissection of the Superficial Layer of the Neck

Step 1. Flip up the platysma muscle.

Cut off the superior margin of the platysma muscle and flip it up to the base of the mandible. Dissect the blood vessels and nerves located on the deep side of the platysma muscle during the flip-up. Pay particular attention to the superficial branches of the cervical plexus.

Step 2. Observe the structures in the superficial layer of the neck.

Observe the external jugular vein running longitudinally on the surface of the sternocleidomastoid muscle, descending to pass through the deep fascia, and draining into the subclavian vein. The superficial lateral cervical lymph nodes are distributed around the external jugular vein.

Observe the following superficial branches of the cervical plexus around the midpoint of the posterior portion of the sternocleidomastoid muscle.

1. The lesser occipital nerve, ascending along the posterior portion of the sternocleidomastoid muscle to the posterior aspect of the auricle
2. The greater auricular nerve, a large branch, ascending vertically along the surface of the sternocleidomastoid muscle to the inferior aspect of the auricle
3. The transverse cervical nerve, with one to two branches, running transversely on the surface of the sternocleidomastoid muscle to the central part of the neck

4. The supraclavian nerves, with the anterior, middle, and posterior branches, descending to the area near the clavicle, and innervating the skin over the shoulder and first intercostal space

The anterior jugular vein descends longitudinally on both sides of the midline of the neck. Its inferior end often anastomoses inward to form the jugular venous arch, which lies within the suprasternal space and generally drains outward into the inferior end of the external jugular vein after passing through the deep aspect of the sternocleidomastoid muscle. The superficial anterior cervical lymph nodes may be present near the anterior jugular vein.

7.7.3.4 Peel Off the Investing Fascia

Remove the small amount of adipose and connective tissues filled in the superficial fascia of neck and observe the investing fascia. It is a complete layer of dense connective tissues lying on the superficial layer of the deep fascia. Make a longitudinal incision on the midline of the neck to cut open the investing fascia and then peel it off posteriorly to the anterior portion of the sternocleidomastoid muscle. At the anterior portion of the trapezius muscle, cut off the investing fascia and peel it off anteriorly to the posterior portion of the sternocleidomastoid muscle. Observe the investing fascia where it fuses at the hyoid bone and linea alba cervicalis, and the capsule of the submandibular gland and sternocleidomastoid muscle sheath it forms.

7.7.3.5 Dissect the Anterior Triangle of the Neck

Step 1. Observe the submental triangle.

Identify the anterior bellies of the digastric muscles on both sides. The submental triangle is a space between them and the hyoid bone. Observe the submental lymph nodes within the submental triangle.

Step 2. Observe the boundary and contents of the submandibular triangle.

Outline the posterior belly of the digastric muscle to expose the boundary of the submandibular triangle, and then observe the contents inside.

The submandibular gland is situated within the submandibular triangle, and its anterior and posterior ends may extend beyond the boundary. The capsule of the submandibular gland is formed by the investing fascia, which can be peeled off. The submandibular lymph nodes are located between the surrounding area of the submandibular gland and the base of the mandible.

Lift the posterior end of the submandibular gland forward. The facial artery, running on its deep side, curves upward over the inferior margin of the mandible anterior to the insertion of the masseter muscle and finally reaches the face. The facial vein lies behind the facial artery and descends. The submandibular duct arises from the anterior portion of the submandibular gland. Observe the course of the submandibular duct.

Identify the hypoglossal nerve and lingual nerve, which are situated inferiorly and superiorly between the deep side of the submandibular gland and the surface of the hyoglossus muscle, respectively.

Step 3. Observe the boundary and contents of the carotid triangle.
Outline the superior belly of the omohyoid muscle to expose the boundary of the carotid triangle. Identify the greater horn of the hyoid bone as the anatomical landmark and observe the following structures.

The hypoglossal nerve and the lingual artery curve forward between the greater horn of the hyoid bone and the posterior belly of the digastric muscle.

The superior thyroid artery and its accompanying superior laryngeal nerve are located below the greater horn of the hyoid bone. The superior thyroid artery descends to the superior pole of the thyroid gland. The internal branch of the superior laryngeal nerve, accompanied by the superior laryngeal artery, pierces the thyrohyoid membrane to enter the larynx. The external branch of the superior laryngeal nerve continues to move forward and downward to the cricothyroid muscle.

The upper one-third part of the carotid sheath is at the posterior part of the carotid triangle. There are deep lateral cervical lymph nodes around the carotid sheath and the superior root of the ansa cervicalis can be found on the surface of the sheath.

Step 4. Dissect and observe the muscular triangle.
Cut off the infrahyoid muscles and the pretracheal fascia behind it on the superior border of the manubrium, and lift them upward to observe the contents of the pretracheal space and muscular triangle.

Loose spaces exist around the trachea and esophagus. The pretracheal space is anterior to the trachea, containing the inferior thyroid vein and thyroid plexus. Observe the thyroid ima artery and the upper end of the thymus (in infants), if present. The recurrent laryngeal nerve lies within the laryngotracheal groove.

Observe the capsule of the thyroid gland, position of the lateral lobes, anatomical relationship between the isthmus and tracheal rings, and the presence or absence of conical lobes. Identify the superior thyroid artery superior to the lateral lobes and the inferior thyroid artery lateral to the lower third of the lateral lobes, and observe their anatomical relationship with the recurrent laryngeal nerve behind the lateral lobes. Fiber bundles in the central part of the lateral lobes and the isthmus that connect with the cricoid cartilage and trachea are known as the suspensory ligament of the thyroid gland. Lift the lateral lobes anteromedially and identify the parathyroid glands between the true and false capsules on the posterior side, and note their position and number. Generally, the superior parathyroid glands are situated at the junction of the upper and middle thirds on the posterior side of the lateral lobes, and the inferior parathyroid glands are located near the inferior thyroid artery.

Observe the adjacent structures of the thyroid gland, including the larynx and trachea posterior to the lateral lobes, carotid sheath on the anterolateral side, and sympathetic trunk on the posterior side.

7.7.3.6 Dissect the Occipital Triangle

Remove the anterior portion of the trapezius muscle and the inferior belly of the omohyoid muscle to observe the boundary of the occipital triangle and the accessory nerve passing through it. The accessory nerve pierces the sternocleidomastoid muscle at the upper third on the posterior portion, obliquely descends backward, and finally reaches the lower third of the anterior portion of the trapezius muscle. The deep lateral cervical lymph nodes are distributed around the accessory nerve.

7.7.3.7 Dissect the Sternocleidomastoid Area

Step 1. Cut off and raise up the sternocleidomastoid muscle.

Remove the anterior and posterior portions of the sternocleidomastoid muscle, cut off the sternal head and clavicular head on the inferior end, and raise them up. Preserve the superficial branches of the cervical plexus on the surface and posterior side of the sternocleidomastoid muscle. Free the omohyoid muscle that is attached to the sternocleidomastoid muscle via an intermediate tendon, and the accessory nerve on the deep side, and preserve them.

Step 2. Observe the structures on the deep side of the sternocleidomastoid muscle.

Find the ansa cervicalis and its superior and inferior roots on the surface of the carotid sheath, and observe their position and the muscles they innervate. Observe the number and size of the deep lateral cervical lymph nodes around the carotid sheath.

Cut open the carotid sheath and free the common carotid artery and internal carotid artery. Observe the anatomical relationship between the internal and external carotid arteries. The internal jugular vein lies on the lateral side of the common carotid artery, and the facial vein and superior and middle thyroid veins drain into it. The vagus nerve and its cervical cardiac branches lie posterior to the space between the common carotid artery and internal jugular vein. Observe the carotid sinus at the origin of the internal carotid artery, and find the carotid sinus nerve of the glossopharyngeal nerve at the posterior side of the carotid bifurcation that connects to the carotid body.

Cut open the prevertebral fascia posterior to the carotid sheath. Identify the cervical sympathetic trunk and cervical sympathetic ganglia on the surface of the longus colli muscle, and observe the location, number, and branches of the cervical sympathetic ganglia.

7.7.3.8 Dissect the Root of the Neck

Step 1. Remove the surrounding structures of the scalenus anterior muscle at the root of the neck and the prevertebral fascia on its surface.
Step 2. Observe the structures at the root of the neck.

On the anterior side of the scalenus anterior muscle, the phrenic nerve longitudinally descends, and the subclavian vein horizontally runs inward. The subclavian vein and internal jugular vein unite to form the venous angle. On the left side, the thoracic duct passes through the internal jugular vein posteriorly, curves forward, and drains into the venous angle. The left cervical trunk, left subclavian trunk, and left bronchial mediastinal trunk connect with the thoracic duct. Lymphatic trunks may also drain directly into the venous angle or the adjacent internal jugular vein or subclavian vein. The right lymphatic duct drains the right venous angle, which is difficult to find.

The scalene interspace lies between the scalenus anterior and medius muscles, in which the subclavian artery (in the anterior and inferior space) and brachial plexus (in the posterior and superior space) pass through and travel to the axilla.

The triangle of the vertebral artery is a space between the medial portion of the scalenus anterior muscle and the longus colli muscle. Observe the vertebral arteries and veins on the deep side, most of which ascend and pass through the transverse process foramen of the sixth cervical vertebra (C6).

Observe the position and the surrounding structures of the cupula of the pleura that is situated medial to the scalenus anterior muscle.

7.8 Summary

There are many important landmarks in the neck, and it is of great clinical significance to know their anatomical positions and how to palpate them. For example, the hyoid bone is a vital landmark for the localization of blood vessels and nerves. The cricoid cartilage, at the level of the sixth cervical vertebra (C6), is a landmark for the junction between the larynx and trachea, and between the pharynx and esophagus. The middle cervical ganglion and carotid tubercle also lie at the level of C6.

The sternocleidomastoid muscle is an important landmark of the neck and forms the muscular triangle along with the omohyoid muscle and digastric muscle. Injuries to the sternocleidomastoid muscle may cause torticollis. The scalenus anterior muscle is another muscular landmark, with many important blood vessels and nerves passing through its surrounding area.

The skin of the neck is thin, and the platysma muscle present in the superficial fascia of the neck is different from that in other areas. The muscles of the neck are arranged in layers and contribute to the formation of many muscular triangles in the neck that contain glands, organs, blood vessels, and nerves. Therefore, muscular triangles can be used to localize corresponding blood vessels and nerves.

From superior to deep, the fascia of the neck includes the superficial cervical fascia and the superficial (investing fascia), intermediate (pretracheal fascia), and deep layers (prevertebral fascia) of the deep cervical fascia. The deep fascia forms the carotid artery sheath, capsule of the thyroid gland and submandibular gland, sternocleidomastoid muscle sheath, and trapezius muscle sheath. The distribution of each layer of the cervical fascia and the structures they cover varies significantly. Fascial compartments of the neck are formed between two layers of the cervical fascia, including the suprasternal space, pretracheal space, parapharyngeal space, retropharyngeal space, and prevertebral space. Loose connective tissues fill these compartments, providing passageways for the spread of inflammation.

The organs of the neck mainly include the respiratory tract, upper part of the digestive tract, and endocrine glands. The thyroid gland is characterized by its important function, complicated surrounding structures, and rich blood supply. Arteries supplying the thyroid gland accompany or intersect with the nerves innervating the larynx, and care should be taken to avoid injuring the nerves during arterial ligation. The thyroid gland is adjacent to the trachea, esophagus, carotid sheath, and sympathetic trunk. Its enlargement can compress adjacent organs such as the trachea, esophagus, etc., thus causing corresponding clinical symptoms.

The trachea is superficial at the upper part and deeper at the lower part. The thyroid isthmus lies anterior to the second to fourth tracheal rings, with structures within the pretracheal space situated inferiorly. A head-tilt/chin-lift posture is used during tracheotomy to ensure the trachea is closer to the body surface, and the layers it passes through should be carefully considered. The anterior jugular vein, thyroid isthmus, inferior thyroid vein, and the azygos thyroid venous plexus should be protected.

The neck is supplied by the branches of the external carotid and subclavian arteries. Venous blood is drained into the internal jugular, subclavian, and brachiocephalic veins. The internal jugular vein is connected to the carotid artery sheath, and its patent lumen can facilitate venous reflux. However, its lumen is difficult to close, which can lead to embolism in cases of injury to the internal jugular vein. The subclavian vein is a common site for intubation, and precautions should be taken to prevent air embolism due to its firm adhesion to surrounding tissues.

Lymph from the head and neck drains into the deep lateral cervical lymph nodes, and at the root of the neck, it drains through the cervical trunk into the thoracic duct on the left side and the right lymphatic duct on the right side, respectively. This pathway is a major route for cancer cell metastases. For example, nasopharyngeal cancer often leads to enlargement of the jugulodigastric lymph nodes, while tongue cancer may cause enlargement of the juguloomohyoid lymph nodes. Abdominal tumors, particularly gastric cancer, can result in enlargement of the left supraclavicular lymph nodes.

The cranial nerves IX, X, and XI along with branches of the cervical plexus innervate the neck. The trunks of the branchial plexus are primarily located superior to the midpoint of the clavicle, which is a common site for supraclavicular brachial plexus block.

7.9 Clinical Application of Key Anatomical Structures of the Neck

The neck connects the head with the torso and upper limbs. Major organs of the neck include the thyroid gland, parathyroid glands, submandibular gland, larynx, trachea, and esophagus. Important blood vessels and nerves that connect the head and chest also run within the cervical fasciae, including the common carotid artery, internal jugular vein, vagus nerve, cervical sympathetic nerve, and thoracic duct. It is important to be very familiar with the anatomy and adjacent relationships of these structures to avoid damage during surgical procedures. In this section, taking radical thyroidectomy for thyroid cancer (including thyroidectomy and neck lymph node dissection) as an example, the separation and protection of key anatomical structures in the neck during surgical operations will be specifically described.

1. Position

   In a supine position, the shoulder is elevated by placing an O-shaped or U-shaped soft pillow underneath, creating a head-tilt/chin-lift posture. This position fixes the head and fully exposes the thyroid gland (Fig. 7.16a). For lateral neck dissection, the patient is placed in a supine position with the head turned to the contralateral side.
2. Skin incision

   Make a transverse arc-shaped incision along the skin tension line approximately two fingers' breadth above the sternal jugular notch.

Confirm the position of the first cervical transverse line, which is usually superior to the thyroid cartilage, laryngeal prominence, jugular notch, and sternocleidomastoid muscle (Fig. 7.16b). This is a vital landmark for selecting skin incisions and determining the range of donor site for flap reconstruction.

The skin incision for thyroidectomy should be 4.0–6.0 cm long and not exceed the anterior portion of sternocleidomastoid muscles on both sides (Fig. 7.16c). For thyroidectomy combined with lateral neck dissection, the skin incision should be extended laterally to the posterior portion of sternocleidomastoid muscles on both sides, following the dermatoglyphic pattern.

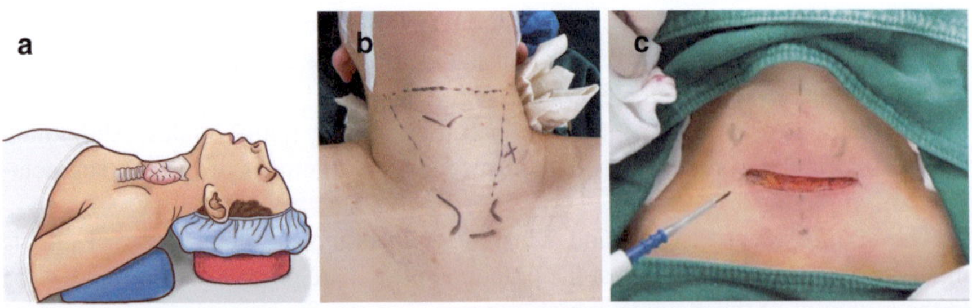

Fig. 7.16 Radical surgery for thyroid cancers. (**a**) Position. (**b**) Anatomical landmarks. (**c**) Skin incision for thyroidectomy

3. Separation of the skin and subcutaneous tissues
   Start from cutting open the skin, superficial fascia, and platysma muscle to free the skin flap on the surface of the investing fascia.

The anterior jugular vein is located within the investing fascia. Protect the integrity of the investing fascia and anterior jugular vein during the separation of the skin flaps within the fascial spaces of the neck. These structures can be ligated and cut off if necessary. The extensive venous drainage of the neck provides reflex compensation, which helps prevent adverse consequences.

The separation range of the skin and subcutaneous tissues should extend from the superior portion of the thyroid cartilage to the jugular notch and laterally to the sternocleidomastoid muscle.

4. Separation of infrahyoid muscles and exposure of the thyroid gland
   The infrahyoid muscles, also known as the strap muscles, include the sternohyoid, omohyoid, sternothyroid, and thyrohyoid muscles.

The cervical linea alba is formed by the convergence of the investing fascia in the midline, an avascular region that serves as the optimal surgical approach to the anterior neck.

Cut through the cervical linea alba, extending superior to the upper margin of the thyroid cartilage and inferiorly to the jugular notch (Fig. 7.17).

The anterior jugular veins lie on either side of the cervical linea alba, often form communication branches near the suprasternal fossa, and cross the linea alba in an H-shaped pattern. When incising the cervical linea alba, the relevant venous vessels should be ligated to prevent hemorrhage.

Bluntly separate the sternothyroid muscle from the surface of the thyroid gland, revealing the thyroid gland with loose connective tissues between them.

In cases of significantly enlarged thyroid volume, such as grade II–III hyperthyroidism, the sternohyoid and sternothyroid muscles can be transected to facilitate exposure of the gland.

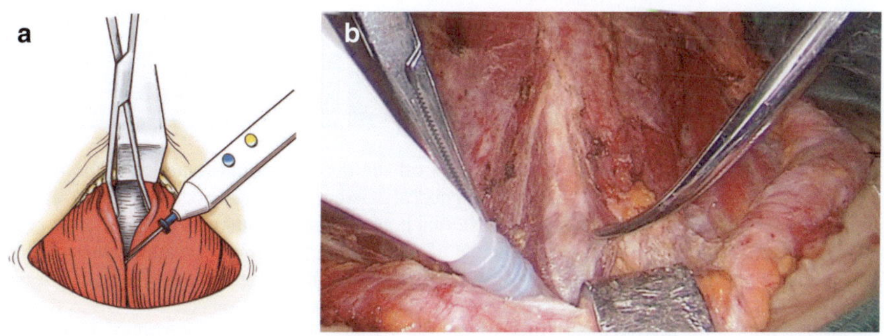

Fig. 7.17 (**a**) Schematic illustration; (**b**) Intraoperative view. The cervical linea alba is longitudinally divided from the superior margin of the thyroid cartilage to the jugular notch, with the strap muscles separated to expose the thyroid region

7.10 Removal of the Thyroid Gland

7.10.1 Dissect and Free the Thyroid Isthmus

Start from dissecting the thyroid isthmus and ligating and severing the inferior thyroid vein below it. Then cut the isthmus along the contralateral edge of the trachea (Fig. 7.18a), and free it upward to facilitate the removal of the cone-like lobes of the thyroid gland (Fig. 7.18b).

7.10.2 Dissect the Superior Pole of the Thyroid Gland

Gently pull the superior pole of the thyroid lateral lobe downward and outward and carefully separate the cricothyroid space using mosquito forceps. Divide the blood vessels of the superior pole close to the thyroid gland, taking care to protect the external branch of the superior laryngeal nerve (Fig. 7.18c, d). Preserve the posterior branch of the superior thyroid artery to maintain blood supply to the superior

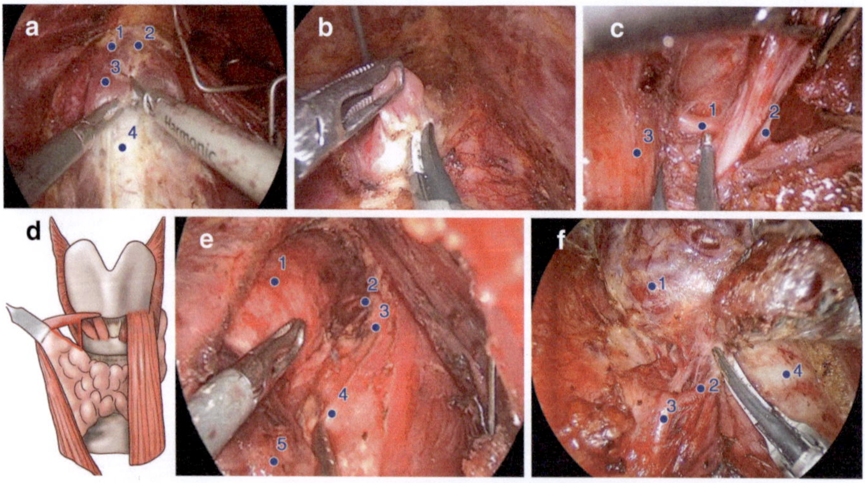

Fig. 7.18 Removal of the thyroid gland. (**a**) Cut off the thyroid isthmus anterior to the thyroid gland (1. pyramidal lobe; 2. prelaryngeal lymph nodes; 3. isthmus; 4. trachea). (**b**) Free and remove the pyramidal lobe. (**c, d**) Dissection of the external branches of the superior laryngeal nerve (Fig. **c**: 1. superior laryngeal nerve; 2. superior pole of the thyroid gland; 3. cricothyroid muscle). (**e**) Dissection of parathyroid glands (1. trachea; 2. right recurrent laryngeal nerve; 3. right inferior parathyroid gland; 4. right superior parathyroid gland; 5. cricothyroid muscle). (**f**) Dissection of the inferior pole of the thyroid gland (thyroid: thyroid gland; *ITA* inferior thyroid artery, *P* pharynx, *T* trachea, *RLN* recurrent laryngeal nerve)

parathyroid glands. Keep the superior parathyroid glands and their blood supply in situ close to the thyroid gland (Fig. 7.18e).

7.10.3 Expose the Recurrent Laryngeal Nerve and Free the Inferior Pole of the Thyroid Gland

Gently pull the thyroid gland medially and carefully separate the branches of the inferior thyroid artery along the capsule of the thyroid gland to expose and protect the recurrent laryngeal nerve. Using mosquito forceps, delicately dissect the loose connective tissues closely attached to the nerve in parallel to expose the nerve course. The inferior thyroid artery serves as a valuable guide for identifying the recurrent laryngeal nerve, which often passes between its branches. After exposing the recurrent laryngeal nerve, ligate the branches of the inferior thyroid artery and free the inferior pole of the thyroid gland, and preserve the inferior parathyroid glands and their blood supply in situ (Fig. 7.18f).

7.10.4 Removal of the Thyroid Gland

Expose the anterior wall of the trachea, pull the superior and inferior poles of the thyroid gland anteromedially, and cut off the middle thyroid vein. Then further expose the full course of the recurrent laryngeal nerve. Completely resect the thyroid gland from below upward. When dissecting the suspensory ligament of the thyroid gland near the point where the recurrent laryngeal nerve enters the larynx, take care to protect the nerve.

7.11 Central Lymph Node Dissection (Fig. 7.19)

7.11.1 Boundary of Central Lymph Node Dissection

The central lymph node dissection is delimited superiorly by the hyoid bone, inferiorly by the thymus, and laterally by the medial aspect of the carotid sheath, encompassing the pretracheal, paratracheal, and prelaryngeal lymph nodes (or Delphian lymph nodes). On the right side, the central lymph nodes are classified into levels VIa and VIb, located superiorly and posteriorly to the recurrent laryngeal nerve, respectively.

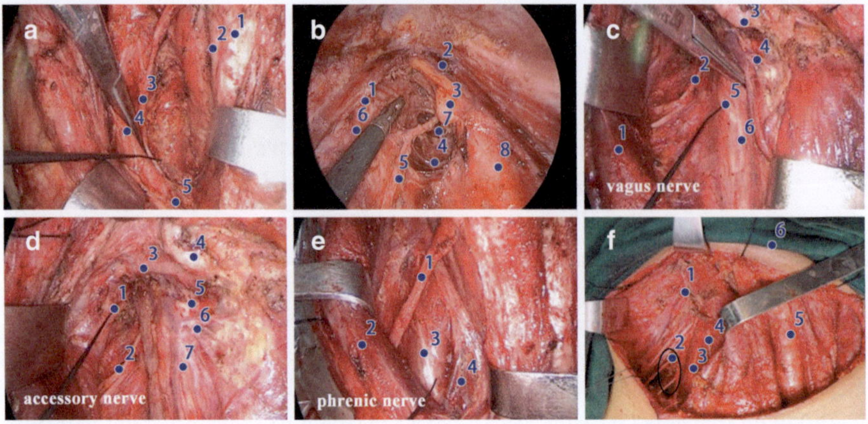

Fig. 7.19 Central lymph node dissection. (**a**) Lymph nodes in the areas of the trachea (1), esophagus (2), recurrent laryngeal nerve (3), carotid sheath (4), and anomalous coronary artery (5). (**b**) Lymph nodes in the areas of the trachea (1), thymus (2), inferior parathyroid gland (3), esophagus (4), recurrent laryngeal nerve (5), level VIa on the surface of the recurrent laryngeal nerve (6), level VIb on the deep side of the recurrent laryngeal nerve (7), and common carotid artery (8). (**c**) Lymph nodes in the areas of the sternocleidomastoid muscle (1), branches of the cervical plexus (2), submandibular gland (3), internal jugular vein (4), vagus nerve (5), and carotid sheath (6). (**d**) Lymph nodes in the areas of the accessory nerve (1), branches of the cervical plexus (2), digastric muscle (3), submandibular gland (4), hypoglossal nerve (5), facial nerve (6), and internal jugular vein (7). (**e**) Lymph nodes in the areas of the omohyoid muscle (1), sternocleidomastoid muscle (2), phrenic nerve (3), and lymphatic vessels (4). (**f**) Lymph nodes in the areas of the sternocleidomastoid muscle (1), branches of the cervical plexus (2), brachial plexus (3), phrenic nerve (4), trachea (5), and submandibular gland (6)

7.11.2 *Procedures*

7.11.2.1 Medial Boundary

Dissect the lymphoid and adipose tissues on the surface of the trachea along the midline of the neck.

7.11.2.2 Lateral Boundary

Perform skeletonizing dissection of lymphoid and adipose tissues along the anterior portion of the thymus, medial to the carotid sheath, and anterior and posterior to the recurrent laryngeal nerve. Protect the inferior parathyroid glands and their blood supply.

7.11.2.3 Inferior Boundary

Elevate the tissues within the central area of the neck and dissect lymph nodes downward to the level of the suprasternal notch. Posterior lymphoid and adipose tissues to the recurrent laryngeal nerve are dissected during the right central lymph node dissection.

7.12 Lateral Lymph Node Dissection

7.12.1 Boundary of Lateral Lymph Node Dissection

The lateral lymph node dissection is delineated superiorly by the digastric muscle, inferiorly by the supraclavicular notch, medially by the medial aspect of the carotid sheath, and laterally by the anterior portion of the trapezius muscle, encompassing lymph nodes and soft tissues at levels II–V.

7.12.2 Procedures

Release the skin from the lower margin of the mandible to the supraclavicular notch, and extend laterally to the anterior portion of the trapezius muscles on both sides.

Liberate and expose the sternocleidomastoid muscle along its anterior aspect. Incise the carotid sheath to expose the internal jugular vein, vagus nerve, and common carotid artery. Proceeding from medial to lateral and inferior to superior, dissect lymphoid and adipose tissues at levels IV, III, and II situated posterior to the internal jugular vein and lateral to the vagus nerve.

Release the posterior aspect of the sternocleidomastoid muscle and locate the accessory nerve posterior to the muscle within the posterior neck triangle. Start from the posterior part of the sternocleidomastoid muscle, and completely free the accessory nerve toward the trapezius muscle.

From posterior to anterior, dissect lymphoid and adipose tissues within the posterior neck triangle along the trapezius muscle, and separate them from the deep muscles. Remove lymphoid and adipose tissues above the cervical plexus while preserving its branches.

7.13 Surgical Suture

Begin by completely arresting bleeding.

Next, suture the cervical linea alba continuously, but not the area 1.0–2.0 cm below. Postoperative bleeding into the subcutaneous tissues can delay the onset of dyspnea.

Finally, suture the platysma muscle, subcutaneous tissues, and skin layer by layer.

Chapter 8
Regional Anatomy of the Thoracic Cavity and Its Clinical Application

Yizhi Zuo, Zhi Li, Jun Wang, and Xiangxiang Zheng

8.1 Regional Anatomy of the Thoracic Cavity

8.1.1 Boundary

The thoracic cavity is formed by the thoracic wall and diaphragm. It superiorly connects the neck via the superior thoracic inlet and inferiorly separates from the abdominal cavity via the diaphragm. A sagittal mediastinum lies in the central part of the thoracic cavity and contains two pleural cavities and lungs laterally. The major contents in the thoracic cavity include the pleura, trachea and main bronchi, lungs, heart, pericardium and pericardial cavity, great vessels of the heart, esophagus, lymph nodes, thoracic duct, and nerves.

8.1.2 Pleural Cavity and Lungs

8.1.2.1 Pleura and Pleural Cavity

Structures of the Pleura

The pleura is divided into visceral and parietal pleurae. The visceral pleura covers the surface of the lungs. The parietal pleura covers the inner surface of the thoracic wall, upper surface of the diaphragm, and side surface of the mediastinum, which can be subdivided into the costal pleura, diaphragmatic pleura, mediastinal pleura,

Y. Zuo (✉) · Z. Li · J. Wang · X. Zheng
Nanjing Medical University, Nanjing, China
e-mail: zuoyizhi@njmu.edu.cn; drwangjun@njmu.edu.cn

Q. Ding et al. (eds.), *Clinically Oriented Regional Anatomy*,
https://doi.org/10.1007/978-981-95-9888-5_8

and cupula of the pleura (or cervical pleura) based on the anatomical position it covers. The cupula of the pleura surrounds the apex of the lungs and is formed by the costal pleura and mediastinal pleura protruding toward the base of the neck through the superior thoracic inlet. The endothoracic fascia superior to the cupula of the pleura plays a structurally supportive role. The visceral and parietal pleurae are connected at the root of the lung, forming a potential space with a negative pressure, known as the pleural cavity. The pleural cavity is a space filled with 1.0–2.0 ml of pleural fluid that encloses the lungs, which favors respiratory movements. The central part of the mediastinal pleura surrounds the root of the lung and extends to the visceral pleura, forming a double-layered mesentery-like band beneath the root of the lung known as the pulmonary ligament, serving as an important landmark for lung surgeries.

The thickness of the parietal pleura and its attachments vary greatly. It becomes the thickest on the bilateral sides of the spine but has the loosest attachment here. It becomes loosely attached with the first to third costal cartilages; at the pericardium, diaphragm, and the area below the seventh rib, the attachment is tight and the pleura is thin and difficult to remove.

Projection Lines of the Parietal Pleura on the Surface

These projection lines correspond to the reflections in the parietal pleura as it passes from one wall of the pleural cavity to another (Figs. 8.1 and 8.2).

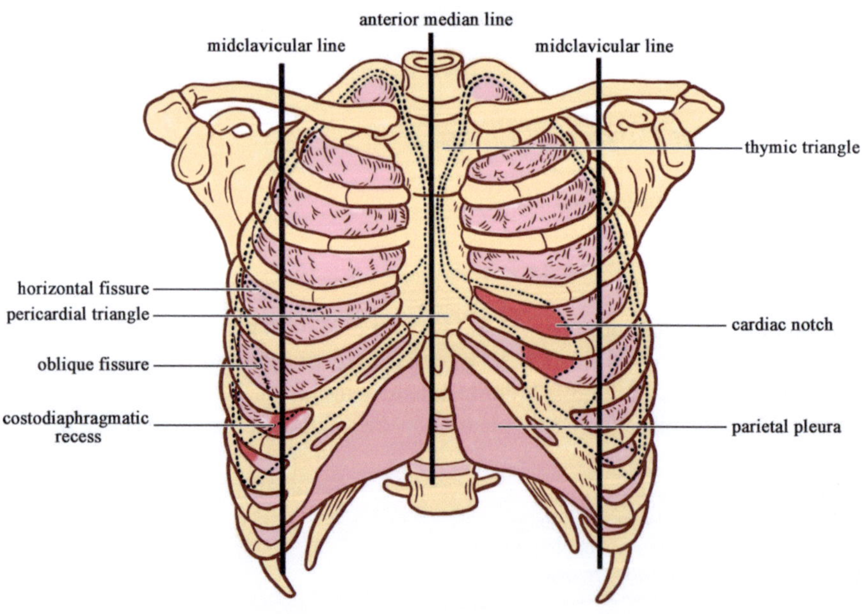

Fig. 8.1 Surface projections of the lungs and pleura in an anterior view

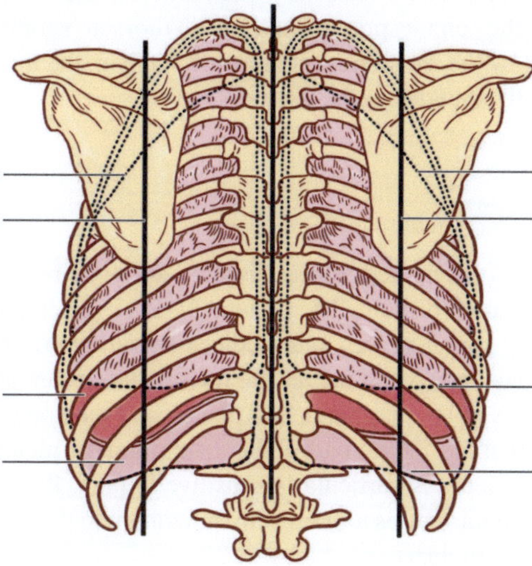

Fig. 8.2 Surface projections of the lungs and pleura in a posterior view

Anterior Border of the Pleura

The pleura is anteriorly bordered by the anterior portion of the mediastinal pleura and the line of costal pleural reflection. On both sides, this border arises from the cupula of the pleura 2.5 cm above the medial third of the clavicle. The anterior border of the bilateral pleurae descends obliquely and medially, courses behind the manubrium after passing through the posterior aspect of the sternoclavicular joint, and draws close at the level of the second sternocostal joint to vertically descend along the midline with a slight turn to the left. The anterior border of the left pleura directs into the inferolateral part at the fourth sternocostal joint and extends to the inferior border of the pleura at the midpoint of the sixth left costal cartilage. The right anterior border of the pleura turns right to extend to the inferior border at the sixth right costal cartilage. The anterior borders of the pleurae on both sides are separated above the plane of the second costal cartilage, forming an inverted triangular space posterior to the manubrium, namely, the thymus triangle. Pericardial triangle points upward to the fourth costal cartilage. The entry for pericardial puncture is usually set between the fourth and fifth left intercostal spaces next to the sternum, where the pericardium is directly attached to the anterior thoracic wall. However, the anatomical structure of the inferior pleural space varies and is absent in 6.0% of the population.

Inferior Border of the Pleura

The pleura is inferiorly bordered by the inferior portion of the costal pleura and the line of diaphragmatic pleural reflection. The inferior borders of the left and right pleurae extend from the midpoint of the sixth costal cartilage and the posterior aspect of the sixth sternocostal joint, respectively. Both turn outward and then backward and inward. The inferior border of the pleura extends to the 8th, 10th, and 11th ribs at the midclavicular line, midaxillary line, and scapular line, respectively, and reaches the level of the spinous process of the 12th thoracic vertebra in the posterior midline. Influenced by the anatomical position of the liver, the inferior border of the right pleura is slightly superior to the left side.

Innervation of the Pleura

The visceral pleura is innervated by the visceral sensory fibers of the pulmonary plexus, with a high pain threshold. The parietal pleura is innervated by the somatic sensory fibers of the spinal nerves and receives sensations from the phrenic and intercostal nerves. The intercostal nerves are mainly distributed at the costal pleura and surrounding areas of the diaphragmatic pleura, and the branches of the phrenic nerve are distributed at the central part of the diaphragmatic pleura and mediastinal pleura. The parietal pleura is particularly sensitive to pain. Pleurisy, an inflammation of the parietal pleura, causes a sharp pain radiating into the thoracic and abdominal walls, neck, and shoulder.

Pleural Recesses

Pleural recesses are semicircular pleural cavities formed by the reflection of the parietal pleura. Due to this structure, the lungs do not lodge into it during inspiration. The costodiaphragmatic recess (or phrenicocostal sinus) is a semicircular space formed by the reflection between the costal and diaphragmatic parietal pleurae, extending backward and downward from the xiphoid process to the bilateral sides of the spine. It becomes deeper in the posterior part, serving as the lowermost portion of the pleural cavity. The lungs expand into this recess during forced inspiration but do not get filled completely (Figs. 8.1 and 8.2). Exudate from pleural inflammation often accumulates here. Thoracentesis is usually performed in the eighth or ninth intercostal space between the posterior axillary line and the scapular line to extract the pleural effusion, thus alleviating the compression on the lungs. The costomediastinal recess is another pleural recess formed by the reflection between the costal and mediastinal parietal pleurae in front of the anterior portion of the lungs. It is larger on the left side and situated medial to the cardiac notch.

Clinical Significance of the Pleura

The negative pressure within the pleural cavity exerts a decisive role in alveolar expansion. Pleural disorders result in pneumothorax due to the air entering the space, disappeared negative pressure, and lung collapse and may even be fatal for mediastinal flutter.

The pleura receives a rich blood supply. After lobectomy, the pleura is usually used to cover the main bronchi and its branches.

Position, Lobes, and Segments of the Lung

The lungs are conical in shape, situated within the thoracic cavity on both sides of the mediastinum and superior to the diaphragm, and are divided into the left lung and the right lung. The right lung is separated into the superior lobe, middle lobe and inferior lobe by the horizontal fissure and oblique fissure, while the left lung possesses only the oblique fissure and is divided into the superior lobe and inferior lobe. The structural unit smaller than the pulmonary lobe is the pulmonary segment. Adjacent pulmonary segments are separated by connective tissue, which ensures their morphological and functional independence. Generally, the right lung consists of 10 pulmonary segments, and the left lung consists of 8 pulmonary segments.

Hilum and Root of the Lung

The hilum of the lung is located at the center of mediastinal surface of the lung, where the main bronchi and pulmonary blood vessels, lymphatic vessels, and nerves pass through. The root of the lung is a group of structures that are enclosed by the pleura and merged at the hilum. Structures passing through the hilum of lung include the superior pulmonary vein, pulmonary artery, and main bronchi from anterior to posterior. Through the left hilum, it contains the left pulmonary artery, left main bronchus, and left inferior pulmonary vein from superior to inferior. The left superior pulmonary vein lies anterior to the left main bronchus. Through the right hilum, it contains the right superior lobar bronchus, right pulmonary artery, right intermediate bronchus, and right inferior pulmonary vein from superior to inferior. The right superior pulmonary vein lies anterior to the middle and inferior lobar bronchi (Figs. 8.3 and 8.4). The phrenic nerve and pericardiophrenic artery and vein lie anterior to the root of the lung, and the vagus nerve and pulmonary ligament respectively lie posterior and inferior. The superior vena cava and right atrium lie superiorly, and the arch of the azygos vein posteriorly and superiorly crosses over the root of the right lung. The aortic arch crosses superiorly over and the thoracic aorta passes anteriorly to the root of the left lung. Inferior pulmonary veins on both sides lie at the lowermost portion of the hilum and are enclosed by the pulmonary

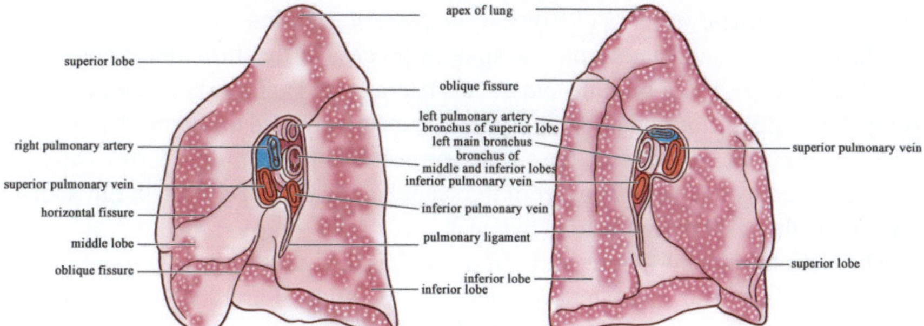

Fig. 8.3 Mediastinal surface of the lung

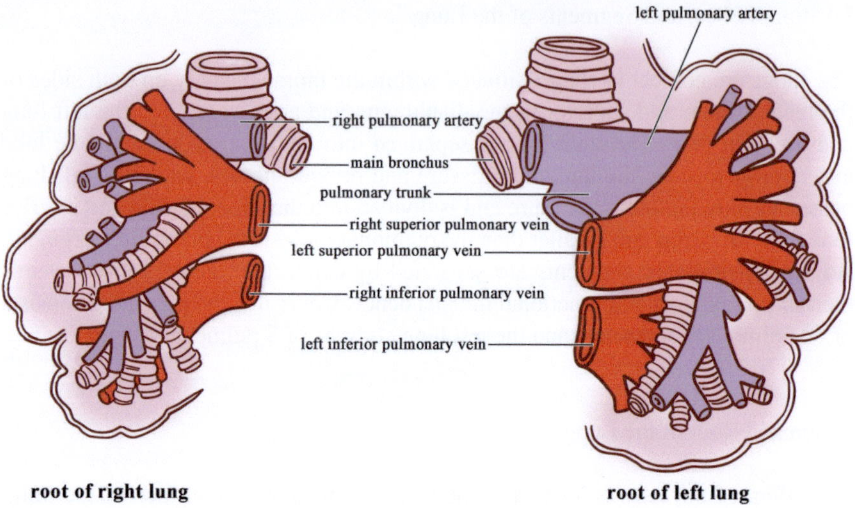

Fig. 8.4 Structures passing through the root of the lung

ligaments. They should be ligated after cutting open the pulmonary ligaments during lobectomy.

Surface Projections of the Lung

The anterior border of the lung is basically projected on the anterior line of pleural reflection.

The apex of the lung is projected on the cupula of the pleura. The highest point is anteriorly marked 2.5 cm above the medial third of the clavicle and posteriorly marked at the level of the spinous process of the seventh cervical spine (C7). The inferior border of the lung is projected above the inferior line of pleural reflection. It extends from the end of the anterior portion of both lungs and travels laterally to the sixth rib along the midclavicular line, the eighth rib along the midaxillary line, and the tenth rib along the scapular line and reach the level of the spinous process of the tenth thoracic vertebra (T10) near the posterior midline.

The oblique fissure starts from the spinous process of the third thoracic vertebra (T3) along the posterior midline and travels laterally and anteriorly to the fourth rib along the scapular line and midaxillary line, respectively, and the sixth rib along the midclavicular line. In addition, the surface projection of the oblique fissure can also be determined by the medial border of the scapula with the upper limb in full abduction and both hands placed behind the neck.

The right horizontal fissure starts from the fourth right sternocostal joint, at the level of the fourth rib, and laterally extends to the midaxillary line, where it meets the projection line of the oblique fissure (Figs. 8.1 and 8.2).

The hilum and root of the lung are projected anteriorly on the anterior side of the second to fourth intercostal spaces and posteriorly at the level of the spinous processes of the fourth to sixth thoracic vertebrae (T4–T6).

8.1.3 Mediastinum

The mediastinum refers to all the organs and soft tissues that are situated between the left and right mediastinal pleurae, mainly containing the pericardium, heart, large vessels of the cardiac base, trachea, main bronchi, esophagus, thoracic duct, nerves, lymphatic vessels, lymph nodes, thymus, and connective tissue. It is bounded anteriorly by the sternum and costal cartilage, posteriorly by the thoracic spine, and laterally by the left and right mediastinal pleurae. The mediastinum superiorly connects with the neck via the superior thoracic inlet and inferiorly extends to the diaphragm. Separated by the plane extending from the sternal angle to the fourth and fifth thoracic vertebrae (T4–T5), the mediastinum is divided into the superior and inferior parts based on the four-compartment model. The inferior mediastinum can be further subdivided into three parts by the pericardium. The anterior mediastinum lies between the sternum and pericardium, the posterior mediastinum lies between the pericardium and spine, and the middle mediastinum contains the pericardium and its contents (Fig. 8.5).

8.1.3.1 Superior Mediastinum

The major structures contained in the superior mediastinum can be divided into six layers (Figs. 8.6, 8.7, and 8.8).

Layer 1. Thymus and the anterior portion of the bilateral pleurae.

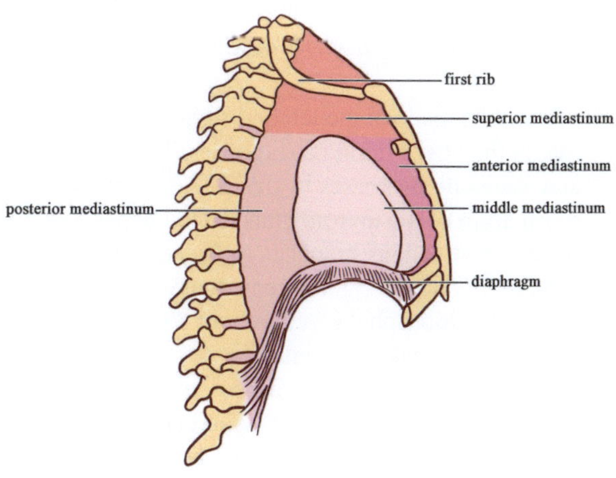

Fig. 8.5 Compartments of the mediastinum

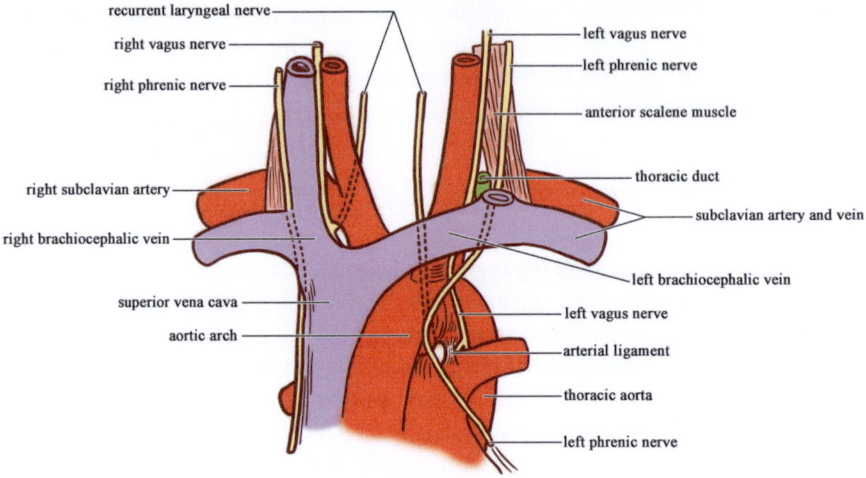

Fig. 8.6 Structures in the superior mediastinum

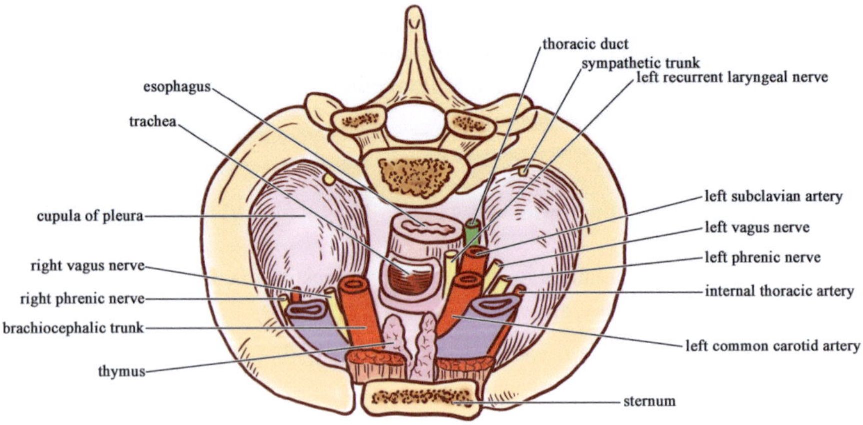

Fig. 8.7 The superior mediastinum at the level of T1 in a superior view

The thymus is made of the left and right lobes with different sizes. It plays a critical role in the host's immune responses. The thymus becomes the largest in puberty and gradually decreases in size. In newborns, the thymus extends from the inferior margin of the thyroid gland to the upper portion of the pericardium.

Layer 2. Great venous branches (left and right brachiocephalic veins and superior vena cava) and the right phrenic nerve.

The right brachiocephalic vein, about 3.0 cm long, descends vertically behind the right sternoclavicular joint. The left brachiocephalic vein, about 7.0 cm long, arises from the posterior aspect of the left sternoclavicular joint, obliquely descends toward the right side, and crosses over the anterior aspect of the three main branches of the aortic arch. The superior vena cava is formed by the left and right brachiocephalic veins posterior to the inferior margin of the first right costal

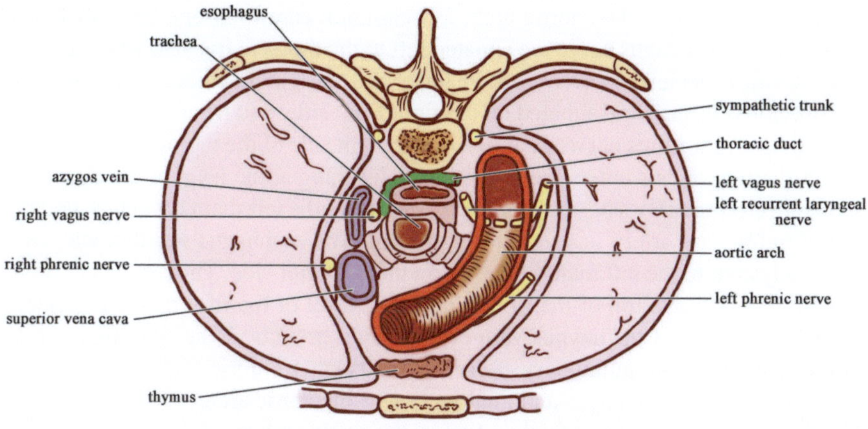

Fig. 8.8 The superior mediastinum at the level of T4 in a superior view

cartilage. It descends to pierce the pericardium on the right side of the aortic arch and ascending aorta below the anterior aspect of the first and second intercostal spaces and ends in the right atrium. The superior vena cava receives the azygos vein above the root of the right lung. The right phrenic nerve descends from the anterior aspect of the right superior vena cava.

Layer 3. Great arterial branches (aortic arch and its branches), pericardiophrenic vessels, left phrenic nerve, and left vagus nerve.

The aortic arch lies behind the manubrium. It arises from the ascending aorta at the second right sternocostal joint and continues into the thoracic aorta inferior to the fourth left thoracic vertebra (T4). From right to left, the aortic arch ascends to branch off the brachiocephalic trunk, left common carotid artery, and left subclavian artery. The pericardiophrenic vessels, left phrenic nerve, and left vagus nerve descend from right to left in front of the aortic arch. The pulmonary trunk and its branches, arterial ligament, left recurrent laryngeal nerve, and left main bronchus travel inferiorly to the aortic arch. The arterial ligament is a fibrous connective tissue cord that connects with the inferior margin of the aortic arch and the origin of the left pulmonary artery, as a vestige of the ductus arteriosus during the embryonic period. The triangle of ductus arteriosus is bounded anteriorly by the left phrenic nerve, posteriorly by the left vagus nerve, and inferiorly by the left pulmonary artery, which contains the arterial ligament. The left recurrent laryngeal nerve ascends around the aortic arch on the left side of the arterial ligament, serving as a landmark for identifying the ductus arteriosus during surgery.

Layer 4. Thoracic trachea, main bronchi and surrounding lymph nodes, and right vagus nerve.

The thoracic trachea is 5.0 cm long and situated in the center of the superior mediastinum, posterior to the manubrium. At the level of the sternal angle, the thoracic trachea is divided into the left and right main bronchi. The aortic arch, brachiocephalic trunk, left brachiocephalic vein, origin of the left common carotid artery, and thymus are situated anterior to the trachea, and the esophagus lies posterior to it. The aortic arch, left common carotid artery, left subclavian artery, and left vagus nerve are situated left to the thoracic trachea, while left and posterior is the left recurrent laryngeal nerve. The right brachiocephalic vein and superior vena cava are situated on the right front side, and the arch of the azygos vein and right vagus nerve are found on the right side of the thoracic trachea. The left main bronchus enters the hilum of the left lung at the level of the sixth thoracic vertebra (T6). The aortic arch crosses above the left main bronchus, and the left pulmonary artery lies superiorly in front. The esophagus and thoracic aorta are adjacent to the left main bronchus on the posterior side. The right main bronchus enters the hilum of the right lung at the level of the fifth thoracic vertebra (T5). The arch of the azygos vein posteriorly crosses over the right main bronchus, and the right pulmonary artery lies on its anteroinferior side.

Layer 5. Thoracic esophagus and final section of the aortic arch.

The thoracic esophagus and final section of the aortic arch are described in the section of inferior mediastinum.

Layer 6. Thoracic duct, azygos vein and accessory hemiazygos vein, posterior intercostal vessels, intercostal nerves, and sympathetic trunks.

Above the level of the fourth and fifth thoracic vertebrae (T4–T5), the thoracic duct is situated between the esophagus and left mediastinal pleura, ascends to the root of the neck, crosses over the cupula of the left pleura, and drains into the left venous angle. The posterior intercostal vessels, intercostal nerves, and thoracic sympathetic trunks are situated on both sides of the spine. The accessory hemiazygos vein and azygos vein lie on the left and right side of the spine, respectively.

8.1.3.2 Inferior Mediastinum

The inferior mediastinum can be subdivided into the anterior, middle, and posterior mediastinum. It can also be structurally divided into four layers. Layer 1 is the anterior mediastinum, layer 2 is the middle mediastinum, and layers 3–4 are the posterior mediastinum. Layer 4 is the extension of layer 6 of the superior mediastinum (Fig. 8.9).

Anterior Mediastinum

The anterior mediastinum, or prepericardial space, is a space between the sternum and anterior surface of pericardium. It contains a small amount of loose connective tissues, anterior mediastinal lymph nodes, and branches of the internal thoracic artery.

Middle Mediastinum

The middle mediastinum contains the pericardium, heart, large vessels of cardiac base, phrenic nerves, pericardiophrenic vessels, cardiac plexus, and lymph nodes.

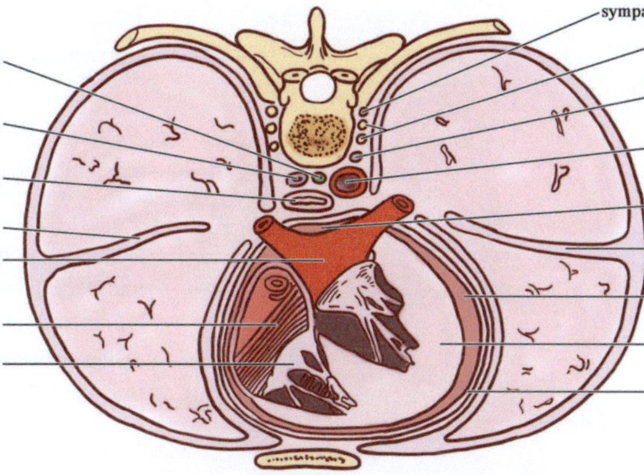

Fig. 8.9 The inferior mediastinum at the level of T8 in a superior view

Pericardium

The pericardium is a two-layer fibrous membrane sac that encloses the heart and great vessels of the ventricles. The outer layer is a fibrous pericardium that superiorly attaches to the root of great vessels of the ventricles and extends to the outer adventitial layer. The inferior part of the outer layer tightly connects with the central tendon of the diaphragm. The inner layer is serous pericardium that is divided into the parietal and visceral serous pericardium. The parietal serous pericardium at the root of great vessels of the ventricles is continuous with the visceral serous pericardium and covers the surface of the heart. The pericardial cavity is a closed space between the parietal and visceral serous pericardium and contains a small amount of serous fluid. The transverse sinus of pericardium is the pericardial space delimited by the ascending aorta and pulmonary trunk with superior vena cava and left atrium (Fig. 8.10). During open heart surgery, blood flow in the aorta and pulmonary artery can be temporarily interrupted through the transverse pericardial sinus. The anteroinferior sinus of pericardium is the lowermost part of the pericardial cavity and formed by the extension of the anterior wall of the parietal serous pericardium to the inferior wall above the diaphragm. In cases of pericardial effusion, the fluid usually builds up in the anteroinferior sinus of pericardium. The oblique sinus of pericardium is a pericardial sac obliquely ascending to the right side and situated between the left and right pulmonary veins, inferior vena cava, and posterior wall of the pericardium, behind the left atrium. The sternopericardial ligaments on the superior and inferior parts of the anterior wall of the pericardium are connective tissues that attach to the sternum, serving to fix the pericardium. The main bronchus, esophagus, thoracic aorta, thoracic duct, azygos vein, and hemiazygos vein lie posterior to the pericardium. The mediastinal pleurae are adjacent to the pericardium on bilateral sides. The phrenic nerve and pericardiophrenic vessels descend between the pericardium and the mediastinal pleura.

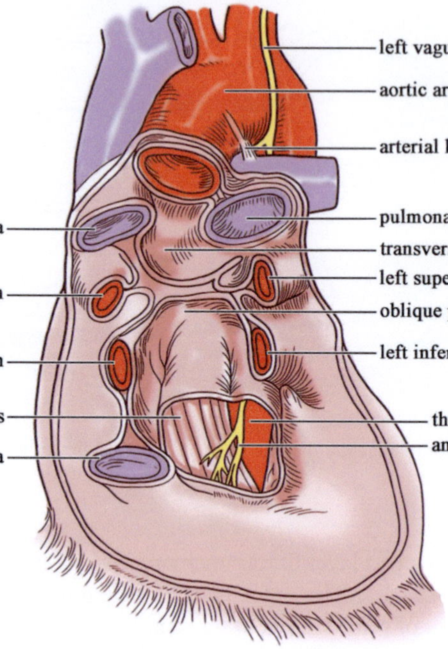

Fig. 8.10 Pericardium and pericardial sinuses

Heart

The heart is situated inside the middle mediastinum, at the level of the inferior part of the sternum posterior to the third to sixth left costal cartilages. The right ventricle and part of the left ventricle lie on the anterior side of the heart. Beneath the pericardium, the anterior wall of the heart in the inferior pleural space (or pericardial triangle) is adjacent to the left half of the body of sternum and fourth to sixth costal cartilages on the left side. Intracardiac injections into the right ventricle are usually performed through the fourth to fifth intercostal space, adjacent to the left margin of the sternum, thus preventing damages to the pleura and lungs that cover the remaining part of the heart. The left atrium and part of the right atrium lie on the posterior side of the heart. Beneath the pericardium, the posterior wall of the heart is adjacent to the esophagus, thoracic aorta, main bronchi, and left vagus nerve. Therefore, the left atrial impression can be observed on the esophageal X-ray scan and serves as a marker for predicting the early-stage left atrial enlargement.

The surface projections of the heart are determined by the four points and their connections (Fig. 8.11).

The top-left point is projected on the inferior border of the second left costal cartilage, 1.2 cm away from the sternum; the bottom-left point is projected in the fifth left intercostal space, 1.0–2.0 cm medial to the left midclavicular line or 7.0–9.0 cm away from the anterior median line; the top-right point is projected on

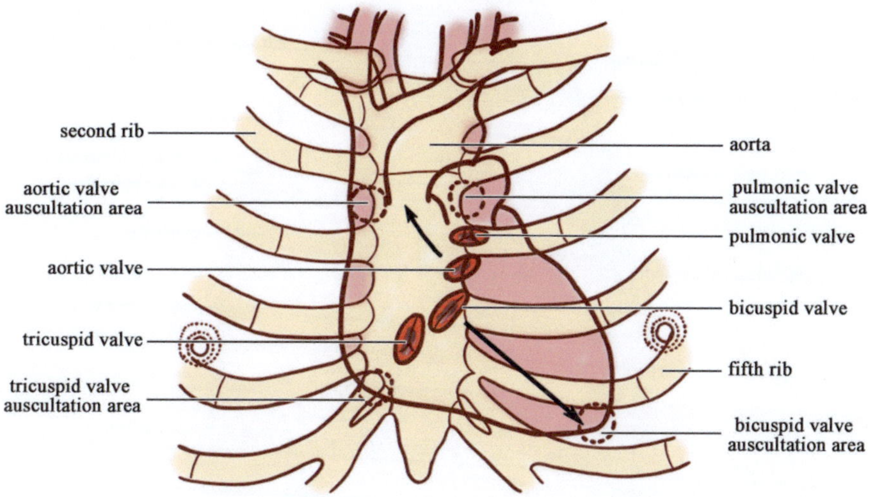

Fig. 8.11 Surface projections of the heart

the superior border of the third right costal cartilage, 1.0 cm away from the sternum; the bottom-right point is projected at the sixth right sternocostal joint. The surface projections of the heart valves differ with sites for heart auscultation (Fig. 8.11).

Phrenic Nerve

The phrenic nerve enters the thoracic cavity through the superior thoracic aperture (or thoracic inlet). The left phrenic nerve descends between the left common carotid artery and left subclavian artery and passes in front of the aortic arch. The right phrenic nerve descends along the right side of the right brachiocephalic vein and superior vena cava. Both the left and right phrenic nerves travel anteriorly to the root of the lung, pass between the mediastinal pleura and pericardium, and descend to the diaphragm. The phrenic nerve supplies motor fibers to the diaphragm and sensory fibers to the pleura, pericardium, diaphragm, and peritoneum below the diaphragm. Sensory fibers of the right phrenic nerve also provide innervations to the liver, gallbladder, and common bile duct.

Posterior Mediastinum

The posterior mediastinum is situated posterior to the pericardium and anterior to the 5th to 12th thoracic vertebrae (T5–T12), mainly containing the thoracic part of esophagus, thoracic aorta, thoracic duct, azygos vein, hemiazygos vein and accessory hemiazygos vein, and thoracic sympathetic trunk (Figs. 8.7, 8.8, 8.9, 8.12, 8.13, 8.14, 8.15, and 8.16).

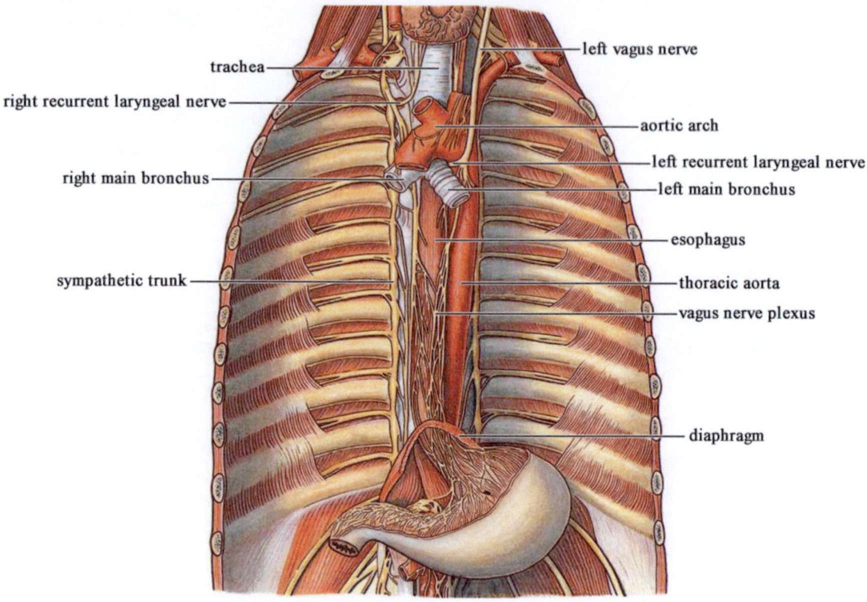

Fig. 8.12 Contents in the posterior mediastinum

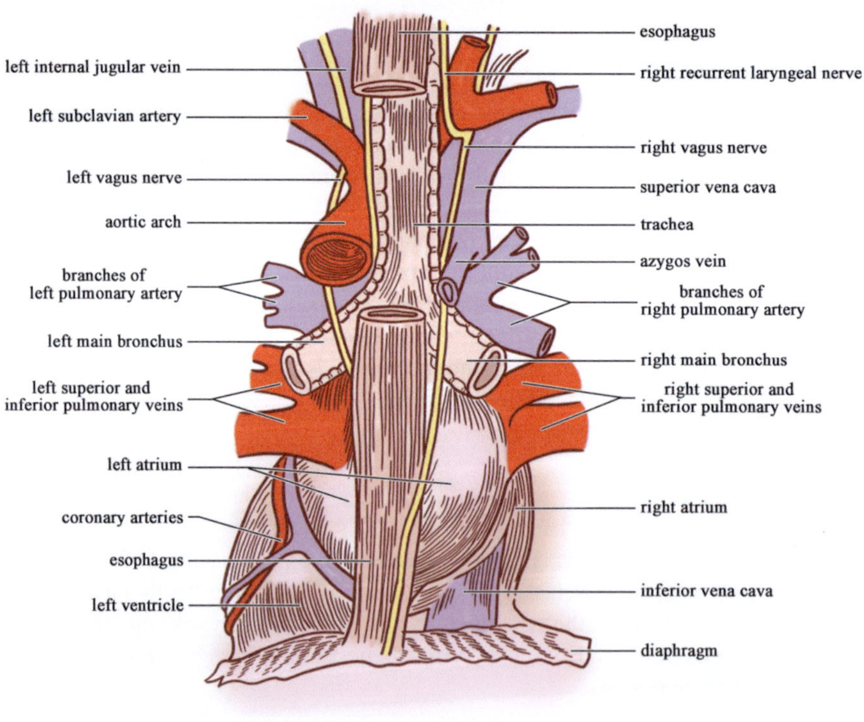

Fig. 8.13 The heart in a posterior view

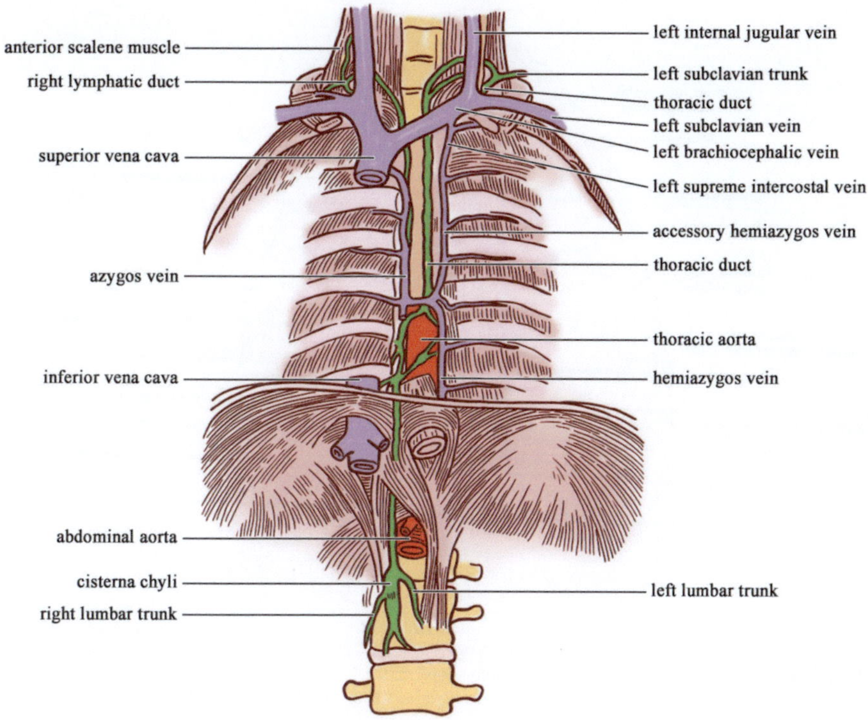

Fig. 8.14 Thoracic duct and azygos vein

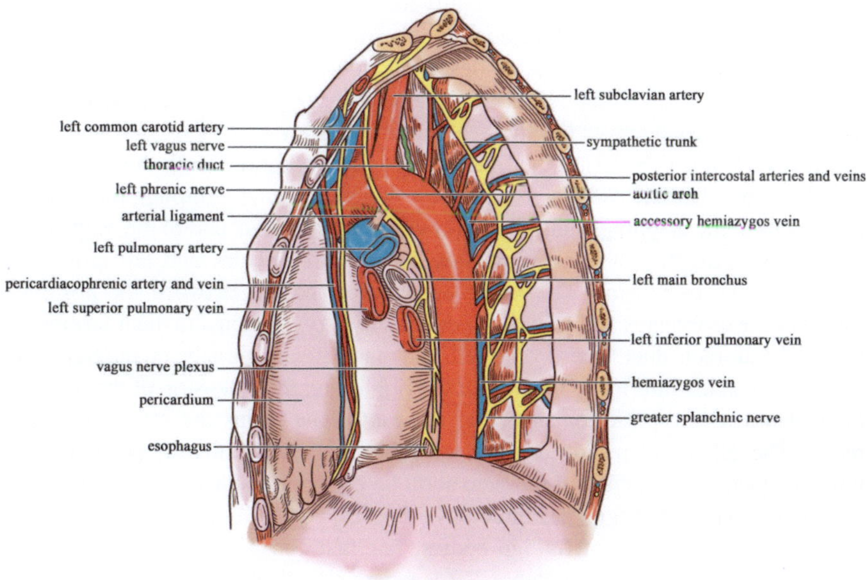

Fig. 8.15 The mediastinum in the left-side view

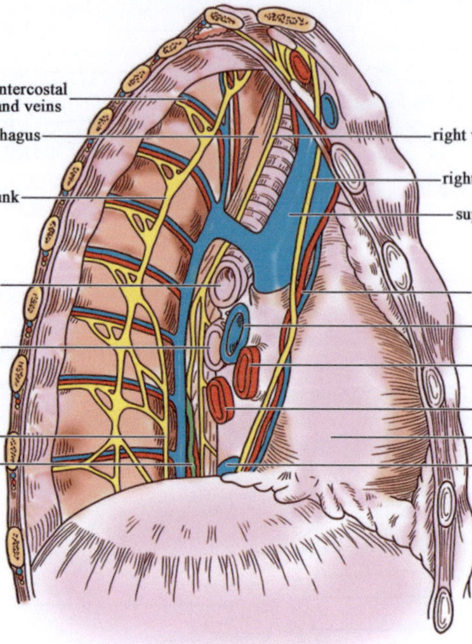

Fig. 8.16 The mediastinum in the right-side view

Thoracic Esophagus

The thoracic esophagus is situated slightly left to the midline, between the trachea and spine in the superior mediastinum. On the right side of the final section of the aortic arch, the thoracic esophagus descends along the right side of the thoracic aorta, gradually turns to the left at the level of the seventh thoracic vertebra (T7), and obliquely crosses over the thoracic aorta at the level of the eighth and ninth thoracic vertebrae (T8–T9) to the front left. At the level of the tenth thoracic vertebra (T10), the thoracic esophagus enters the abdominal cavity through the esophageal hiatus of the diaphragm and continues with the abdominal part of the esophagus.

From superior to inferior, the trachea, left main bronchus, and left atrium lie anterior to the esophagus. The retroesophageal space lies between the posterior aspect of the esophagus and spine and contains the azygos vein and the inferior portion of the thoracic duct. The azygos vein and mediastinal pleura lie on the right side of the esophagus. Inferior to the root of the right lung, the extension of the mediastinal pleura to the posterior aspect of the esophagus forms the retroesophageal recess. The left common carotid artery, left subclavian artery, superior portion of the thoracic duct, aortic arch, and thoracic aorta lie on the left side of the retroesophageal recess. The esophagus has three physiological constrictions, as common sites for esophageal retention of foreign bodies. The first constriction is situated at the level of the sixth cervical vertebra (C6), where the pharynx continues with the esophagus; the second is situated posterior to the left main bronchus, at the level of the lower border of the fourth thoracic vertebra (T4); the third is situated at the level of the tenth thoracic vertebra (T10), where the esophagus passes through the diaphragm via the esophageal hiatus.

Thoracic Aorta

The thoracic aorta starts from the aortic arch on the left side of the inferior border of the fourth thoracic vertebra (T4), descends along the left side of the spine, and turns to the anterior aspect of the spine and posterior aspect of the esophagus. At the level of the 12th thoracic vertebra (T12), the thoracic aorta passes through the aortic hiatus of the diaphragm and continues with the abdominal aorta. The superior portion of the left anterior thoracic aorta is covered by the mediastinal pleura, and the esophagus, thoracic duct, and azygos vein lie on the right side of the thoracic aorta. The inferior portion of the thoracic aorta is adjacent to the esophagus, hemiazygos vein, and thoracic duct on the anterior, posterior left, and posterior right side, respectively.

Thoracic Duct

The thoracic duct arises from the cisterna chyli anterior to the first lumbar vertebra (L1), ascends on the posterior right of the abdominal aorta, and enters the posterior mediastinum through aortic hiatus of the diaphragm. Posterior to the esophagus, it ascends along the anterior aspect of the spine on the right side between the thoracic aorta and azygos vein. At the level of the fourth to fifth thoracic vertebrae (T4–T5), the thoracic duct gradually crosses over the midline from the posterior aspect of the thoracic aorta and esophagus to the anterior aspect of the spine on the left side, enters the root of the neck through the superior thoracic inlet, and drains into the left venous angle.

Azygos Vein

The azygos vein originates from the right lumbar ascending vein. It passes behind the right diaphragmatic foot and the right side of the 12th thoracic vertebra and enters the thoracic cavity. It ascends along the right anterior side of the vertebrae behind the esophagus to the 4th thoracic vertebra level, arches forward across the upper part of the right pulmonary root, and then injects into the superior vena cava. Along the way, it collects the blood from the posterior intercostal veins, esophageal veins, and bronchial veins.

Hemiazygos Vein

The hemiazygos vein originates from the left lumbar ascending vein. It ascends along the left anterior side of the vertebrae to the 8th thoracic vertebra level, then crosses to the right side and enters the azygos vein. It collects the blood from the lower part of the left posterior intercostal veins, esophageal veins, and the accessory hemiazygos vein.

Accessory Hemiazygos Vein

The accessory hemiazygos vein descends along the left side of the vertebrae and injects into the hemiazygos vein, or crossing in front of the spine to inject into the azygos vein. It collects the blood from the posterior intercostal veins in the upper part of the left side.

Thoracic Sympathetic Trunk

The thoracic sympathetic trunk is situated on the bilateral sides of the spine, posterolateral to the azygos and hemiazygos veins. It contains 11–12 pairs of thoracic sympathetic ganglia and interganglionic branches. The superior portion of the thoracic sympathetic trunk is situated anterior to the costal head and posterior intercostal vessels, and the inferior portion gradually moves to the medial side. Postganglionic nerve fibers from the first to fifth thoracic ganglia are involved in the formation of the cardiac, pulmonary, and esophageal plexuses. The branches of the sixth to ninth thoracic ganglia contribute to the formation of the greater splanchnic nerve, and the lesser splanchnic nerve derives from the branches of the 10th to 12th thoracic ganglia. Both pass through the diaphragm, enter the abdominal cavity, and terminate on the celiac ganglion and aorticorenal ganglion. Postganglionic nerve fibers of the 8th to 12th thoracic ganglia help to form the celiac plexus.

8.1.3.3 Mediastinal Lymph Nodes

The mediastinal lymph nodes mainly include the anterior mediastinal lymph nodes, posterior mediastinal lymph nodes, and tracheobronchial lymph nodes.

Anterior Mediastinal Lymph Nodes

The anterior mediastinal lymph nodes are situated anterior to the superior vena cava, brachiocephalic vein, aortic arch and its branches, and pericardium. Lymphatic vessels of the anterior pericardium, heart, mediastinal pleura, diaphragm, and liver drain to the anterior mediastinal lymph nodes. The efferent vessels of the anterior mediastinal lymph nodes are involved in the formation of the bronchomediastinal trunk.

Posterior Mediastinal Lymph Nodes

The posterior mediastinal lymph nodes are situated posterior to the pericardium, surrounding the thoracic esophagus and thoracic aorta. Lymphatic vessels of the posterior pericardium, adjacent areas of the thoracic esophagus and thoracic aorta, and liver drain into the posterior mediastinal lymph nodes. The efferent vessels of the posterior mediastinal lymph nodes directly drain into the thoracic duct.

Lymph Nodes of the Trachea, Bronchi, and Lungs

Lymph nodes of the trachea, bronchi, and lungs are situated on both sides of the trachea, surrounding the tracheal bifurcations and main bronchi. Having a large number, they mainly include the paratracheal lymph nodes, superior and inferior tracheobronchial lymph nodes, and bronchopulmonary or hilar lymph nodes. Lymph nodes of the lungs, main bronchi, thoracic trachea, and esophagus drain into them. The efferent vessels anastomose those of the anterior mediastinal lymph nodes to form the left and right bronchomediastinal trunks, which drain into the thoracic duct and right lymphatic duct, respectively.

8.1.3.4 Lateral View of the Mediastinum

Left-Side View

The root of the left lung lies in the middle part of the mediastinum on the left side. A bulge is formed by the pericardium on the anteroinferior part of the root of the left lung. The arc-shaped aortic arch superior to the bulge crosses over the root of the left lung, where the left common carotid artery and left subclavian artery arise. The aortic arch descends posteriorly to the left and continues with the thoracic aorta that is situated posterior to the root of the left lung and pericardium. The left sympathetic trunk and greater splanchnic nerve are situated posterior to the thoracic aorta. The thoracic duct and the superior portion of the esophagus lie posterior to the left subclavian artery, and the inferior portion of the esophagus lies between the inferior half of the pericardium and thoracic aorta. The left vagus nerve descends anterior from the aortic arch on the left side, passes through the posterior aspect of the root of the left lung, and reaches the anterior aspect of the esophagus. The phrenic nerve and pericardiophrenic artery and vein descend from the anterior aspect of the aortic arch on the left side, pass through the anterior aspect of the root of the left lung, travel along the pericardium, and reach the diaphragm (Fig. 8.15).

Right-Side View

The root of the right lung lies in the middle part of the mediastinum on the right side. A bulge is formed by the pericardium on the anteroinferior part of the root of the right lung, which is smaller than that on the left side. Superior to the bulge, the superior vena cava and the right brachiocephalic vein lie at the level of the sternoclavicular joint. The inferior vena cava lies inferior to the posterior border of the bulge. The right phrenic nerve and the pericardiophrenic artery and vein can be observed on the right side of the superior vena cava and pericardium, anterior to the root of the right lung. The esophagus, azygos vein, right sympathetic trunk, and greater splanchnic nerve are situated posterior to the root of the right lung; the right brachiocephalic vein, arch of the azygos vein, superior vena cava, trachea, and esophagus are found superior; and the inferior vena cava lies inferior (Fig. 8.16).

8.1.4 *Anatomy of the Thoracic Cavity*

8.1.4.1 Objective

Learn the structures and arrangements of the root and hilum of the lung, lines of pleural reflection, surface projections of the lung, and major contents in the mediastinum and its surrounding structures

8.1.4.2 Dissection Procedures

Cut Open the Anterior Wall of the Thoracic and Abdominal Cavities and Observe the Structures in the Inner Side of the Thoracic Cavity

Step 1. Cut open the soft tissues in each intercostal space sequentially along the lateral third of the clavicle to the midaxillary line and downward to the iliac crest. Insert the fingers into the skin incision to separate the parietal pleura and expose the cut ribs. Note that the cutting point of the first rib must be medial to the insertion of the scalenus anterior muscle.

Step 2. Cut off the clavicle with a hand saw or dissociate the sternoclavicular joint. Then cut off the subclavian muscle attached to the medial half of the clavicle and the ribs in sequence using the rib scissors.

Step 3. Cut open the abdominal muscles without damaging the peritoneum.

Step 4. Cut off the sternohyoid and sternothyroid muscles superior to the sternum, bluntly separate the soft tissues posterior to the sternum, and cut off the intrathoracic blood vessels near the manubrium.

Step 5. Raise up the anterior wall of the thoracic cavity and separate the parietal pleura at the meantime. Keep the parietal pleura intact.

Step 6. Bluntly dissect the origin of the diaphragm at the costal arch.

Step 7. Separate the parietal peritoneum and keep the umbilicus on the peritoneum.

Step 8. Remove the thin layer of intrathoracic fascia on the inner surface of the anterior wall of the thoracic cavity, and observe the innermost intercostal muscles, transversus thoracis muscle, internal thoracic artery and vein, and lymph nodes of the anterior thoracic cavity. The innermost intercostal muscles are only situated on the central part of the intercostal space, and their muscle fibers course as the same as the internal intercostal muscles. They can cross by one or more intercostal spaces. The transversus thoracis muscle originates from the posterior aspect of the inferior body of the sternum and inserts into the posterior aspect of the third to sixth ribs. It has four bundles of muscular fiber that diverge radially. Cut apart the transversus thoracis muscle along the course of the internal thoracic artery and vein until they continue as the superior epigastric and musculophrenic arteries. Observe the anterior intercostal arteries and perforators within the intercostal spaces (Fig. 8.17). There are one to two parasternal lymph nodes around the intrathoracic blood vessels anterior to each intercostal space.

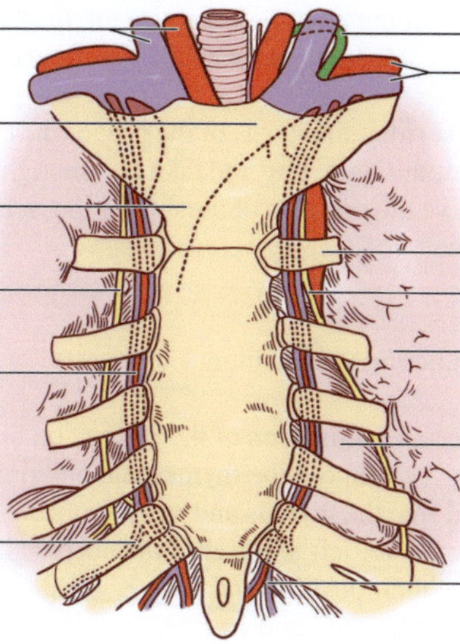

Fig. 8.17 Thoracic vessels

Dissection of the Pleura, Pleural Cavity, and Lungs

Step 1. Cut open the costal pleura along the midclavicular line 3.0–4.0 cm long and insert the knife handle into the pleural cavity. Explore the anterior and inferior lines of pleural reflections and observe their position and relationship with landmarks.

Step 2. Delineate the superior and inferior pleural spaces, and observe their position and size.

Step 3. Measure the distance from the left margin of the sternum to intrathoracic blood vessels at the fourth to fifth left intercostal space. Observe the pericardial triangle and think about the site for intracardiac injections.

Step 4. Extend the pleural incision longitudinally, and observe the distribution of the diaphragmatic, mediastinal, costal, and pulmonary pleurae. Insert your fingers into the pleural cavity to explore the cupula of the pleura upward, and localize its position and surface projection. Explore the costodiaphragmatic recess downward, and observe its position, formation, and shape.

Step 5. Pull the anterior portion of the lung outward with your hands to expose the root of the lung and the inferior pulmonary ligament, and observe the surrounding structures of the pulmonary ligament.

Step 6. Observe the position and shape of the lungs within the pleural cavity, and localize the surface projections of the anterior and inferior portions of the lung, apex of the lung, oblique fissure, and horizontal fissure.

Step 7. Expose the root of the lung by tearing off the pleura around it using a forceps. Expose the pulmonary artery, superior and inferior pulmonary veins, main bronchi, and lymph nodes. Be careful to protect the aortic arch and arch of the azygos vein that cross over the left and right main bronchi.

Step 8. Observe the components of the root of the lung and their position and arrangement, and compare the arrangement differences in the root of the left and right lungs.

Step 9. Explore the surrounding areas of the root of the right lung using your hands. Cut off the root of the right lung and take out the right lung while the left lung is preserved. Observe the contents of the root of the right lung at the hilum, and put them back in situ.

Dissection of the Superior Mediastinum

Step 1. Separate the anterior portion of the pleurae on both sides of the midline and push them laterally to expose the thymus and anterior mediastinal lymph nodes.

Step 2. Observe and free the thymus and anterior mediastinal lymph nodes. Expose the right phrenic nerve, left and right brachiocephalic veins, and superior vena cava, and observe their position and course.

Step 3. Expose the aortic arch and its branches, left phrenic nerve, and left vagus nerve deeply on the left side of the superior vena cava, and observe their location and course. Observe the boundary and contents of the triangle of ductus arteriosus.

Step 4. Separate the trachea and bronchi on the deep side between the branches of the aortic arch, and observe the paratracheal and tracheobronchial lymph nodes. Identify the right vagus nerve on the right side of the trachea.

Step 5. Organize the revealed structures in the superior mediastinum and restore their original anatomical relationships. Observe the structures in each layer of the superior mediastinum and their anatomical relationships. Note that the esophagus and superior portion of the thoracic duct are left to be removed during the dissection of the posterior mediastinum.

Dissection of the Inferior Mediastinum

Step 1. Expose the anterior and lateral sides of the pericardium. Identify the pericardiophrenic vessels and phrenic nerves on both sides, and observe their positions and courses.

Step 2. Anterior to the pericardium, pericardiophrenic vessels, and phrenic nerves and 1.5 cm above the diaphragm, make an inverted V-shaped incision using a scalpel toward the root of the aorta. Cut open the anterior wall of the pericardium, and insert your fingers into the pericardial cavity to check the parietal and visceral serous pericardium and their extensions. Observe the shape of the heart on the sternocostal surface and the position of the transverse, oblique, and antero-inferior sinuses of the pericardium. Do not dissect the heart.

Step 3. Remove the right lung and observe the distribution of the right mediastinal pleura. Explore the presence or absence of the retroesophageal recess with your fingers.

Step 4. Tear off part of the mediastinal pleura on the right side of the mediastinum, inferior to the root of the right lung, and push the esophagus to the left side. Identify the thoracic duct running between the azygos vein and the thoracic aorta, and trace the position and course of the superior portion of the thoracic duct upward. Be careful to dissect the thoracic duct due to the thin wall.

Step 5. Expose the structures around the left lung and turn it inward and upward. Tear off the mediastinal pleura posterior to the root of the lung to expose the thoracic aorta and the anterior esophagus on the right side. Observe the anatomical relationship between the thoracic aorta and esophagus, and separate them below the root of the left lung. Identify the esophageal and bronchial branches, and observe the number and origin.

Step 6. Trace the thoracic part of esophagus. Observe the adjacent relationship of the thoracic part of esophagus with the left main bronchus, left atrium, and retroesophageal recess.

Step 7. Free a small part of the pleura on the lateral side of the thoracic vertebrae. Expose the posterior intercostal arteries and veins, intercostal nerves, sympathetic trunks, and the greater and lesser visceral nerves, and observe their position and course. The first and second posterior intercostal arteries originate from the superior intercostal artery, a branch of the costocervical trunk. The remaining posterior intercostal arteries and subcostal arteries originate from the posterior wall of the thoracic aorta. Trace the posterior intercostal arteries and observe the course of its main trunk and branches arise from the surrounding area of the costal angles. The uppermost two to three pairs of posterior intercostal veins drain into the ipsilateral brachiocephalic vein, and the remaining drain into the azygos venous system. Observe the course of the azygos vein, and trace the reflux of the hemiazygos and accessory azygos veins. Observe the course of the intercostal nerves and their relationship with the posterior intercostal vessels. Expose the sympathetic trunks on both sides. Observe the number of the thoracic sympathetic ganglia (paravertebral ganglia) on each side, the gray and white communicating branches between the sympathetic trunk and intercostal nerves, and the origin and course of the greater and lesser visceral nerves.

8.1.5 Summary

The thoracic cavity is surrounded by the thoracic wall and diaphragm. The dome of the diaphragm inferiorly protrudes toward the thoracic cavity, and the apex of the lung superiorly connects with the neck via the superior thoracic inlet. As a result, the shape and volume of the thoracic cavity are inconsistent with those of the bony thorax. The heart and lungs are the most important organs in the thoracic cavity, and the pleural cavity and mediastinum are the major structures inside.

The pleural cavity is surrounded by the pleura. Each part of the parietal pleura extends to its subdivisions, forming the pleural recesses. Among them, the costodiaphragmatic recess is the largest pleural recess that lies lowermost. The bottom of the costodiaphragmatic recess is situated posterior to the costal arch. Therefore, the costal arch can be cut off during the upper abdominal surgery to prevent the damage to the pleura. The lowermost part behind the costodiaphragmatic recess is inferior to the level of the 12th costovertebral joint and contacts with the diaphragm to separate from the kidneys. Hence, the pleura should be protected during renal surgeries. Pleural effusions first build up in the costodiaphragmatic recess, which is the optimal site for drainage.

The mediastinum is surrounded by loose connective and adipose tissues and contains a group of structures between the left and right mediastinal pleurae. It is divided into the left and right pleural cavities. The major contents in the mediastinum include the heart, great vessels of the heart, trachea, and esophagus. Areolar tissue spaces formed by loose connective tissues laterally communicate with the interstitium via the root of the lung and superiorly connects with the retroesophageal (retropharyngeal space), prevertebral, and pretracheal spaces. Along the surrounding area of the trachea, gas can enter the mediastinum from rupture of alveoli and causes pneumomediastinum. Gas of pneumomediastinum can extend toward the neck, and infections in the neck can spread to the mediastinum.

Surrounding structures of the esophagus are complex and vary greatly in different portions of the esophagus. The esophagus is anteriorly adjacent to the trachea, left main bronchus, aortic arch, pericardium (left atrium), esophageal branches of the vagus nerve, and anterior vagal trunk and posteriorly to the spine, thoracic aorta (inferior to the ninth thoracic vertebra), right posterior intercostal arteries, azygos vein, inferior portion of the thoracic duct, esophageal branches of the vagus nerve, and posterior vagal trunk. It is adjacent to the mediastinal pleura, pleural cavity, and azygos vein on the right side and the final section of the aortic arch, thoracic aorta, superior portion of the thoracic duct, and left recurrent laryngeal nerve on the left side.

The heart is situated in the middle mediastinum and covered by the pericardium. Pericardiophrenic vessels and phrenic nerve lie between the lateral sides of the pericardium and mediastinal pleura. Hiccups occur due to phrenic nerve irritation in patients with acute pericarditis. The anteroinferior sinus of pericardium is situated anteroinferior to the pericardium, where the excessive fluid builds up to cause pericardial effusion. It is the optimal site for pericardiocentesis.

8.2 Clinical Application of Key Anatomical Structures of the Thoracic Cavity

8.2.1 Anatomy of the Sternum and Its Clinical Application

The sternal angle connects with the second costal cartilage on either side, serving as an important landmark for counting ribs (Fig. 8.18). In the normal breathing at rest, the sternal angle is posteriorly corresponded to the spinous process of the fourth thoracic vertebra. The plane of the sternal angle marks the level of a series of features, including the boundary of the superior and inferior mediastinum, junction of the bilateral pleurae approaching to the midline, superior margin of the heart, inferior margin of the aortic arch, tracheal bifurcation and superior portion of the hilum,

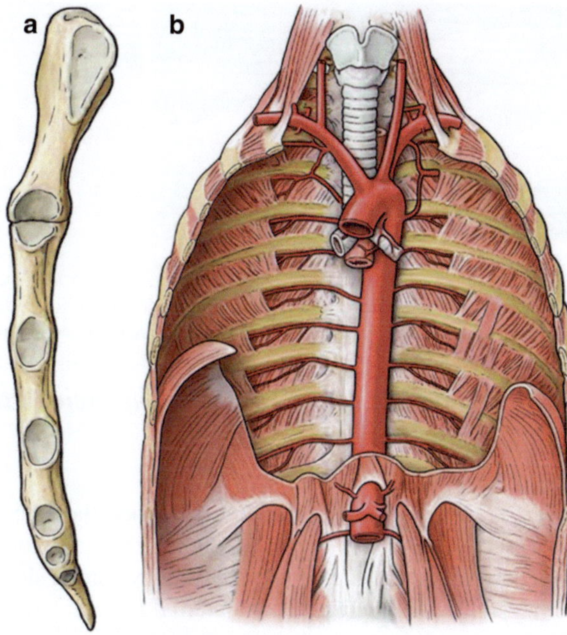

Fig. 8.18 Anatomy of the key structures in the thoracic cavity. (**a**) Left-side view of the sternum. (**b**) Distributions and courses of intercostal arteries

passage of the left main bronchus across the esophagus, and passage of the thoracic duct ascending from right to left. The ventricles are situated deep at the lower third of the body of sternum, where the extracardiac compressions can be performed. Acting as a pump, the sternum moves downward to squeeze the heart and then elastically reset to expand the thoracic cavity, moving by 5.0–6.0 cm on the sagittal plane.

8.2.2 Anatomy of the Ribs and Intercostal Spaces and Its Clinical Application

The costal angle is superficial and palpable and is the optimal site for performing the intercostal nerve block. It lies on the lateral side of the erector spinae and leaves the posterior midline from the superior to inferior thorax. The costal angles of the second and tenth ribs are 6.0 cm and 10.0 cm lateral to the spinous processes, respectively, and those of the remaining ribs lie on the line connecting the above two points. Intercostal vessels and nerves enter the costal groove at the costal angle and run between the internal and innermost intercostal muscles. From superior to inferior, the veins, arteries, and nerves are arranged in the costal groove. The intercostal arteries often branch off near the costal angle and ascend along the superior border of the lower rib (Fig. 8.19). The thoracentesis needle is advanced at the superior border of the lower rib posterior to the costal angle, or in the middle of the intercostal space anterior to the costal angle, thus preventing damages to the intercostal vessels and nerves.

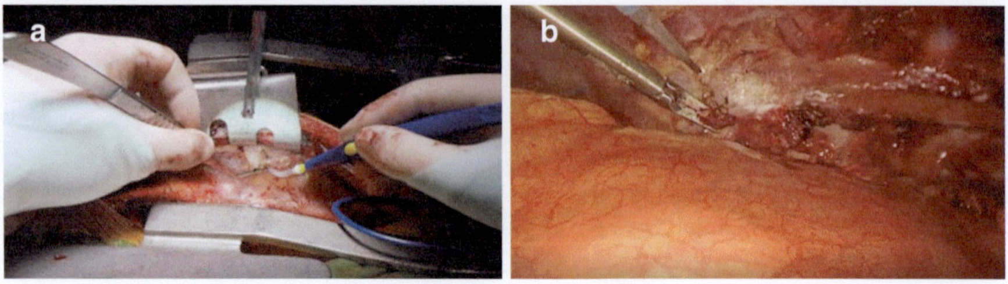

Fig. 8.19 Puncture site for intercostal nerve block. (**a**) A midline incision into the sternum. Free the internal thoracic artery from inside to outside. (**b**) A single left intercostal space incision for minimally invasive surgery. Free the internal thoracic artery from outside to inside

8.2.3 Anatomy of the Internal Thoracic Artery and Its Clinical Application

Along both sides of the sternum, the internal thoracic artery descends posterior to the first to sixth costal cartilages close to the anterior wall of the thoracic cavity, with the distance of 12.0–15.0 mm from the lateral side of the sternum. At the level of the sixth costal cartilage, the internal thoracic artery bifurcates as the superior epigastric and musculophrenic arteries. The transversus thoracis muscle lies between the internal thoracic artery inferior to the third and fourth intercostal spaces and the parietal pleura. Therefore, the transversus thoracis muscle is a landmark for freeing the internal thoracic artery from inside to outside. The internal thoracic artery is exposed only after cutting open the transversus thoracis muscle (Fig. 8.19a). Owing to the protection of the transversus thoracis muscle, dissection of the internal thoracic artery from outside to inside does not cause damages to the pleura and parietal pericardium (Fig. 8.19b). Ligation of the internal thoracic vessels is usually performed within the anterior aspect of the second and third intercostal spaces due to the existence of a space wide enough. The needle insertion site for pericardiocentesis should be close to the sternum, thus preventing damages to the internal thoracic artery (Fig. 8.20).

8.2.4 Anatomy of the Pleura and Its Clinical Application

The anterior boundaries of the lines of pleural reflections approach to each other or overlap in the intermediate portion but leave apart in the inferior portion. An up-pointing triangular space between the lines of pleural reflections on bilateral sides does not cover the pleura, which is known as the pericardial triangle. The anterior aspect of the pericardium lacks the covering of the pleura that directly contacts with the sternum and posterior portion of the costal cartilages, which is known as the bare area of the pericardium. The left xiphocostal angle is the junction of the xiphoid process and left costal arch, serving as a common site for pericardiocentesis

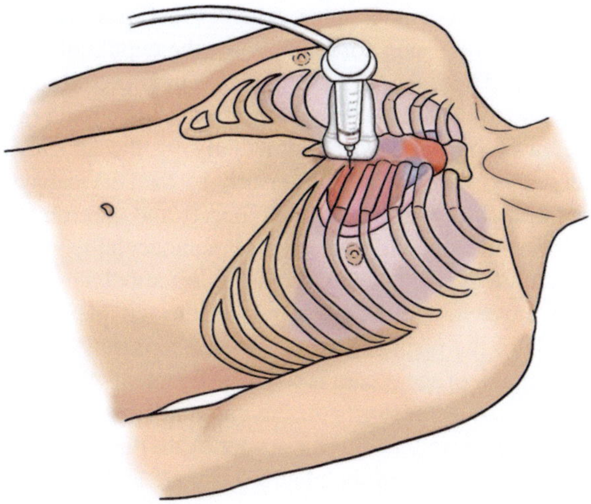

Fig. 8.20 Pericardiocentesis next to the sternum

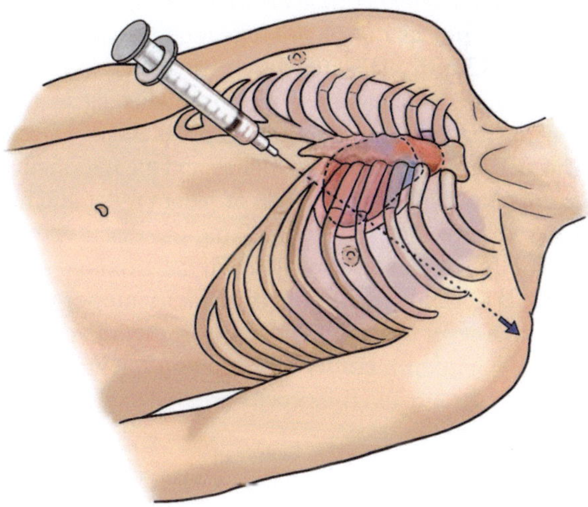

Fig. 8.21 Pericardiocentesis through the approach of the left xiphocostal angle

(Fig. 8.21). The bare area of the pericardium faces the anteroinferior sinus of pericardium and is formed by the extension of the anterior wall of the parietal serous pericardium to the inferior wall above the diaphragm. It is not occupied by the heart either in the systolic phase or the diastolic phase. Serving as the lowermost part of the pericardial cavity, the anteroinferior sinus of pericardium is the optimal site for fluid drainage of pericardial effusion.

The cupula of the pleura protrudes from the superior thoracic inlet and extends to the root of the neck and is prone to injuries and the following pneumothorax due to the complicated adjacent structures and lack of the protection from the thorax. The degree and shape of the cupula of the pleura protruding from the superior thoracic aperture are linked with the shape of the thorax. It becomes cone-shaped with the superior end lying 2.0–4.0 cm above the medial third of the clavicle if the thorax is narrow and long, or spherical and superior to the medial half of the clavicle if the thorax is wide and short. Generally, the cupula of the right pleura is inferior to the left side. The right internal jugular vein is preferred to the left one for catheterization due to decreased risks of injuries to the cupula of the pleura. The cupula of the pleura is surrounded anteromedially by the subclavian artery and vein, phrenic nerve, and vagus nerve; posteriorly by the cervical sympathetic trunk and the anterior branch of the first thoracic nerve; and anterolaterally by the scalene muscles. The brachiocephalic trunk, right brachiocephalic vein, and trachea lie medial to the cupula of the right pleura, and the left subclavian artery and left brachiocephalic vein travel medial to the cupula of the left pleura. Surrounding structures of the cupula of the pleura should be protected during puncture or brachial plexus block. The cupula of the pleura is fixed by ligaments formed by the thickening of the connective tissues posterior to the cupula of the pleura as well as the scalene fascia extending from the anterior aspect of the first thoracic vertebra (T1) to the medial side of the cupula of the pleura. They are cut off during pneumonolysis of the lung apex to disrupt the negative pressure of the pleural cavity, thus collapsing the lung apex from the cupula of the pleura (Fig. 8.22).

The inferior line of pleura reflection presents a close relationship with the kidneys and 12th rib. The kidneys are situated on both sides of the spine, posterior to the peritoneum. They are posteriorly adjacent to the lateral portions of the diaphragm, quadratus lumborum, and psoas major muscles. The 12th rib courses over the superior pole of the right kidney and the intermediate pole of the left kidney. On the dorsal side, the inferior line of pleura reflection intersects the intermediate part of the 12th rib horizontally, making the distal end of the 12th rib inferior to the inferior line of pleura reflection, and the proximal superior end. Therefore, the 12th rib needs to be localized from superior to inferior prior to the surgery, thus preventing a high-level incision to damage the pleura and the following artificial pneumothorax. The inferior border of the lines of pleura reflections at the right xiphocostal angle and the left and right costovertebral angles lie below the inferior border of the

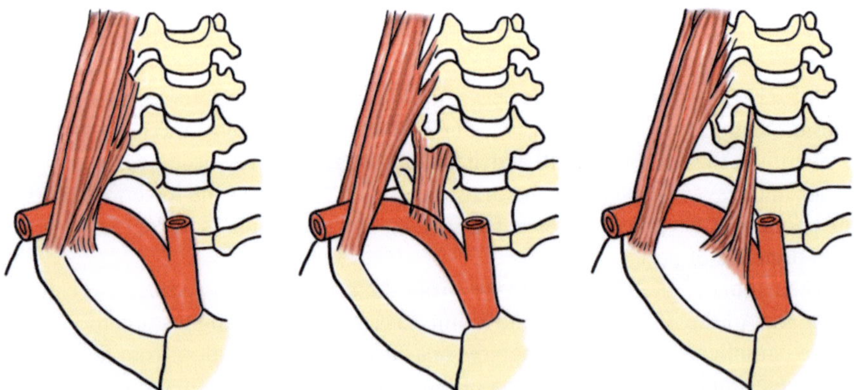

Fig. 8.22 Ligaments that fix the cupula of the pleura

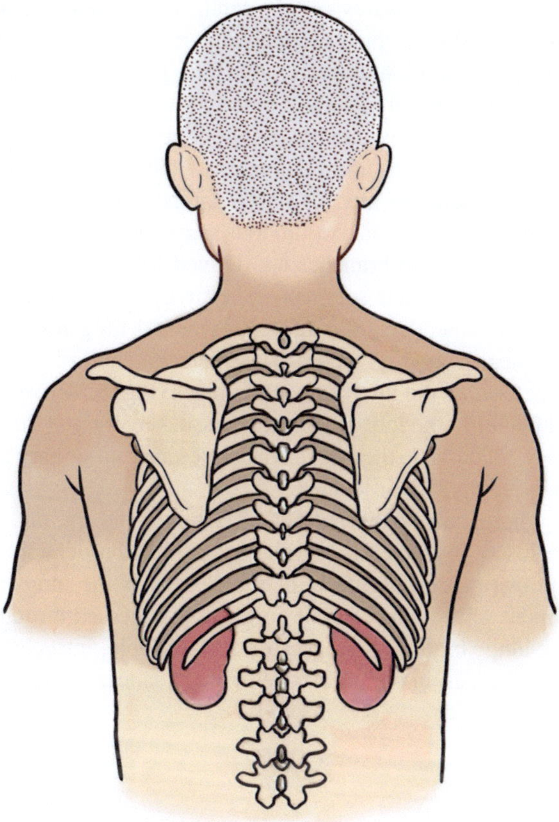

Fig. 8.23 The costovertebral angle

costal arch. Approximately one-third of the population has the right pleura crossing the right xiphocostal angle downward. Therefore, skin incisions inferior to the right costal arch raise the possibility of damaging the right pleura. The costovertebral angle is the angle formed between the inferior border of the 12th rib and 12th thoracic vertebra (T12) (Fig. 8.23). It faces the posterior aspect of the superior pole of the kidney, and as a result, the pleura should be protected during renal surgeries. The costovertebral angle also serves as the lowermost point of the costodiaphragmatic recess, where the excessive fluid accumulates in cases of pathological pleural effusion. The needle can be inserted through the costovertebral angle to drain the fluid.

8.2.5 Anatomy of the Lungs and Its Clinical Application

Lung fissures are double folds of visceral pleura that divide the lungs into lobes. The left lung is divided into upper and lower lobes by an oblique fissure, and the right lung is divided into upper, middle, and lower lobes by oblique and horizontal fissures. Lung fissures vary in depth. The incomplete development of lung fissures results in fusion into lung parenchyma between adjacent lung lobes. During the surgical separation of incomplete lung fissures, passage of aberrant branches of the intrapulmonary bronchi and blood vessels should be concerned. A complete development of lung fissures favors the lobectomy. Lung segments are centered on the segmental bronchi and composed of the corresponding segmental arteries, veins, and lymphatic vessels. The lung parenchyma between lung segments is separated by interlobular septa. An obvious segmental marker is absent on the surface of the lung. Only small branches are derived from the bronchi and pulmonary arteries at the margins of lung segments. The structure and function of lung segments are relatively independent. Therefore, segmental lung resection is performed to remove lung segments (Fig. 8.24a). The intersegmental veins usually serve as the landmark to determine the intersegmental planes (Fig. 8.24b). Separation of the intersegmental planes in the loose connective tissues by tracing the intersegmental veins usually does not damage the large bronchioles and pulmonary arteries, with a low incidence of bleeding and air leakage.

The origin of the pulmonary arteries and the end of the pulmonary veins are enclosed by the pericardium, a section called intrapericardial segments. Intrapericardial segments of the vessels of the lungs are usually long. Therefore, vessels of the lungs can be surgically processed through the pericardial cavity during lung surgeries (Fig. 8.24c). For example, intrapericardial process of vessels of the lungs, as an option in cases of lung cancer with the infiltration of the hilum, can

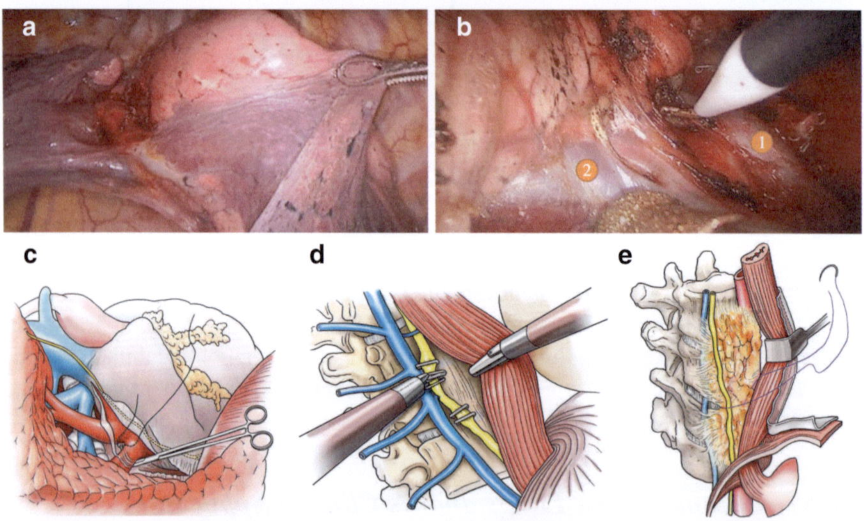

Fig. 8.24 Segmental lung resection. (**a**) Segmental lung resection. (**b**) Segmental lung resection and separation between intersegmental planes (*1*, *2*. intersegmental arteries). (**c**) Surgical process of the pulmonary veins through the pericardial cavity. (**d**) Clamping of the thoracic duct above and below the leakage. (**e**) Ligation of large pieces of tissues above the diaphragm for thoracic duct repair

remarkably increase the surgical resection rate of lung cancer. Briefly, cut open the pericardium 1.0 cm anterior to the phrenic nerve and make an incision upward to the plane above the pulmonary trunk. Then separate the pulmonary arteries and pericardial reflections downward to the plane below the inferior pulmonary vein. The superior and inferior spaces of the pulmonary veins are easy to pass through, which can be processed by vascular sutures circumferentially or a linear cutter. A part of the atrial walls can be removed in cases of lung cancer with infiltration into or obstruction of pulmonary veins, or even the left atrium wall.

8.2.6 Anatomy of the Esophagus and Its Clinical Application

The full-length esophagus varies in diameter. It has three constrictions and two dilations formed due to the anatomical characteristics and influences of adjacent organs. The first constriction lies at the junction of the pharynx and esophagus and is the upper esophageal sphincter formed by the cricopharyngeal muscle and cricoid cartilage encircling the opening of the uppermost esophagus. It usually blocks the passage of the fiberscope. The second constriction, or bronchoaortic constriction, lies at the bronchial bifurcation, where the aortic arch and left main bronchus cross in front. It does not influence swallowing or the passage of the fiberscope. However, a vascular ring encircling the esophagus and trachea formed by congenital abnormally developed aortic arch, or the presence of the right aberrant subclavian artery would cause constriction of the esophagus. The third constriction lies at the esophageal hiatus where the esophagus passes through the diaphragm, and is formed by the circular muscle layer of the abdominal esophagus and the surrounding muscle fibers that constitute the esophageal hiatus. Spasmodic contractions of muscles at the third constriction result in the esophageal achalasia. Two dilations present between three constrictions of the esophagus. The three constrictions are of great physiological significance. In a resting state, the superior and inferior ends of the esophagus, or the first and third constrictions, are closed. The first constriction prevents the air inhaled from the pharynx from entering the esophagus, and the third constriction prevents gastric contents from refluxing into the esophagus. The first and third constrictions of the esophagus are physiological, and the second one is nonfunctional and does not influence the passage of food. The constrictions are common sites for esophageal retention of foreign bodies. The mechanical stimulation of hard food and the corrosive effect of chemicals further cause damages, perforations, and ulcers here or even result in the pathological changes like cicatricial constrictions and diverticular diseases and high risk of malignancies.

The thoracic part of esophagus lacks a distinct outer serosal layer and a clear boundary with the surrounding connective tissues. Due to the close contact with the organs in the mediastinum through connective tissues, esophagus cancer with the involvement of the muscle layer and adventitia is prone to affecting adjacent organs. Most part of the esophagus contacts with the mediastinal pleurae on both sides. The left side of the esophagus contacts with the left mediastinal pleura above the aortic arch, with only the superior portion of the thoracic duct passing through. The contact with the mediastinal pleura disappears from the plane of the aortic arch to that of the seventh thoracic vertebra (T7). Inferior to the plane of T7, the left side of the esophagus is covered by the left mediastinal pleura again. The two parts covered by the left mediastinal pleura are known as the superior and inferior triangles of the esophagus. The superior triangle of the esophagus is bounded by the left subclavian artery, superior portion of the aortic arch, and spine. During the resection of the left cervical esophagus cancer and anastomosis above the aortic arch, the esophagus is lifted up through the superior triangle to pass through the aortic arch. The inferior triangle of the esophagus is bounded by the pericardium, thoracic aorta, and diaphragm. During the resection of the left cervical esophagus cancer, the esophagus is first separated from this triangle after entering the thoracic cavity. Except for the arch of azygos vein, all structures on the right side of the esophagus contact with the right mediastinal pleura and extend to the posterior side of the esophagus to approach or attach to the left mediastinal pleura, forming the meso-esophagus. Therefore, a perforation in the middle or lower part of the esophagus may cause pleural effusion or pneumothorax on the right side. Surgeries for the lower part of the esophagus through the left thoracic approach may damage the right pleural cavity. The esophagus is adjacent to the left atrium below the level of the fifth thoracic vertebra (T5). The enlargement of the left atrium may compress the esophagus. In a barium meal examination, the degree of left atrial enlargement caused by mitral valve stenosis can be observed on X-ray scans. The aortic arch crosses the left wall of the esophagus at the level of the fourth thoracic vertebra (T4) to its left border, and the esophagus lies on the right side of T4. The inferior portion of the thoracic aorta gradually approaches to the midline. The esophagus lies anterior to the thoracic aorta and then turns to the left front. Therefore, a high-level aortic aneurysm can push the esophagus backward, while a low-level aortic aneurysm pushes it to the left. Areolar tissue spaces between the esophagus and trachea in the superior mediastinum is poorly developed or absent, leading to the difficulty in separating the esophagus and trachea in upper esophageal surgery. The retroesophageal space is situated posterior to the esophagus, between the pleura and internal thoracic fascia. A clear boundary on the lateral side of the retroesophageal space is lacked. The retroesophageal space communicates superiorly with the prevertebral fascia of the neck and continues with the retroperitoneal space through the crus of diaphragm. Areolar tissues are rich in the retroesophageal space, which are conductive to the swallowing function of the esophagus. However, the infection of retroesophageal abscess or fluid easily spreads to nearby structures. The lymphatic drainage of the esophagus arises from the lymphatic network in the esophageal submucosa and drains into the lymph node groups around the esophagus, presenting an extensive connection with the lymph nodes adjacent to the trachea. The collecting lymph channels of the esophagus are segmentally distributed and drain into different regional lymph nodes. However, a small number of them directly drain into the thoracic duct without passing through regional lymph nodes. Clinically, esophagus cancer cells are able to directly metastasize to the thoracic duct without infiltrating regional lymph nodes and further spread to distant organs through the bloodstream, resulting in the rapid metastasis.

8.2.7 Anatomy of the Thoracic Duct and Its Clinical Application

The inferior portion of the thoracic duct is adjacent to the right mediastinal pleura. Superior to the level of the fifth thoracic vertebra (T5), the ascending thoracic duct on the left side of the esophagus attaches to the left mediastinal pleura. Therefore, damages to the inferior portion of the thoracic duct may cause chylothorax on the right side, and those to the superior portion cause chylothorax on the left side. The full-length thoracic duct accompanies with the esophagus. Abundant areolar tissues exist between the inferior portion of the thoracic duct and esophagus. However, they approach to each other at the level of the aortic arch due to the less areolar tissues, where the risk of thoracic duct injuries is high in surgeries for the esophagus. In cases of thoracic duct injuries that can be visualized by naked eyes, the thoracic duct can be directly clamped above and below the leakage if present (Fig. 8.24d); otherwise, a large pierce of tissue around the esophagus, spine, pericardium, and aorta can be clamped above the diaphragm (Fig. 8.24e). The thoracic duct not only collects the efferent of lymph nodes of the thoracic cavity but also forms a plexus of lymphatic vessels through lymph node groups and lymphatic vessels they connect. Extensive collateral lymphatic anastomoses exist between the branches of the thoracic duct or between the thoracic duct and the right lymphatic duct. Communicating anastomoses of the thoracic duct with the azygos and intercostal veins are also observed. Ligation of the thoracic duct at any site generally would not cause serious lymphatic stasis. The structure of the thoracic duct is similar to that of a vein, the wall of which is also divided into the intima, media, and adventitia. However, it has a thinner wall with a boundary blurred between two layers. The intima of the thoracic duct protrudes into the lumen to form a valve, which is more common at the venous angle where the thoracic duct drains into. There are also two valves to prevent the flow of venous blood into the thoracic duct. Suture repair of the damaged thoracic duct is difficult due to its unique anatomical structures. In case of venous congestion, the increased venous pressure causes the dilation of the thoracic duct, due to the valve regurgitation and obstructed lymphatic reflux, which may even cause chylothorax or chyloabdomen. There are no valves in the lymphatic vessels that drain into the thoracic duct. The obstruction of the thoracic duct therefore results in the lymphatic reflux, through which the inflammatory or tumor cells spread.

8.2.8 Anatomy of the Thoracic Sympathetic Trunk and Its Clinical Application

The sympathetic preganglionic nerve fibers that originate from the upper thoracic spine (first to fifth thoracic vertebrae) enter the sympathetic trunk at the corresponding thoracic segments in the form of white communicating branches. Some fibers ascend in the sympathetic trunk and fuse to travel continuously as the stellate ganglion or other cervical ganglions that provide the sympathetic innervation of the head, neck, and upper limbs. Upper thoracic sympathectomy is currently an effective therapeutic strategy for palmar and craniofacial hyperhidrosis and facial flushing (Fig. 8.25). The Horner's syndrome is the most complication associated with stellate ganglion injuries in the upper thoracic sympathectomy. The stellate ganglion is situated at the level of the transverse process of the seventh cervical vertebra (C7) and neck of the first rib, anterior to the anterior rami of the eighth cervical nerve. The Horner's syndrome can be prevented if the white communicating branches originate from the first thoracic nerve and the sympathetic trunk above it are not cut off. On the lateral side of the upper thoracic sympathetic trunk, there are some nerve fibers that originate from the spinal nerves, travel upward, and combine with the higher spinal nerve (or its extensions of the brachial plexus or intercostal nerve) or sympathetic trunk ganglion. These collateral fibers are mainly situated on the lateral side of the sympathetic trunk above the third thoracic cord. To achieve acceptable surgical outcomes of the upper thoracic sympathectomy, it is recommended to cut off the sympathetic nerve trunk at the level of the second and third ribs and extend the dissection laterally to a minimum of 15 mm.

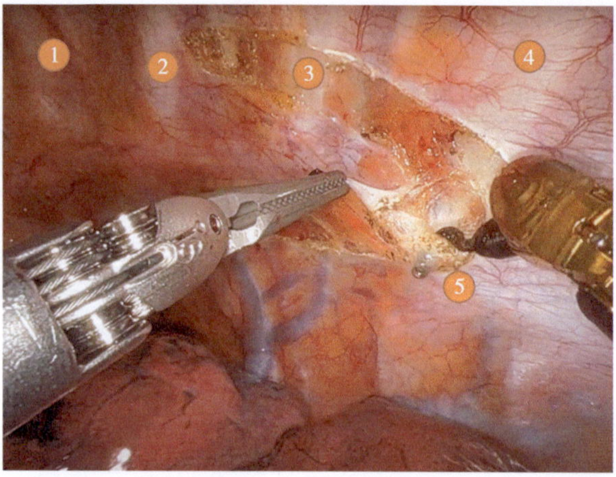

Fig. 8.25 Upper thoracic sympathectomy. *1*. First rib; *2*. second rib; *3*. third rib; *4*. fourth rib; *5*. sympathetic trunk

Chapter 9
Regional Anatomy of the Abdominal Cavity and Its Clinical Application

Jianliang Jin, Hao Xu, Fengyuan Li, and Xiaodong Yang

9.1 Regional Anatomy of the Abdominal Cavity

9.1.1 Summary

9.1.1.1 Boundary

The boundary of the abdominal cavity is inconsistent with the surface area of the abdomen. The abdominal cavity is bounded superiorly by the dome-shaped diaphragm that protrudes into the thoracic cavity, inferiorly by the pelvic inlet that connects to the pelvis, and laterally by the abdominal walls. The dome-shaped roof extends on the left and right sides up to the level of the fourth and fifth intercostal spaces, respectively. The small intestine and other organs in the abdomen usually reside within the lesser pelvis. Therefore, the exact range of the abdominal cavity is much larger than that appears on the abdominal surface.

9.1.1.2 Regions

A total of nine abdominal regions are divided using two horizontal and two vertical lines to help localize, identify, and diagnose abdominal symptoms. Briefly, the upper horizontal line connects the lowest points of the inferior borders of the costal arches on both sides, and the lower horizontal line passes through the anterior superior iliac spines or iliac tubercles on both sides. The two vertical lines pass through the midpoints of the inguinal ligaments on both sides. Consequently, the abdomen

J. Jin (✉) · H. Xu · F. Li · X. Yang
Nanjing Medical University, Nanjing, China
e-mail: jinjianliang@njmu.edu.cn; hxu@njmu.edu.cn; lfyuan@njmu.edu.cn

Q. Ding et al. (eds.), *Clinically Oriented Regional Anatomy*,
https://doi.org/10.1007/978-981-95-9888-5_9

is divided into the left hypochondriac, epigastric, and right hypochondriac regions in the upper abdomen; the left lumbar, umbilical, and right lumbar regions in the middle abdomen; and the left inguinal, hypogastric, and right inguinal regions in the lower abdomen (Fig. 9.1).

The surface projections of major abdominal organs on the anterior abdominal wall are as follows.

The right hypochondriac region contains a larger portion of the right half liver, part of gallbladder, the right colic flexure, and the superior pole of the right kidney.

The epigastric region contains a smaller part of the right half liver and a greater part of the left half liver, the gallbladder, the pylorus, and part of the body of the stomach, a greater part of the duodenum, pancreas, parts of kidneys and adrenal glands, common bile duct, hepatic portal vein, and proper hepatic artery.

The left hypochondriac region contains a smaller portion of the left half liver, the cardia of the stomach, the fundus and a part of the body of the stomach, the tail of pancreas, spleen, left colic flexure, and a part of the left kidney.

The right lumbar region contains the ascending colon, a part of the ileum, and the inferior pole of the right kidney.

The umbilical region contains the greater curvature of the stomach, the transverse colon, the smaller part of the duodenum, part of the jejunum and ileum, left and right ureters, inferior vena cava, and abdominal aorta.

The left lumbar region contains part of the jejunum, the descending colon, and the inferior pole of the left kidney.

The right inguinal region contains the cecum, appendix, and terminal ileum.

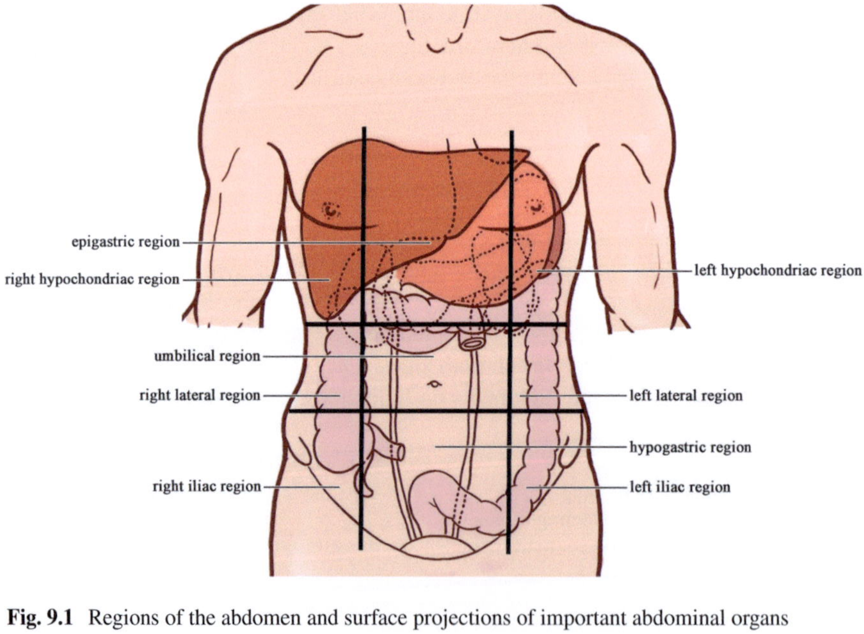

Fig. 9.1 Regions of the abdomen and surface projections of important abdominal organs

The hypogastric region contains part of the small intestine, part of the sigmoid colon, left and right ureters, the full bladder, and uterus during pregnancy.

The left inguinal region contains a larger portion of the sigmoid colon and part of the small intestine.

9.1.2 Peritoneal Cavity

9.1.2.1 Compartments and Spaces of the Peritoneal Cavity

The peritoneum is divided into the visceral and parietal layers, which are continuous with each other. The visceral peritoneum covers the surface of the abdominal organs, while the parietal peritoneum lines the abdominal wall, pelvic wall, and diaphragm. The space between the visceral and the parietal peritoneum is called the peritoneal cavity and is divided into the supracolic and infracolic compartments by the transverse mesocolon. The supracolic compartment contains the liver, gallbladder, spleen, stomach, and the superior part of the duodenum; the infracolic compartment contains the ascending part of the duodenum, jejunum, ileum, cecum, appendix, and colon. The supracolic and infracolic compartments communicate through a narrow gap between the anterior aspect of the greater omentum and anterior abdominal wall. Inflammation can cause in the adherence of the greater omentum to the peritoneum of the anterior abdominal wall, thus isolating the supracolic and infracolic compartments and limiting the spread of inflammation.

Supracolic Compartment

The supracolic compartment, or subphrenic space, is situated between the diaphragm and the transverse mesocolon, which is a common site for subphrenic abscesses. The subphrenic space is further subdivided into the suprahepatic and infrahepatic spaces by the liver.

The compartments of the peritoneal cavity are described as follows (Fig. 9.2).

Suprahepatic Space

The suprahepatic space is situated superior to the liver and inferior to the diaphragm and is divided into the right and left suprahepatic spaces by the longitudinal falciform ligament. The left suprahepatic space is further subdivided into the left anterior and left posterior suprahepatic spaces by the left triangular ligament. The anterior and posterior layers of the right coronary ligament lie posterior to the right lobe of the liver, and its posterior layer is very close to the posterior portion of the liver. Moreover, the right triangular ligament is short in length. The right suprahepatic space is therefore not subdivided. The bare area of the liver, or the subphrenic extraperitoneal space, lies between the two layers of the coronary ligament, inferior

Fig. 9.2 Compartments of the peritoneal cavity in the sagittal plane

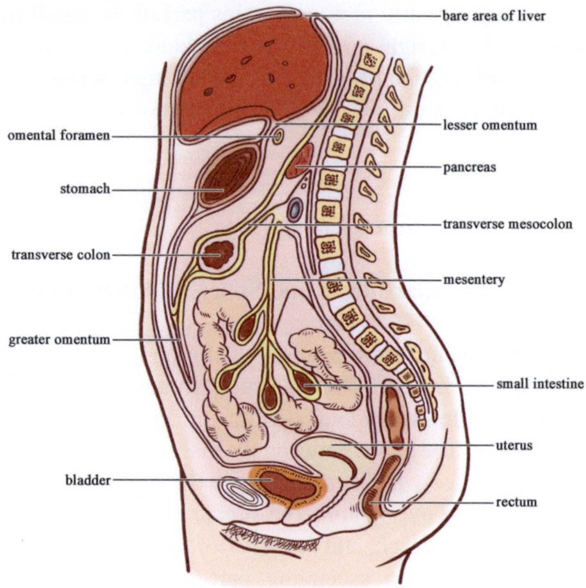

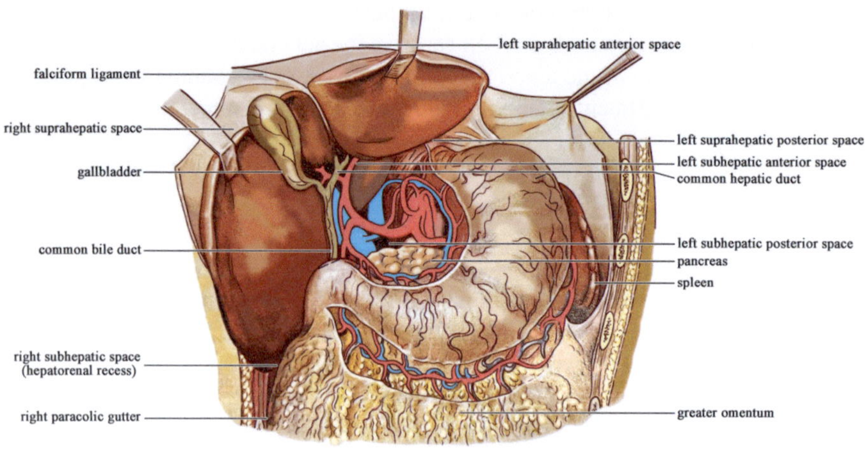

Fig. 9.3 Suprahepatic space

to the diaphragm. Inflections of liver abscesses spread from the bare area of the liver to the thoracic cavity by invading the diaphragm (Fig. 9.3).

Infrahepatic Space

The infrahepatic space is situated between the liver and transverse mesocolon and is divided into the right and left infrahepatic spaces by the round ligament of the liver (or ligamentum teres). The hepatorenal recess is a right infrahepatic space situated between the inferior part of the right lobe of the liver and the superior pole of the right kidney, appearing as the lowermost point of the peritoneal cavity in the supine position. The left infrahepatic space is divided into the left anterior and left posterior infrahepatic spaces (or omental bursa) by the lesser omentum and the stomach (Fig. 9.4).

Boundary of the Omental Bursa

The omental bursa is bounded superiorly by the caudate lobe of the liver and peritoneum inferior to the diaphragm; inferiorly by the fusion of the second and third layers of the greater omentum; anteriorly by the lesser omentum, peritoneum posterior to the stomach, and the anterior two layers of the greater omentum from superior to inferior; and posteriorly by the posterior two layers of the greater omentum, the transverse mesocolon, and the peritoneum covering the pancreas, left kidney, and left adrenal gland from inferior to superior. It is adjacent to the spleen, the gastrosplenic ligament, and the lienorenal ligament on the left side and communicates with the right infrahepatic space and hepatorenal recess through the omental foramen on the right side. In adults, the omental foramen is approximately one to two fingers' breadth in size. It is bounded superiorly by the caudate lobe of the liver, inferiorly by the superior part of the duodenum, anteriorly by the hepatoduodenal ligament, and posteriorly by the peritoneum anteriorly covering the inferior vena cava. Due to the deep location of the omental bursa, gastric contents and blood in cases of posterior perforation of gastric ulcers are limited inside, transferred to the right infrahepatic space through the omental foramen, and leaked downward. Therefore, a diagnosis of posterior perforation of gastric ulcers should be distinguished from other acute abdominal diseases, such as appendicitis (Fig. 9.5).

Seven spaces surround the liver, and an accumulation of infected fluid in these spaces is known as the subphrenic abscess, most frequently in the right suprahepatic space, followed by the right infrahepatic space. Drainage of fluid accumulated in the suprahepatic space is difficult due to its narrowness.

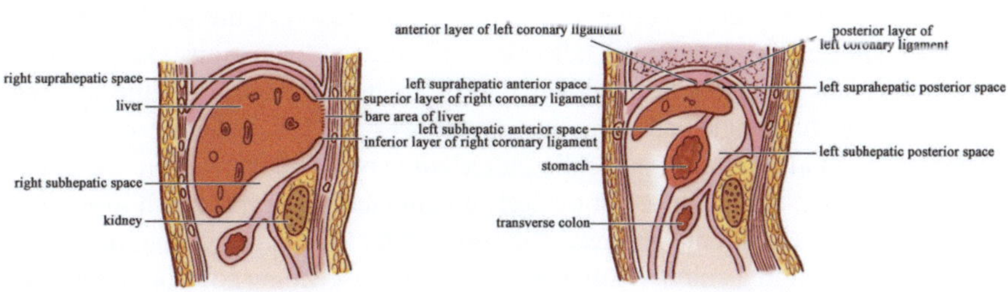

Fig. 9.4 Infrahepatic space

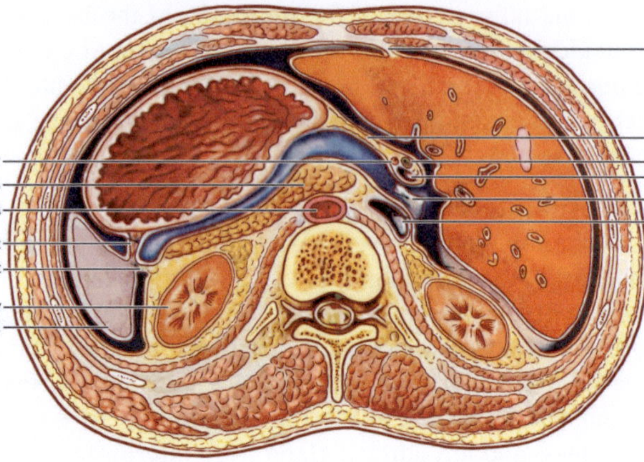

Fig. 9.5 Omental bursa and boundaries of the omental foramen

Infracolic Compartment

The infracolic compartment is a part of the peritoneal cavity situated inferior to the transverse mesocolon. It is further subdivided into the left and right paracolic gutters and the left and right mesenteric sinuses by the root of the mesentery and the ascending and descending colons. The right paracolic gutter, or the lumbar space of the ascending colon, lies on the right side of the ascending colon, serving as an important passageway from the right suprahepatic space and right iliac fossa to the pelvic cavity. In cases of perforated appendicitis, the pus spreads upward through the right paracolic gutter to the right infrahepatic space and hepatorenal recess or right suprahepatic space through the right paracolic gutter or downward to the pelvic cavity with the position changes. Gastric contents, inflammatory exudates, and blood in patients with posterior perforation of gastric ulcers can spread from the omental bursa to the right infrahepatic space and hepatorenal recess through the omental foramen and further to the right iliac fossa and even the pelvic cavity through the right paracolic gutter. The left paracolic gutter, or the lumbar space of the descending colon, lies on the left side of the descending colon. The phrenicocolic ligament is situated inferolateral to the spleen and continues from the left colic flexure to the diaphragm, crossing superiorly over the left paracolic gutter. The accumulated fluid in the left paracolic gutter only spreads downward to the pelvic cavity. Therefore, the incidence of the left subphrenic infection is much lower than that of the right subphrenic abscess. The right mesenteric sinus, or the mesenteric space of the ascending colon, is situated between the ascending colon and right side of the mesentery root. It is almost a closed space containing less fluid. An excessive fluid within the right mesenteric sinus leaks into the left mesenteric sinus through the space between the duodenojejunal flexure and the root of the transverse mesocolon. The left mesenteric sinus, or the mesenteric space of the descending colon, is situated between the descending colon and the left side of the root of the mesentery and inferiorly communicates with the pelvic cavity. The fluid accumulated in the

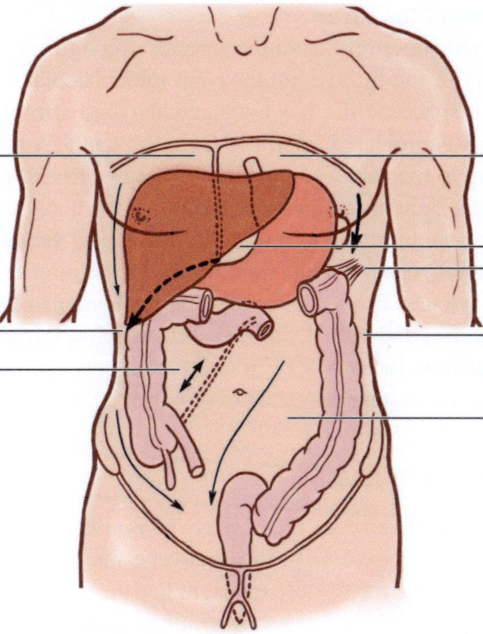

Fig. 9.6 Communications inside the peritoneal cavity

left mesenteric sinus directly leaks into the pelvic cavity, while that in the right mesenteric sinus indirectly leaks into the pelvic cavity through the left mesenteric sinus (Fig. 9.6).

9.1.2.2 Organs in the Peritoneal Cavity

Liver

Location, Surrounding Structures, and Projections

The greater part of the liver is mainly situated in the right hypochondriac and epigastric regions, while the lesser part is situated in the left hypochondriac region. The liver, situated between the left and right costal arches, attaches to the anterior abdominal wall. It is superiorly adjacent to the right costophrenic recess, the base of the right lung, and the inferior border of the heart through the diaphragm. Therefore, liver abscesses can invade the pleural cavity and right lung by penetrating the diaphragm. The visceral surface of the liver is adjacent to the right adrenal gland, right kidney, superior part of the duodenum, right colic flexure, and lesser curvature of the stomach. Therefore, gastric and duodenal ulcers result in adhesions between the stomach wall and duodenum to the visceral surface of the liver.

Surface Projections of the Liver

The liver is projected superiorly from the seventh rib on the right midaxillary line, extending obliquely to the fifth rib on the right midclavicular line. It then turns to the fifth intercostal space on the left midclavicular line after passing through the xiphisternal joint. It is projected inferiorly from the tenth rib on the right midaxillary line, extending to the cartilage junction of the eighth and ninth ribs along the inferior border of the right costal arch and turning to the upper third of the line connecting the xiphisternal joint and umbilicus until it meets the insertion of the superior projection of the liver on the left side. In adults, the inferior border of the liver on the right midclavicular line is above the inferior border of the costal arch, contacting with the anterior abdominal wall 2.0–3.0 cm below the xiphoid process. The liver is larger in relative to body size in childhood, and its inferior border on the right midclavicular line is generally 2.0 cm or closer below the costal arch.

Porta Hepatis and Hepatic Pedicle

The porta hepatis, or transverse fissure of the liver, is situated on the visceral surface of the liver, within the transverse groove between the left and right longitudinal grooves. It allows passage for the left and right hepatic ducts, left and right hepatic portal veins, left and right hepatic arteries, lymphatics, and nerves. The above structures are enclosed by connective tissue to form the hepatic pedicle that runs within the hepatoduodenal ligament. The common hepatic duct and proper hepatic artery sit anterior to the porta hepatis on the right and left side, respectively, and the hepatic portal vein is located posterior to them in the center. From superior to inferior, the junction of the left and right hepatic ducts, hepatic portal vein, and bifurcation of the proper hepatic artery sit within the porta hepatis, with the lowermost point at the level of the cystic duct joining with the common bile duct. The common bile duct is situated on the right side of the hepatoduodenal ligament and proper hepatic artery, right front of the hepatic portal vein. The hepatic portal vein and proper hepatic artery should be protected during the exposure of the common bile duct (Fig. 9.7).

Vessels, Nerves, and Lymphatics of the Liver

Arteries

The proper hepatic artery branches into two arteries near the porta hepatis that supply the liver. In addition, the inferior phrenic artery, left gastric artery, and superior mesenteric artery sometimes branch off arteries that supply the liver as the supplements or alternatives.

Veins

The hepatic portal vein, which serves as the functional blood vessel of the liver, is formed by the confluence of the superior mesenteric and splenic veins posterior to the neck of the pancreas. It travels posteriorly to the common bile duct and proper hepatic artery within the hepatoduodenal ligament, dividing into the left and right branches to supply the venous blood to the left and right lobes of the liver. The

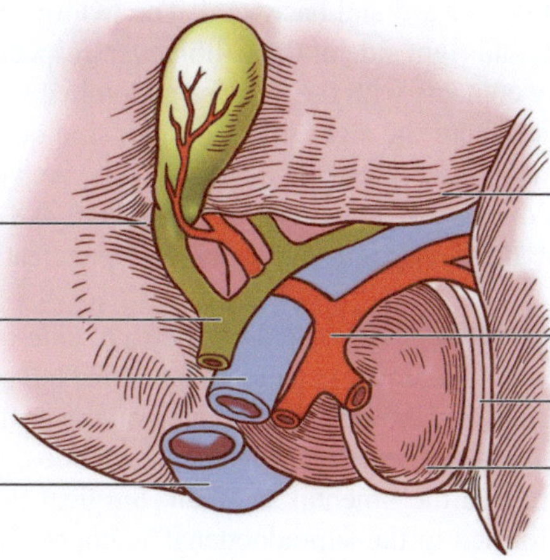

Fig. 9.7 The porta hepatis

hepatic portal vein is usually 6.0–8.0 cm in length and 1.0–1.2 cm in diameter. The left, middle, and right hepatic veins penetrate the parenchyma of the liver superior to the groove for vena cava and drain the venous blood from the liver into the inferior vena cava, which is also known as the second hepatic hilum.

Nerves

The liver is innervated by the celiac plexus and the anterior trunk of the vagus nerve. Nerve fibers of the celiac plexus enclose the innate hepatic artery and hepatic portal vein, forming the hepatic plexus that enters through the porta hepatis into the liver. Sensory fibers of the right phrenic nerve travel downward to provide innervation to the liver.

Lymphatic Vessels

The lymphatic vessels of the liver mainly drain into the hepatic lymph nodes. Those at the porta hepatis are arranged along the proper hepatic artery and finally drain into the abdominal lymph nodes.

Gallbladder and Common Bile Duct

Location, Surrounding Structures, and Projections

The gallbladder is situated within the right anterior longitudinal fissure on the visceral surface of the liver, which is also known as the gallbladder fossa. It superiorly connects to the liver via the loose connective tissue, and both move up and down with breathing. The inferior aspect of the gallbladder is covered by the peritoneum. It needs to be sutured after cholecystectomy to prevent bleeding, bile leakage, and adhesions; this process is known as the suturing of the peritoneum attached on the gallbladder bed. The gallbladder is adjacent to the superior part of the duodenum and transverse colon downward and backward. The pylorus and right colic flexure are located on the left and right side of the gallbladder, respectively. The base of the gallbladder anteriorly contacts with the anterior abdominal wall. The gallbladder is projected to the point where the right midclavicular line or the lateral side of the right rectus abdominis muscle intersects the right costal arch (Fig. 9.8).

The common bile duct is 7.0–8.0 cm in length and 0.6–0.8 cm in diameter and is divided into the supraduodenal, retroduodenal, retropancreatic, and intraduodenal segments.

The supraduodenal segment is situated on the right side of the hepatoduodenal ligament. It is adjacent to the proper hepatic artery on the left side, the hepatic portal vein on the rear left side, and the omental foramen on the posterior side. The posterior wall of the supraduodenal segment of the common bile duct can be accessed by inserting your fingers into the omental foramen. Surgical procedures for the bile duct are usually performed in the supraduodenal segment. The surrounding structures, including the gastroduodenal artery, proper hepatic artery, and right gastric artery, should be carefully protected during the incision of the supraduodenal segment.

The retroduodenal segment is situated posterior to the superior part of the duodenum, traveling downward in front of the inferior vena cava and on the right side of the hepatic portal vein.

The retropancreatic segment usually travels posteriorly to the head of the pancreas, within the groove between the pancreatic head, descending part of the duodenum, and common bile duct. It is covered by a thin layer of the pancreatic tissue. Cancers in the head of the pancreas or chronic pancreatitis that compress the retropancreatic segment of the common bile duct may cause obstructive jaundice.

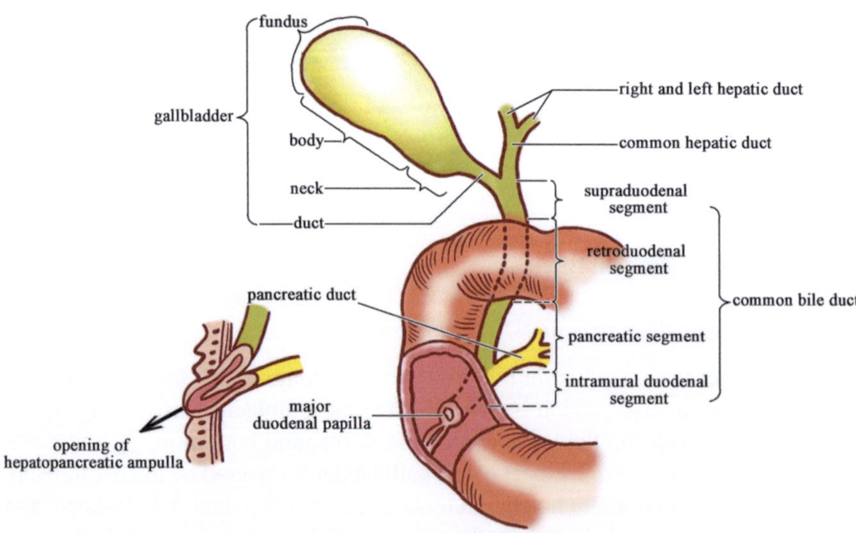

Fig. 9.8 Segments of the common bile duct

The intraduodenal segment is 1.5–2.0 cm long and obliquely travels across the posteromedial wall of the middle part of the descending duodenum. The hepatopancreatic ampulla is formed by the union of the distal end of the intraduodenal segment and pancreatic duct and opens at the major duodenal papilla. The thickening of the annular smooth muscle at the end of the hepatopancreatic ampulla, common bile duct, and main pancreatic duct forms the hepatopancreatic sphincter, or sphincter of Oddi, which regulates the release of bile and pancreatic fluids. Obstruction in the hepatopancreatic ampulla due to stones, tumors, or sphincter of Oddi dysfunction causes obstructive jaundice and acute pancreatitis by inducing the reflux of bile or pancreatic fluids.

Blood Vessels, Nerves, and Lymphatics of the Gallbladder

Arteries

The cystic artery is situated in Calot's triangle, which is bounded by the cystic duct, common hepatic duct, and the visceral surface of the liver. It usually originates from the right hepatic artery (70–80%) or variably from the proper hepatic artery, left hepatic artery, gastroduodenal artery, or a double cystic artery. The variant cystic artery often travels to the gallbladder neck anterior to the common hepatic duct or common bile duct and should be carefully explored during the surgeries for the gallbladder or common bile duct.

Veins

One or two branches of the cystic vein accompany with the cystic artery and drain into the main trunk of the hepatic portal vein or its right branch. Occasionally, a large cystic vein descends parallel to the common bile duct and drains into the superior mesenteric vein and should be concerned during surgeries for the common bile duct.

Lymphatic Vessels and Nerves

The lymphatic vessels of the gallbladder drain into the hepatic lymph nodes. The nerves of the gallbladder often travel along with the arteries and are mainly derived from the hepatic plexus (Fig. 9.9).

Spleen

Location and Surrounding Structures

The spleen is situated deep in the left hypochondriac region, between the fundus of the stomach and diaphragm. It lies superiorly at the level of the 9th rib, inferiorly at the level of the 11th rib, and along the axis of the 10th rib. There are two to three deep splenic notches on the superior portion of the spleen, serving as important landmarks for the palpation. The spleen is not palpable below the costal arch, unless in cases of splenomegaly. An enlarged spleen can be palpable on the right side of the midline or even below the level of the umbilicus (known as the

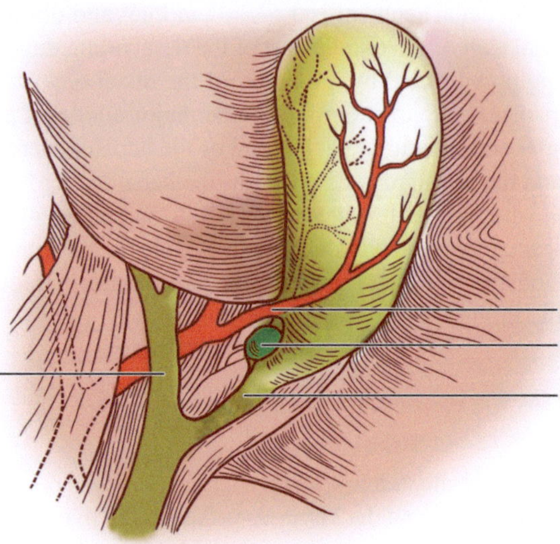

Fig. 9.9 Calot's triangle and cystic artery

megalosplenia). The spleen is lateral to the diaphragm. On the medial side, the splenic hilum, a depression containing blood vessels, lymphatic vessels, and nerves, attaches to the tail of the pancreas. The spleen is inferoposterior to the left adrenal gland and left kidney on the inferoposterior side and inferior to the left colic flexure (Fig. 9.10).

Ligaments of the Spleen

The spleen is an intraperitoneal organ that connects with the surrounding structures through the following four ligaments (Figs. 9.11 and 9.12).

Gastrosplenic Ligament

The gastrosplenic ligament extends between the greater curvature and fundus of stomach and the splenic hilum. It contains the short gastric artery and vein and the left gastroepiploic artery and vein. Protect the stomach, spleen, and blood vessels of them during the ligation of the gastrosplenic ligament.

Splenorenal Ligament

The splenorenal ligament is a posteromedial extension of the peritoneum, extending from the splenic hilum to the anterior aspect of the left kidney. It contains the arteries, veins, lymphatic vessels and nerves of the spleen, and tail of the pancreas. The spleen can only be lifted up after ligating the splenorenal ligament. During splenectomy procedures, the structures within the splenorenal ligament must be carefully protected.

Fig. 9.10 Location of the spleen

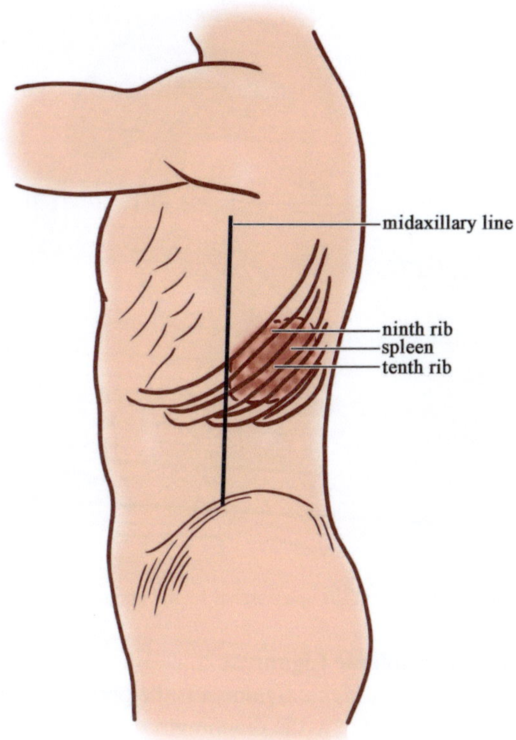

Fig. 9.11 Ligaments of the spleen in the transverse section passing through the splenic hilum

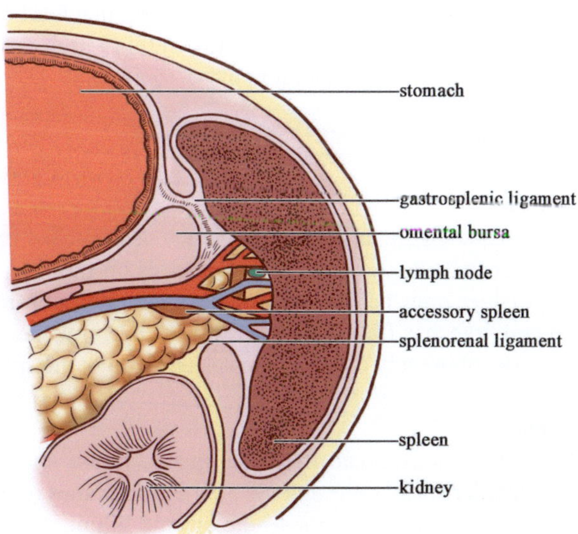

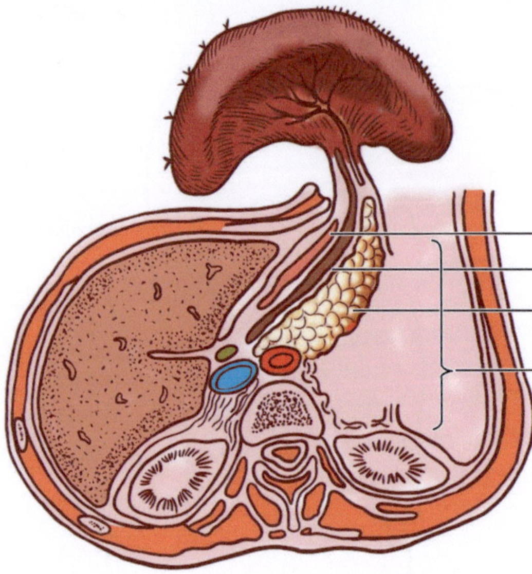

Fig. 9.12 Cut off the splenorenal ligament and lift up the spleen through the incision

Phrenicosplenic Ligament
The phrenicosplenic ligament is the peritoneal fold that connects the posterior border of the spleen to the diaphragm.

Splenocolic Ligament
The splenocolic ligament is a short ligament that lies between the anterior border of the spleen and left colic flexure. Be careful to protect the colon during the ligation of the splenocolic ligament for splenectomy.

Blood Vessels, Nerves, and Lymphatics of the Spleen

Arteries
The splenic artery, as the largest branch of the celiac trunk, travels on the left side, superior to the body of the spleen. It gives off downward branches to the pancreas, two to three branches of posterior gastric arteries upward at the middle segment, and several branches traveling between two layers of the splenorenal ligament on the left side, ultimately reaching the spleen through the splenic hilum.

Veins
Several veins originate from the splenic hilum and drain into the splenic vein, which is larger than the splenic artery. Sometimes, the splenic vein may leave the spleen superior or inferior to the splenic hilum, without passing through it. The splenic vein travels inferiorly to the splenic artery and posteriorly to the body of the pancreas, joins with the superior mesenteric vein, and drains into the hepatic portal vein.

Nerves

The splenic plexus, which accompanies the splenic artery, provides innervation to the spleen.

Lymphatic Vessels

The lymphatic vessels of the spleen drain into the splenic lymph nodes and subsequently into the abdominal lymph nodes.

Stomach

Location, Surrounding Structures, and Projections

When moderately filled, the stomach is mainly situated in the left hypochondriac region, with a smaller portion extending into the epigastric region. The anterior wall of the stomach is adjacent to the diaphragm on the left side and the inferior part of the left lobe of the liver on the right side. The remaining part of the anterior wall contacts the anterior abdominal wall, where the stomach can be palpated. This area is referred to as the free area of the anterior wall of the stomach. Structures adjacent to the posterior wall of the stomach, including the pancreas, left adrenal gland, left kidney, and transverse mesocolon separated by the omental bursa, are known as the stomach bed. The pancreas is adjacent to the posterior wall of the stomach. Therefore, posterior gastric ulcers can adhere to the pancreas and cause penetrating ulcers. The positions of the cardia and pylorus of the stomach are usually constant. The cardia is located on the left side of the 11th thoracic vertebra (T11). The pylorus is situated on the right side of the first lumbar vertebra (L1) or, in some cases, the third lumbar vertebra (L3), approximately 2.0 cm from the midline. A circular groove is present on the surface of the pyloroduodenal junction, through which the prepyloric vein (of Mayo) passes. This groove serves as a landmark for identifying the junction between the stomach and duodenum during surgery. Additionally, the junction can be identified by palpating the pyloric sphincter (Figs. 9.13, 9.14, and 9.15).

Ligaments of the Stomach

The stomach connects to the surrounding structures through a series of ligaments formed by the peritoneum. The hepatogastric ligament and hepatoduodenal ligament connect the lesser curvature of the stomach and the superior part of the duodenum to the porta hepatis. The gastrosplenic ligament sits between the superior part of the greater curvature of the stomach and splenic hilum. The gastrocolic ligament lies between the greater curvature of the stomach and transverse colon, posterior to the transverse mesocolon. Adhesions between the gastrocolic ligament and transverse mesocolon may occur near the pylorus. Therefore, caution should be taken to protect the middle colic artery in the transverse mesocolon during the dissection of the gastrocolic ligament. The gastrophrenic ligament is a peritoneal fold that

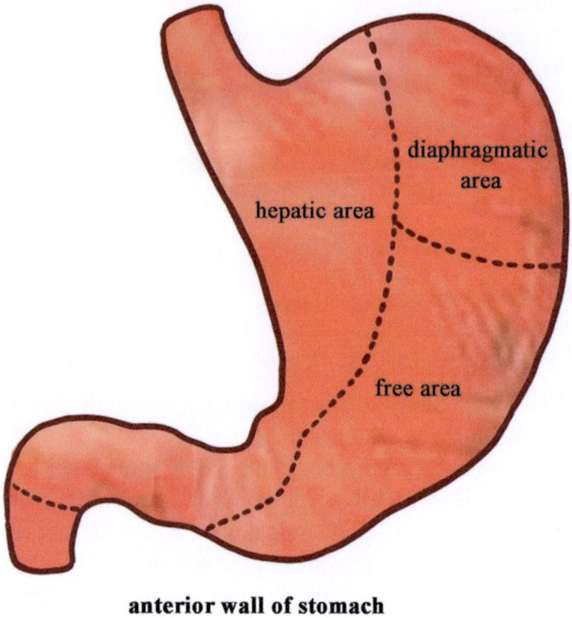

Fig. 9.13 Surrounding structures of the anterior wall of the stomach

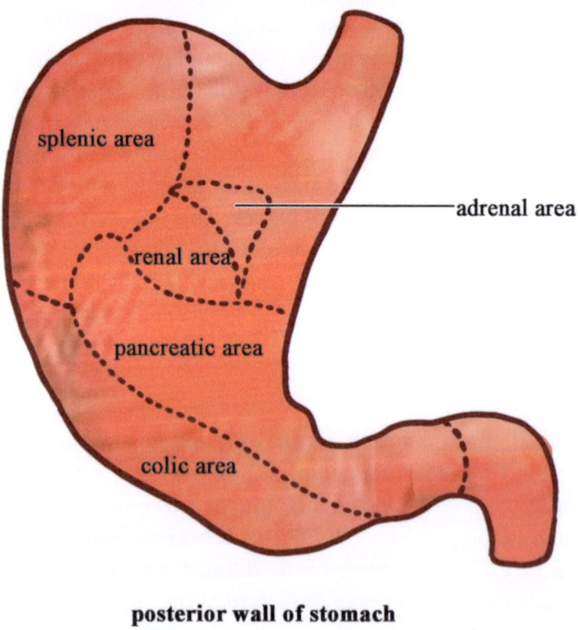

Fig. 9.14 Surrounding structures of the posterior wall of the stomach (stomach bed)

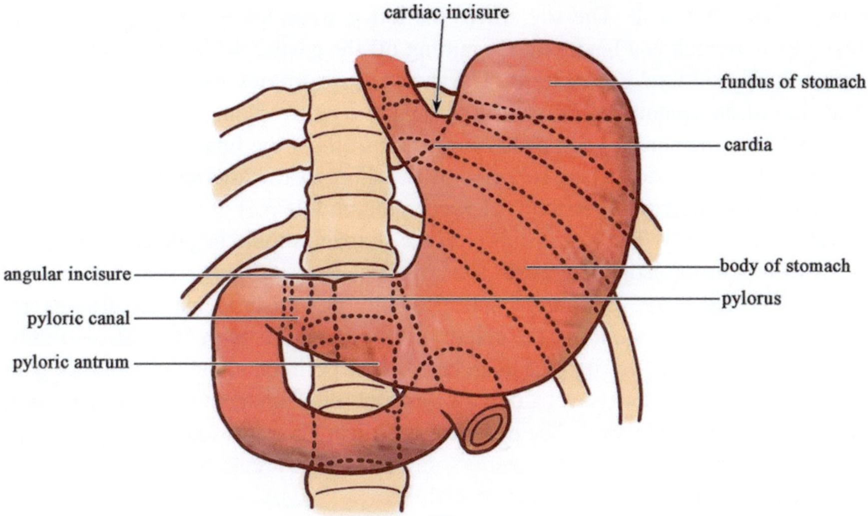

Fig. 9.15 Sections of the stomach and the major structures

connects with the cardia and diaphragm. It needs to be cut before freeing the cardia and esophagus during the total gastrectomy.

Blood Vessels, Nerves, and Lymphatics of the Stomach

Arteries

The arteries supplying the stomach arise from the celiac trunk and its branches, forming two arterial arches along the greater and lesser curvatures of the stomach. They branch off into small arteries that travel to the anterior and posterior walls of the stomach, forming a rich vascular network through anastomoses. Therefore, ligation of a major blood vessel of the stomach would not cause ischemia or necrosis of the gastric wall. The left and right gastric arteries travel between the two layers of the lesser omentum and anastomose with each other to form the arterial arch of the lesser curvature of the stomach. The left gastric artery originates from the celiac trunk and branches off five to six small arteries to the gastric wall. The space between the first two branches serves as the landmark for resecting the gastric wall on the lesser curvature of the stomach during subtotal gastrectomy. Arterial supply to the lesser curvature of the stomach is much denser than that of other parts of the stomach, due to the large left gastric artery with a high arterial pressure and a closer distance between the two ends of the lesser curvature. Gastric ulcers of the lesser curvature usually cause bleeding. The left and right gastroepiploic arteries travel between the first two layers of the greater omentum and anastomose with each other to form a vascular arch. They give off gastric and omental branches at a distance 1.0 to 2.0 cm from the greater curvature of the stomach. The left gastroepiploic artery originates at 2.0–3.5 cm from the splenic hilus and descends through the gastrosplenic ligament. The site where the left gastroepiploic artery gives off the first gastric branch is a landmark for cutting off the gastric wall on the greater curvature during subtotal gastrectomy. The short gastric arteries are three to four small branches of the splenic artery that run through the gastrosplenic ligament. They are distributed in the anterior and posterior gastric walls of the fundus. The lateral and medial sides of the fundus are supplied by the short gastric arteries and branches of the left gastric artery, respectively. However, the middle part of the fundus receives a poor blood supply. The blood supply of the stomach should be preserved as much as possible during esophagogastric anastomosis. The site for anastomoses is cautiously selected to prevent anastomotic leakage. The posterior gastric arteries are two to three small branches of the splenic artery that are seen in 60%–80% of individuals. They ascend through the deep layer of the peritoneum on the posterior wall of the omental bursa and travel along the gastrophrenic ligament to the superior part of the posterior gastric wall. The posterior gastric artery is the main artery that supplies the stomach after subtotal gastrectomy or high gastrectomy, which should be carefully protected during surgical procedures.

Veins

The gastric veins accompany with the arteries and mainly drain into the hepatic portal system. The left gastric vein, or coronary vein, passes to the inferior end of the esophagus and turns to the right to drain into the hepatic portal system. The esophageal branch of the left gastric vein anastomoses the esophageal veins that drain into the azygos vein, forming the portacaval anastomosis. In cases of portal hypertension, the blood flow refluxes from the hepatic portal system to the superior vena cava via the left gastric vein, leading to esophageal and gastric varices and hematemesis or hematochezia in cases of ruptures. The right gastric vein drains into the hepatic portal vein, and the right gastroepiploic vein drains into the superior mesenteric vein. The left gastroepiploic vein, the short gastric veins, and the posterior gastric vein generally drain into the splenic vein (Figs. 9.16 and 9.17).

Lymphatic Vessels

Most lymphatic vessels originating from the gastric wall accompany with the blood vessels of the stomach. Generally, lymphatic vessels of the cardia and lesser curvature of the stomach drain into the left and right gastric lymph nodes. Lymphatic vessels of the greater part of the greater curvature on the right side drain into the right gastroomental and subpyloric lymph nodes. Those on the left side, including the fundus and superior part of the body of the stomach, drain into the left gastroomental and splenic lymph nodes. Lymphatic vessels of the lesser part of the upper half of pylorus drain into the suprapyloric and hepatic lymph nodes.

The efferent lymphatics of the above lymph nodes drains into the celiac lymph nodes, and their efferent lymphatics further form the intestinal trunk and drain into the cisterna chyli. Lymph node metastases of gastric cancer first infiltrate the lymph nodes around the stomach, followed by the invasion of abdominal lymph nodes and organs near the stomach. Advanced gastric cancer can metastasize to the left supraclavicular lymph nodes through the thoracic duct and cause the malignant enlargement (Fig. 9.18).

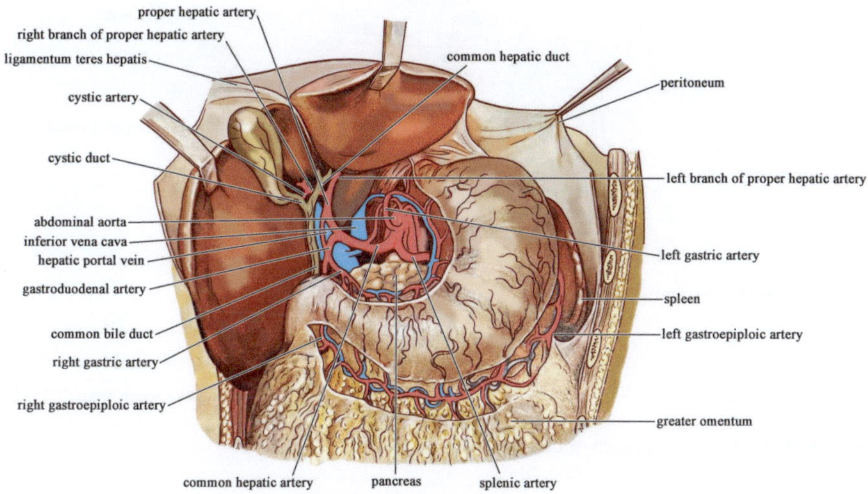

Fig. 9.16 Blood vessels of the stomach in an anterior view

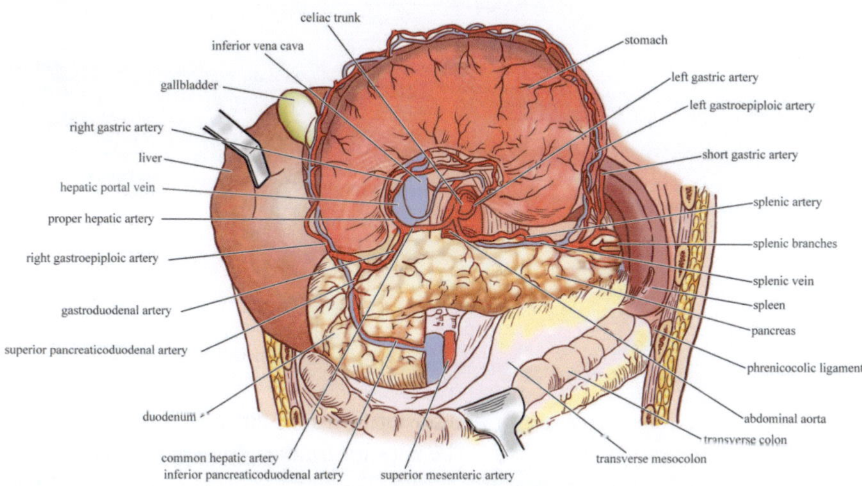

Fig. 9.17 Blood vessels of the stomach in a posterior view

Nerves

The sympathetic nerves of the stomach arise from the sixth to eighth thoracic (T6–T8) spinal cord segments and synapse at the celiac ganglion via the greater splanchnic nerve. The postganglionic fibers from the celiac ganglion are distributed in the stomach alongside the branches of the celiac trunk and are responsible for inhibiting the contraction of smooth muscle in the gastric walls and reducing the secretion of gastric juice (mainly gastric acid and pepsin). The parasympathetic nerves of the stomach arise from the vagus nerve and are responsible for promoting the contraction of smooth muscle and secretion of gastric juice. The

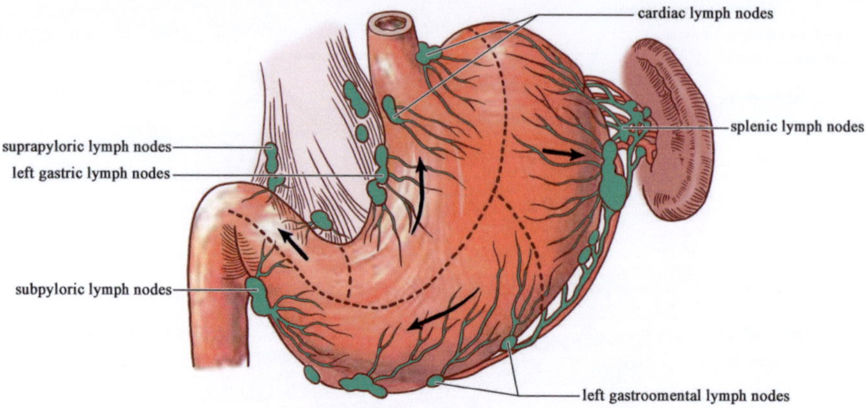

Fig. 9.18 Lymphatic drainage of the stomach

Fig. 9.19 Vagus nerve innervating the stomach

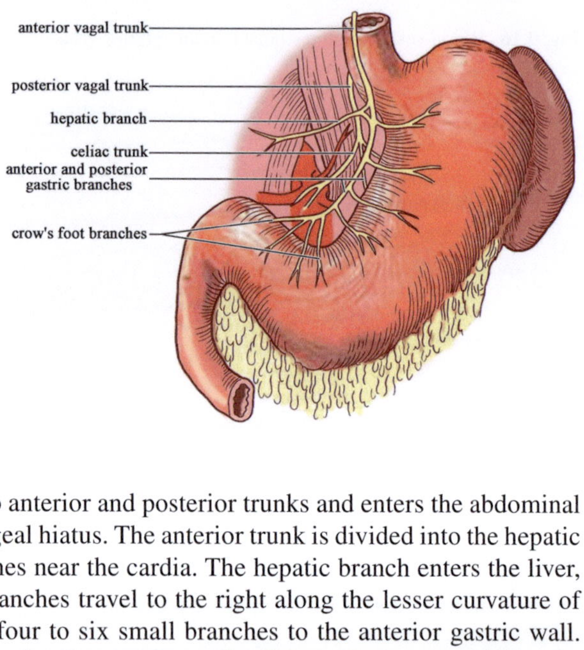

vagus nerve is divided into anterior and posterior trunks and enters the abdominal cavity through the esophageal hiatus. The anterior trunk is divided into the hepatic and anterior gastric branches near the cardia. The hepatic branch enters the liver, and the anterior gastric branches travel to the right along the lesser curvature of the stomach and give off four to six small branches to the anterior gastric wall. The terminal branches supply the anterior wall of the pylorus, resembling the digits of a crow's foot. The posterior trunk of the vagus nerve is mainly divided into the celiac and posterior gastric branches. The celiac branch travels along the left gastric artery to the right of the left gastric artery and participates in the formation of the celiac plexus. The posterior gastric branches travel along the deep part of the lesser curvature of the stomach, branch off to supply the posterior gastric wall, and finally supply the posterior wall of the pylorus, like the digits of a crow's foot as well (Fig. 9.19).

Duodenum

The descending and horizontal parts of the duodenum are situated in the retroperitoneal space. They are described in the following section, with the other two parts of the duodenum together.

Location and Surrounding Structures

The superior part of the duodenum reaches the level of the first lumbar vertebra (L1). It is superior to the omental foramen and hepatoduodenal ligament, inferior to the head of the pancreas, anterior to the quadrate lobe of the liver and gallbladder, and posterior to the hepatic portal vein, common bile duct, and gastroduodenal artery. The superior part of the duodenum tightly contacts with the gallbladder and liver, which may be influenced by duodenal lesions. For example, cholecystitis causes adhesion of the gallbladder to the duodenum.

The descending part of the duodenum is extraperitoneal and situated in the retroperitoneal space on the right side of the first to third lumbar vertebrae (L1–L3). It is anterior to the transverse mesocolon, posterior to the right kidney and superior part of the right ureter, lateral to the ascending colon, medial to the right side of the head of the pancreas, and posteromedial to the descending retropancreatic segment. Protect the descending part of the duodenum during the right hemicolectomy and right nephrectomy.

The horizontal part of the duodenum is extraperitoneal, turning to the left at the level of the third lumbar vertebra (L3). It is posterior to the right ureter, inferior vena cava, the spine and abdominal aorta; anterior to the transverse colon and superior mesenteric artery and vein; superior to the head and neck of the pancreas; and inferior to the jejunal loops and mesentery. The horizontal part of the duodenum sits in the angle formed between the superior mesenteric artery and abdominal aorta. A low origin of the superior mesenteric artery causes compression of the horizontal part of the duodenum, leading to duodenal obstruction, which is known as the superior mesenteric artery syndrome.

The ascending part of the duodenum extends from the third lumbar vertebra (L3) to the second lumbar vertebra (L2) to the left side and sharply turns to the left and descends anteroinferiorly to form the duodenojejunal flexure. The peritoneal fold located below the left border of the duodenojejunal flexure, inferior to the root of the transverse mesocolon is known as the duodenojejunal fold, or ligament of Treitz. It is the landmark for identifying the origin of the jejunum. On the deep side of the duodenojejunal fold, a thin layer of muscle fibers originating from the right crus of the diaphragm that attaches to the duodenojejunal flexure posteroinferiorly contributes to fixing and lifting up the duodenojejunal flexure, this structure, known as the suspensory muscle of the duodenum. Its contraction widens the angle of the duodenojejunal flexure, allowing the valve effect or intestinal lumen closing (Figs. 9.20 and 9.21).

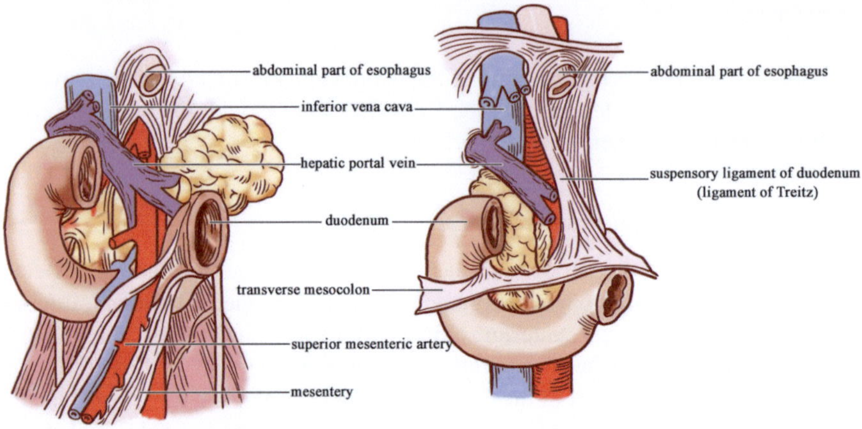

Fig. 9.20 Surrounding structures of the duodenum

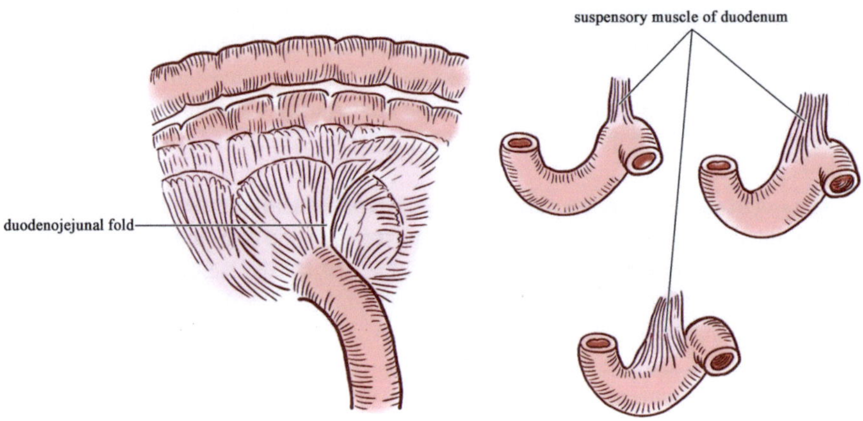

Fig. 9.21 Duodenojejunal fold and suspensory muscle of duodenum

Blood Vessels, Nerves, and Lymphatics of the Duodenum

Arteries

The superior and inferior pancreaticoduodenal arteries are the major arteries supplying the duodenum. The superior pancreaticoduodenal artery originates from the gastroduodenal artery and is divided into anterior and posterior branches descending anteriorly and posteriorly between the duodenum and the head of the pancreas, respectively. The inferior pancreaticoduodenal artery originates from the superior mesenteric artery, and is divided into anterior and posterior branches ascending anteriorly and posteriorly between the duodenum and the head of the pancreas, respectively. It forms the anastomosis with the anterior and posterior branches of the superior pancreaticoduodenal artery and distributes branches to the duodenum and the head of the pancreas (Fig. 9.22).

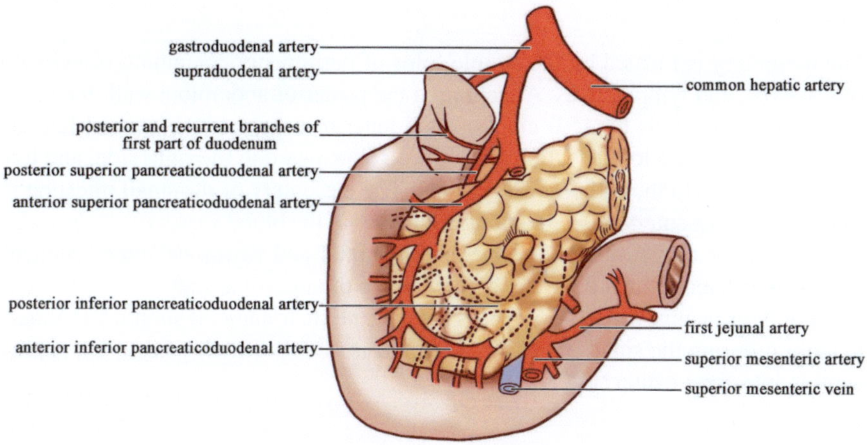

Fig. 9.22 Arteries supplying to the duodenum

Veins

The veins of the duodenum accompany the arteries supplying to it and mainly drain into the superior mesenteric vein.

Nerves

Nerves that innervate the duodenum mainly arise from the celiac plexus and superior mesenteric plexus.

Lymphatic Vessels

Lymphatic vessels of the duodenum drain into the superior and inferior pancreaticoduodenal lymph nodes and are situated between the descending part of the duodenum and the head of the pancreas. Their efferents drain into the right gastroepiploic and superior mesenteric lymph nodes, respectively.

Jejunum and Ileum

Location and Surrounding Structures

The jejunum and ileum occupy the majority of the infracolic compartment. There is no clear boundary between the jejunum and the ileum. Generally, the jejunum constitutes about two-fifths of the proximal part and the ileum constitutes the distal three fifths. The most of the jejunum is situated in the upper left quadrant of the abdomen, and a small part lies in the left iliac fossa. Most of the ileum is situated in the umbilical region and the lower right quadrant of the abdomen, and a small part lies in the pelvic cavity. The jejunum and ileum are anterior to the greater omentum, and posterior to the posterior abdominal wall, including the tissues and organs of the retroperitoneal cavity.

Mesentery

The mesentery is formed by the double folds of peritoneum containing blood vessels, nerves, and lymph nodes. Attaching to the posterior abdominal wall, the radix of mesentery extends by 15.0 cm from the anterior aspect of the second lumbar vertebra (L2) on the left side, obliquely travels downward to the right side, and terminates anterior to the right sacroiliac joint. The mesentery of the small intestine is a fan-shaped mesentery 5.0–7.0 m long. Damages to the blood vessels near the radix impair a broad range of the intestine. The jejunum and ileum are intraperitoneal organs. A triangular area near the attachment of the intestinal mesentery lacks the cover of peritoneum, which is known as the mesenteric triangle. It should be sutured to close it during the small intestinal anastomosis, thus promoting healing and preventing intestinal fistula (Fig. 9.23).

Blood Vessels, Nerves, and Lymphatics of the Jejunum and Ileum

Arteries

The left side of the superior mesenteric artery branches off 12–18 arteries supplying the jejunum and ileum, and their branches anastomose to form the arterial arcades. Generally, type I arterial arcades are situated in the proximal one-fourth, type II–III arterial arcades lie in the middle two-fourths, and type IV arterial arcades are only observed in the distal one-fourth. Type IV arterial arcades distribute straight branches to corresponding intestinal segments. Straight branches in the jejunum are longer than those of the ileum. Anastomoses formed by small and straight blood vessels in the intestinal wall are less abundant. Therefore, a fan-shaped resection of the small intestine and removal of the intestinal wall on the contralateral side of the

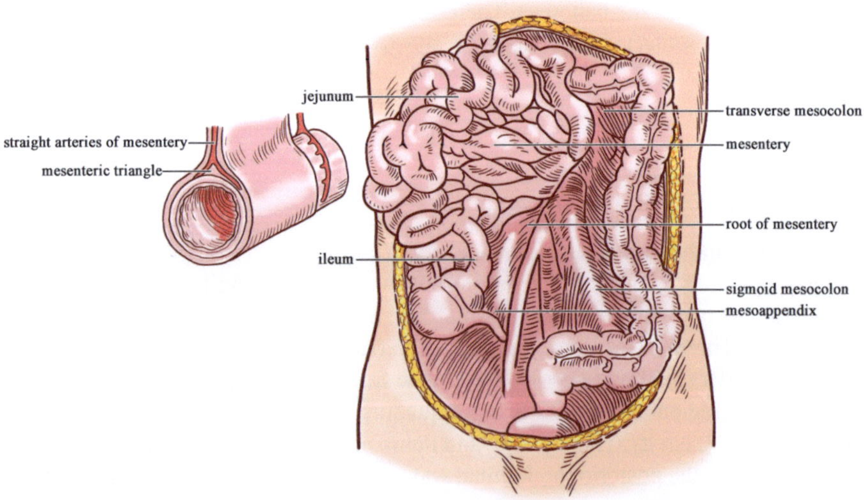

Fig. 9.23 The jejunum, ileum, and mesentery

intestinal mesentery as much as possible are essential to ensure the rich blood flow to the anastomoses and the rapid recovery (Fig. 9.24).

Veins

The veins of the jejunum and ileum accompany with the arteries supplying them and drain into the superior mesenteric vein.

Lymphatic Vessels

Lymphatic vessels of the jejunum and ileum lie between the double folds of the intestinal mesentery. About 100–200 mesenteric lymph nodes are arranged along the arteries supplying to the jejunum and ileum. Their efferent vessels drain into the superior mesenteric lymph nodes at the root of the superior mesenteric artery.

Nerves

Sympathetic nerve fibers that innervate the jejunum and ileum arise from the celiac ganglion and superior mesenteric ganglion, and parasympathetic nerve fibers arise from the vagus nerve. They form the superior mesenteric plexus that branches off nerves to accompany the superior mesenteric artery distributed in the intestinal wall.

Cecum and Appendix

Location and Surrounding Structures

The cecum is usually located in the right iliac fossa. The position of the cecum in childhood is relatively high and gradually descends with age. The cecum is posterior to the iliopsoas muscle separated by the parietal peritoneum, lateral to the right paracolic gutter, medial to the terminal ileum and attached mesentery, and anterior to the abdominal wall of the right inguinal region covered by the greater omentum. The base of the appendix originates from the posteromedial surface of the cecum. It can be bent by varying degrees into hook shaped, spiral shaped, or arc shaped due to the shorter free margin of the mesoappendix than that of the appendix. The location of the appendix varies according to the position of the cecum. The taeniae coli are three

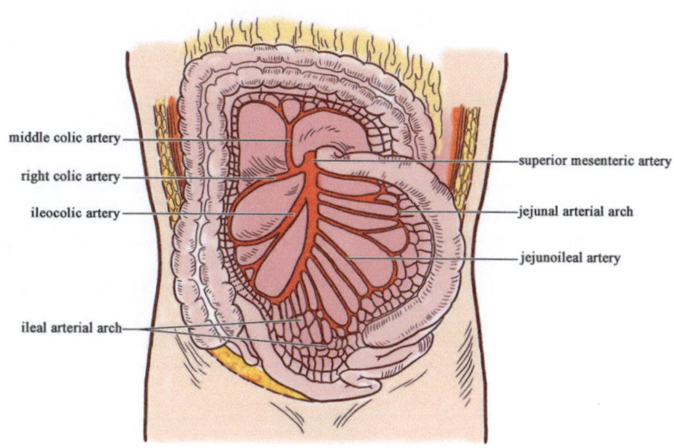

Fig. 9.24 Arteries supplying to the jejunum and ileum

longitudinal smooth muscle bands in the cecal wall and converge at the base of the appendix, serving as the landmark for identifying the base of the appendix. The base of the appendix is identified as the point that is one-third of the distance from the right anterior superior iliac spine to the umbilicus, which is known as the McBurney's point. Obvious tenderness and rebound pain occur at the McBurney's point in cases of acute appendicitis. Due to the position of the vermiform appendix, tenderness in cases of acute appendicitis may occur at the Lanz' point, which is two-thirds of the distance from the left to the right anterior superior iliac spines. The tip of the appendix is variably located, including the preileal (27.97%), pelvic (26.14%), retrocecal (24.05%), retroileal (8.26%), and subcecal (6.14%) positions. In the preileal position, the tip of the appendix faces the upper left, and acute appendicitis causes an obvious tenderness in the right lower quadrant of the abdomen. In the pelvic position, the tip of the appendix faces downward to cross over the superior margin of the lesser pelvis or even descends to the surrounding area of the obturator internus muscle. In cases of acute appendicitis, passive pain is induced when the thigh is inflexion and internal rotation. Right fallopian tube and ovarian lesions in females with the pelvic appendix may be misdiagnosed as appendicitis due to the close anatomical relationship. The retroileal appendix is positioned on the posterior abdominal wall, posterior to the peritoneum and the ileum. The tip of the subcecal appendix faces toward the lower right. The pus of perforated subcecal appendix builds up in the right iliac fossa or floods upward or downward along the right paracolic gutter (Fig. 9.25).

The wall and lumen of the appendix in children differ from those in adults. The appendix in children is funnel shaped, with a thin wall and a large opening, which makes it less susceptible to inflammation or obstruction. Nevertheless, an inflamed appendix in children is associated with a high incidence of perforation. The incidence of obstructive appendicitis is high in adults due to the thick wall and narrow lumen and opening of the appendix.

The ileocecal region comprises the terminal ileum, cecum, and appendix and serves as a site where the ileum connects to the colon. The angle between the ileum and colon in the ileocecal junction, which approaches 90°, is a factor that contributes to the common occurrence of intussusception in this region.

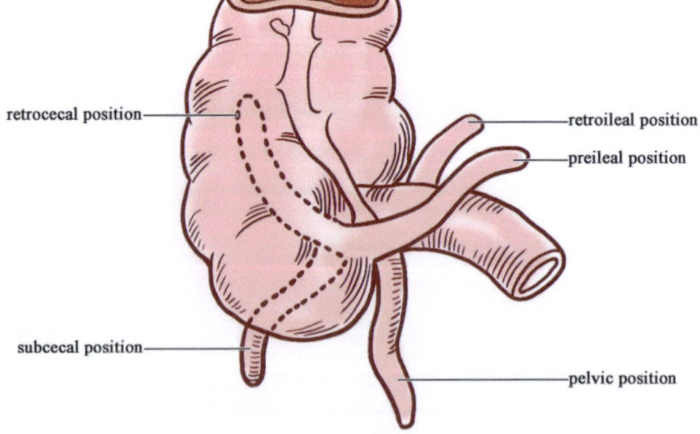

Fig. 9.25 Position of the appendix

Blood Vessels, Nerves, and Lymphatics of the Cecum and Appendix

Arteries

The anterior and posterior cecal arteries, arising from the ileocolic artery, supply blood to the cecum. The appendicular artery, usually with one branch, or occasionally two or more branches, arises from the ileocolic artery as well. It enters the triangular mesoappendix posterior to the terminal ileum and travels toward the tip of the appendix along the free margin of the mesoappendix. It also gives off small branches to supply the base of the appendix (Fig. 9.26).

Veins

The veins of the cecum and appendix accompany the arteries and drain into the ileocolic vein, which in turn empties into the superior mesenteric vein and finally into the hepatic portal vein. Purulent inflammation of the appendix may cause pylephlebitis and pyogenic liver abscess as the septic emboli enter the liver through the venous flow into the hepatic portal vein.

Nerves

The cecum and appendix are innervated by the sympathetic nerves and vagal (parasympathetic) nerve fibers that arise from the superior mesenteric plexus.

Lymphatic Vessels

Lymphatic vessels of the cecum and appendix drain into the superior mesenteric lymph nodes.

Colon

The colon is divided into the four sections of the ascending colon, transverse colon, descending colon, and sigmoid colon.

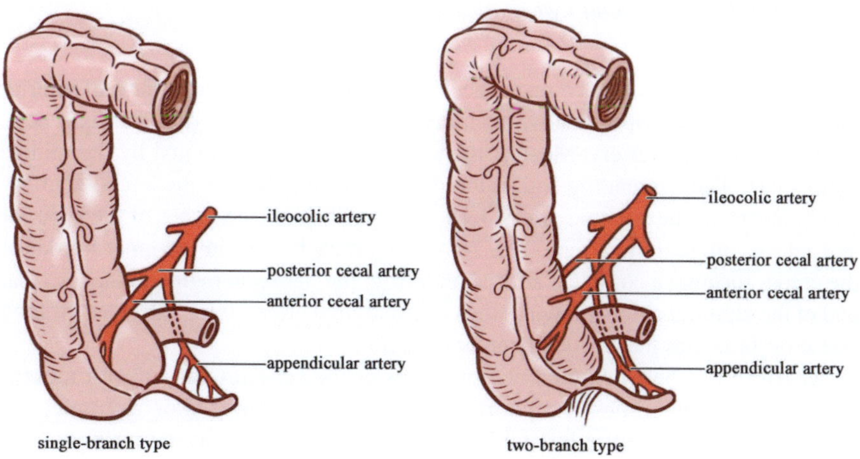

Fig. 9.26 Arteries supplying to the cecum and appendix

Location and Surrounding Structures

The ascending colon is 12.0–20.0 cm long and posterior to the psoas major muscle and the right kidney. It passes upward to the inferior part of the right lobe of the liver and turns left to form the right colic flexure, where it becomes the transverse colon. The right colic flexure sits between the right kidney and liver, with the descending part of the duodenum and fundus of the gallbladder situated superomedial. The transverse colon, measuring 40.0–50.0 cm in length, is situated between the left and right colic flexures. It is posterior to the anterior aspect of the right kidney, duodenum, and pancreas with the attachment of the transverse mesocolon, superior to the stomach, and inferior to the greater omentum. The left colic flexure is bent into an acute angle and therefore located higher than the right colic flexure. It laterally connects with the diaphragm by the phrenicocolic ligament and is anteriorly covered by the costal arch and greater curvature of the stomach. As a result, tumors in the left colic flexure are usually unpalpable. The descending colon, 25.0–30.0 cm long, extends from the left colic flexure, passes downward to the level of the left iliac crest, and transits into the sigmoid colon. Structures posterior to it are similar to those situated behind the ascending colon. The sigmoid colon is an S-shaped loop of the large intestine traveling from the left iliac crest along the left iliac fossa. It crosses anteriorly over the left external iliac vessels, testicular or ovarian vessels, and left ureter, descends into the pelvic cavity, and extends into the rectum at the level of the third sacral vertebra (S3). The sigmoid colon is fixed to the posterior pelvic wall relying on its mesentery (sigmoid mesocolon). Because of its long length and significant mobility of the sigmoid mesocolon, the sigmoid colon can sometimes descend into the pelvic cavity or the right lower quadrant of the abdomen. Redundant sigmoid mesocolon may cause sigmoid volvulus and strangulation.

Blood Vessels, Nerves, and Lymphatics of the Colon

Arteries

The arterial supply to the colon comes from branches of the superior and inferior mesenteric arteries. Specifically, the ascending colon is supplied by the right colic artery and ileocolic artery. Most of the transverse colon is supplied by the middle colic artery. The descending and sigmoid colon are supplied by the left colic artery and branches of the sigmoid artery, respectively. The colic branches of the superior and inferior mesenteric arteries anastomose with each other in the inner border of the colon, forming a complete arterial arch from the ileocecal region to the terminal end of the sigmoid colon known as the colic marginal artery. It further gives off long and short branches that vertically enter the colon.

Anastomoses between the colic branches of the superior and inferior mesenteric arteries sometimes are poorly formed or interrupted. For example, the anastomosis between the left middle colic artery and the ascending branch of the left colic artery at the left colic curvature is weakly formed or even absent.

Injuries to the left middle colic artery may cause necrosis of the left transverse colon. An arcuate collateral branch is absent between the superior rectal artery and sigmoid artery that arises from the inferior mesenteric artery. High ligation of the inferior mesenteric artery above the origin of the superior rectal artery is needed to prevent ischemia and necrosis of the superior part of the rectum (Fig. 9.27).

Veins

The veins of the colon accompany the arteries and drain into the superior and inferior mesenteric veins and finally to the hepatic portal vein.

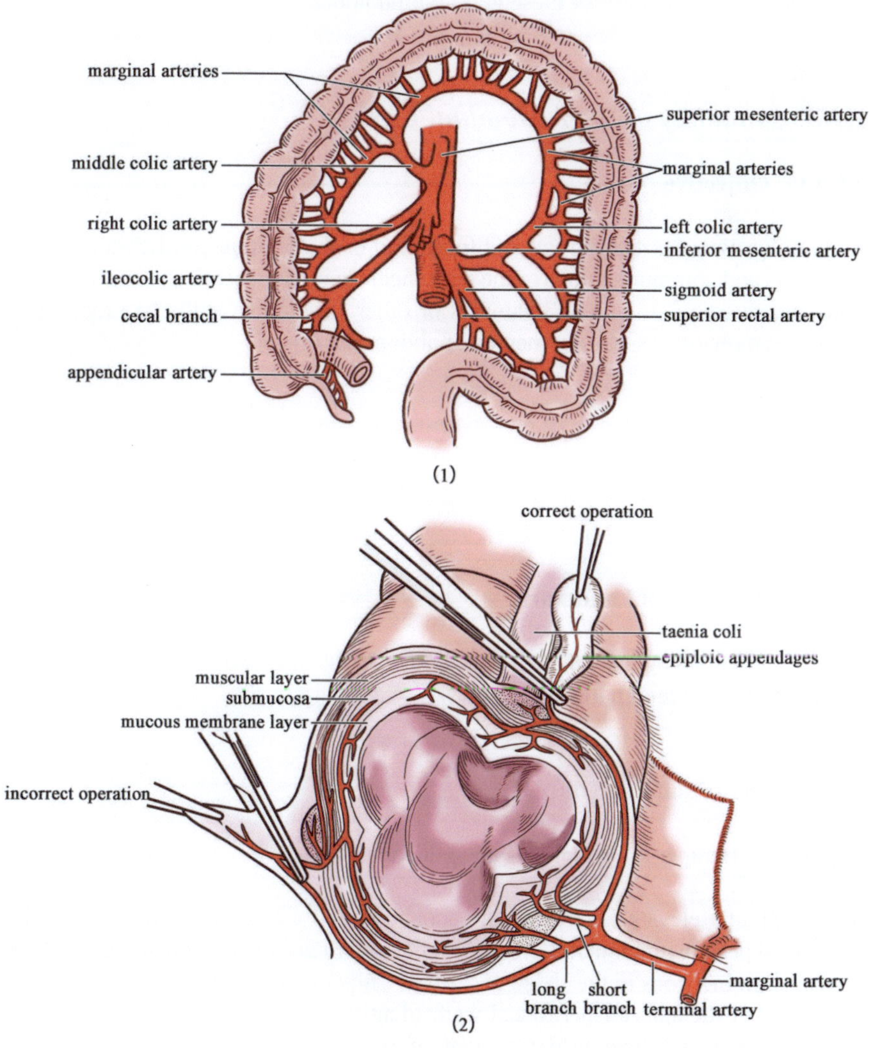

Fig. 9.27 Arteries between the colon and rectum

Nerves
The nerves that innervate the ascending and transverse colon originate from the sympathetic and vagal (parasympathetic) nerve fibers of the superior mesenteric plexus. The nerves that innervate the left colic flexure, descending colon, and sigmoid colon arise from the sympathetic nerve fibers of the inferior mesenteric plexus and pelvic splanchnic nerve fibers.

Lymphatic Vessels
The greater part of the lymphatic vessels of the ascending colon and right transverse colon drains into the superior mesenteric lymph nodes. The lesser part of the lymphatic vessels of the left transverse colon and those of the descending and sigmoid colon drains into the inferior mesenteric lymph nodes.

9.1.3 Anatomy of the Abdominal Cavity

9.1.3.1 Objective

Be familiar with the distribution and formation of the peritoneum. Learn the compartments and communications of the peritoneal cavity and location, surface projections, surrounding structures, ligaments or other structures for the fixation, blood vessels, lymphatic vessels, and nerves of abdominal organs.

9.1.3.2 Position

Supine position.

9.1.3.3 Anatomical Landmarks

Palpate abdominal organs on the human bodies in the nine abdominal regions based on the anatomical landmarks and lines.

9.1.3.4 Dissection Procedures

Explore the Intraperitoneal Organs and Peritoneal Spaces

Step 1. Bluntly elevate the incised thoracoabdominal wall downward and keep the parietal peritoneum intact. Centered on the umbilicus, the peritoneum is cut open with skin incisions in the shape of "大" (a Chinese character). Observe the inner surface of the anterior peritoneal wall. Identify the round ligament of the liver, the median umbilical fold (remnant of the embryonic urachus), the medial umbilical folds (remnants of the obliterated fetal umbilical arteries), and the lateral umbilical folds (containing the inferior epigastric artery and vein). Observe the distribution of the greater omentum.

Step 2. Observe the peritoneal organs and the division of the supracolic and infracolic compartments by the transverse colon.

Step 3. Explore the suprahepatic space. Insert your hands into the left and right suprahepatic spaces from both sides of the falciform ligament. Use fingers to touch the anterior layer of the coronary ligament, with the subphrenic extraperitoneal space, or the bare area of the liver posterior to it. The coronary ligament extends laterally to form the triangular ligament. The right triangular ligament is shorter in length than the left one. Therefore, the left suprahepatic space is subdivided into the left anterior and posterior suprahepatic spaces, while the right suprahepatic space is not subdivided.

Step 4. Explore the infrahepatic space. Expose the infrahepatic space by pushing the liver upward and pulling the stomach downward. The left infrahepatic space lies on the left side of the right margin of the hepatoduodenal ligament. It is further subdivided into the anterior and posterior left infrahepatic spaces, with the former situated anterior to the lesser omentum (hepatogastric ligament and hepatoduodenal ligament) and the latter posterior to it (omental bursa). The right infrahepatic space sits below the right lobe of the liver, and the bulging right kidney is palpable on its deep side. The hepatorenal recess is a peritoneal depression between the liver and right kidney.

Step 5. Explore the stomach and spleen. Insert your hands into the subphrenic space along the anterior wall of the stomach to the upper left side, where the circular thickening of the gastric wall is palpable, that is, the pyloric sphincter. Insert your right hand into the left hypochondrial region to touch the spleen. The splenic notches are palpable on the anterior portion of the spleen. After passing through the posterior portion of the spleen, insert your fingers between the diaphragm and spleen to reach the posterior abdominal wall, and then palpate the superior pole of the left kidney and the splenorenal ligament. Gently pull the stomach to the lower right side, and observe the gastrosplenic ligament between the fundus of the stomach and splenic hilum.

Step 6. Explore the greater omentum. Transversely incise the anterior surface of the greater omentum below the arterial arch of the greater curvature of the stomach. Clamp the greater omentum and stomach above the incision with your index and middle fingers; observe that the anterior surface of the greater omentum is composed of the visceral peritoneum of the anterior and posterior gastric wall folded below the greater curvature of the stomach. Insert your fingers posterior to the anterior surface beneath the incision, and further extend downward to palpate the free margin of the greater omentum at the nonunion part of the anterior and posterior surfaces, that is, the reflection of the anterior and posterior surfaces. The posterior surface turns upward to attach to the transverse colon, where the constitution of the greater omentum by four layers of peritoneum can be observed.

Step 7. Explore the omental bursa. Insert your right hand upward through the incision of the greater omentum into the posterior left infrahepatic space that sits posterior to the stomach and lesser omentum, that is, the omental bursa. The peritoneum that covers the spleen, left kidney, and left adrenal gland, as well as the transverse mesocolon, lies posterior to the inserted hand. The caudate lobe of the liver and diaphragm are palpable above the fingers. The index finger reaches the omental foramen along the lesser curvature of the stomach to the right side, and the posterior right infrahepatic space lies on the right side out of the omental foramen. Insert your left index finger to the left to explore the splenic hilum, where the gastrosplenic and splenorenal ligaments sit anterior and posterior to the index finger, respectively.

Step 8. Explore the large intestine. Turn the greater omentum upward and identify the colon and small intestine based on the three major morphological characteristics of the colon. Lift up the cecum slightly in the right iliac fossa, and observe the location of the appendix and its variation. Observe the anatomical relationship between the base of the appendix and taeniae coli, and the mesoappendix and blood vessels in its free margin. The ascending and descending colons attach to the posterior abdominal wall, lateral to the right and left paracolic gutters, and communicate inferiorly with the pelvic cavity. The right paracolic gutter continues superiorly with the posterior right infrahepatic space (hepatorenal recess) and is separated by the phrenicocolic ligament on the left side. The left colic flexure sits higher than the right one. Peritoneal folds that extend from the left colic flexure to the diaphragm are known as the phrenicocolic ligament, serving to support the spleen. Observe the mesentery that attaches to the transverse and sigmoid colon by lifting them up.

Step 9. Explore the mesentery of the small intestine. Expose the left mesenteric sinus (or the mesenteric space of the descending colon) by pushing the small intestine toward the upper right. This mesentery of the small intestine extends obliquely from the upper left to the anterior aspect of the right sacroiliac joint. The duodenojejunal flexure lies superior to the root of the mesentery of the small intestine, and both are connected by the duodenojejunal fold, or ligament of Treitz, at the left border. Push the small intestine toward the lower left to expose the mesenteric space of the ascending colon. Explore the communication between the left and right mesenteric sinuses, which lies between the roots of mesentery of the small intestine and transverse mesocolon.

Dissect the Supracolic Compartment

Observe the location and surrounding structures of the liver, gallbladder, stomach, and spleen. Observe the duodenum and pancreas during the exposure of the celiac trunk and hepatoduodenal ligament. Cover with the anterior abdominal wall, and mark the surface projections of the inferior margin of the liver, fundus of the gallbladder, pylorus of the stomach, and pancreas on the surface of the abdominal wall.

Dissection of the Blood Vessels, Lymph Nodes, and Nerves of the Stomach

Step 1. Expose the lesser omentum by pulling the anterior margin of the liver upward. Make an incision on the anterior surface of the lesser omentum (hepatogastric ligament) along the middle of the lesser curvature of the stomach, and clean off the left gastric artery along the lesser curvature of the stomach to the left, until reaching the cardia. The left gastric artery gives off the ascending, horizontal, and descending branches to supply the inferior end of the esophagus, the area surrounding the cardia of the stomach, and the gastric wall surrounding the lesser curvature of the stomach to the right, respectively. Dissect the left gastric vein (or coronary vein) and cardia lymph nodes that accompany the left gastric artery. Clean off the right gastric artery along the lesser curvature of the stomach to the right. Observe the prepyloric vein, which may be blurred in a cadaver. Palpate the pyloric sphincter and observe the surrounding lymph nodes. Dissect the gastric branch of the anterior trunk of the vagus nerve and terminal branches that supply the pylorus resembling the digits of a crow's foot.

Step 2. Explore the left and right gastroepiploic arteries 1.0 cm inferior to the middle of the greater curvature of the stomach, and observe their anastomosis. The gastric branch ascends to supply the gastric wall, and the omental branch descends to supply the greater omentum. Clean off the right gastroepiploic artery to the right side until reaching the inferior aspect of the pylorus of the stomach. Observe the lymph nodes accompanying with the right gastroepiploic artery and running below the pylorus. Clean off the left gastroepiploic artery to the left side until reaching the splenic hilum, where the origin from the splenic artery can be observed. The short gastric arteries, with two to four branches, arise from the splenic artery at the splenic hilum and course to the fundus of the stomach along the gastrosplenic ligament. Observe the drainage of the left and right gastroepiploic veins into the splenic vein and superior mesenteric vein, respectively.

Dissection of the Branches of Celiac Trunk and Their Distribution

Step 1. Expose the posterior wall of the omental bursa by lifting up the stomach upward. Observe the bed of the stomach, which has a smooth surface adjacent to the pancreas, left kidney, and adrenal gland, all connected by the peritoneum. Identify the common hepatic artery inferior to the omental foramen. It branches off the proper hepatic artery that ascends to the hepatoduodenal ligament and the gastroduodenal artery that descends through the superior part of the duodenum posteriorly. The latter further splits into the right gastroepiploic artery that travels in the greater omentum below the pylorus of the stomach along the greater curvature and the anterior superior pancreaticoduodenal artery that travels between the head of the pancreas and descending part of the duodenum.

Step 2. Explore the celiac trunk along the identified common hepatic artery, which lies superior to the pancreas and extends to the left. Along this path to the left, expose the origin of the splenic artery. Observe the celiac lymph nodes and celiac plexus that surround the celiac trunk. Incise the peritoneum along the superior margin of the pancreas, and clean off the splenic artery along the celiac trunk to the left. It travels to the left along the superior margin of the pancreas, descends, and branches off the pancreatic branches to supply the pancreas. The posterior gastric arteries, with two to three branches, arise from the splenic artery in the middle segment. Before entering the splenic hilum, it branches off the left gastroepiploic artery that travels to the right in the greater omentum along the greater curvature of the stomach. Observe the course of the splenic artery from the tail of the pancreas to the splenic hilum along the splenorenal ligament and the distribution of lymph nodes surrounding the tail of the pancreas and at the splenic hilum.

Dissection of the Hepatoduodenal Ligament and Gallbladder

Step 1. Incise the hepatoduodenal ligament longitudinally and observe the proper hepatic artery, common bile duct, and hepatic portal vein. The proper hepatic artery lies on the left front, and the common bile duct sits on its right side. The hepatic portal vein is situated posterior and between the proper hepatic artery and common bile duct, where the drainage of the left gastric vein into the hepatic portal vein can be seen.

Step 2. Identify the courses of the proper hepatic artery, common bile duct, and hepatic portal vein upward to the porta hepatis. Explore their left and right branches.

Step 3. Clean off the common bile duct to better observe its anatomical relationship with the gallbladder. Identify the fundus, body, and neck of the gallbladder, as well as the cystic duct. Note that the cystic duct enters the hepatoduodenal ligament and joins the common hepatic duct at an acute angle to form the common bile duct. Expose the cystohepatic triangle, also known as Calot's triangle, which is bounded by the cystic duct, common hepatic duct, and a portion of the visceral surface of the right lobe of the liver. Within this triangle, locate the cystic artery and observe any variations in its position or appearance.

Step 4. Clean off the common bile duct downward, which passes through the superior part of the duodenum posteriorly, descends between the head of the pancreas and descending part of the duodenum, and enters the duodenum medial to its descending part.

Step 5. Clean off the hepatic portal vein and observe its branches and course. The splenic vein travels inferior to the splenic artery and posterior to the body of the pancreas. Be careful to protect the inferior mesenteric vein that drains into the inferior part of the splenic vein. Clean off the hepatic portal vein continuously to the right until fusing with the superior mesenteric vein to form the hepatic portal vein posterior to the neck of the pancreas. It then ascends along the hepatoduodenal ligament.

Dissect the Infracolic Compartment

Observe the positions and surrounding structures of the jejunum, ileum, cecum, appendix, ascending colon, transverse colon, descending colon, and sigmoid colon. Reset the anterior abdominal wall and observe the surface projection of the base of the appendix.

Explore the Superior Mesenteric Artery and Vein

Step 1. Lift up the greater omentum, transverse colon, and transverse mesocolon upward, and push the jejunum and ileum to the left to expose the mesenteric root of the small intestine. Peel off the peritoneum on the right side of the mesenteric root, inferior to the pancreas, and identify the superior mesenteric artery. Trace the superior mesenteric artery upward, which originates from the abdominal aorta and passes through the spleen and posterior aspect of the splenic vein. The dense superior mesenteric plexus is observed around the superior mesenteric artery. Lift up the inferior portion of the pancreas, and identify the hepatic portal vein posterior to the neck of the pancreas. Clean off the superior mesenteric vein on the right side of the superior mesenteric artery downward from the hepatic portal vein.

Step 2. Explore the 12–18 arteries that arise from the left side of the superior mesenteric artery and supply the jejunum and ileum. Observe the branches of the jejunal and ileal arteries, their anastomoses, as well as the straight arteries distributed in the intestinal wall. Observe the nerve plexus and lymph nodes encircling these vessels.

Step 3. Explore the root of the mesentery, the peritoneum of the right posterior abdominal wall, and that inferior to the transverse mesocolon. Dissect the middle colic artery within the transverse mesocolon on the right side of the superior mesenteric artery. Then clean off the origin of the right colic artery and its branches. It may not directly arise from the superior mesenteric artery but from the middle colic artery or ileocolic artery. Clean off the ileocolic artery and its branches. Explore the appendiceal artery near the free margin of the mesoappendix, and trace it upward to observe its origin from the ileocolic artery and entry into the mesoappendix posterior to the ileum.

Explore the Inferior Mesenteric Artery and Vein

Step 1. Lift the jejunum and ileum to the lower right, and pull the sigmoid colon to the lower left. A longitudinal, circular, strip-like bulge can be observed on the left side of the inferior segment of the abdominal aorta, which lies on the posterior abdominal wall and separates by the peritoneum. Trace this structure upward along the main trunk until reaching the posterior aspect of the descending part of the duodenum, where the origin of the inferior mesenteric artery from the abdominal aorta can be observed. The superior segment of the inferior mesenteric artery does not accompany the vein.

Step 2. Peel off the peritoneum of the posterior abdominal wall from the main trunk of the inferior mesenteric artery to both sides of the descending colon and the root of mesentery. Observe the left colic artery traveling to the descending colon and the sigmoid artery traveling to the sigmoid colon by exploring the lateral wall of main trunk of the inferior mesenteric artery on the left side from superior to inferior. Then trace the main trunk of the inferior mesenteric artery downward to identify the terminal branch of the superior rectal artery at the pelvic inlet. Explore the inferior mesenteric vein by tracing the superior rectal vein upward, which drains into the splenic vein posterior to the pancreas. Note that the inferior mesenteric vein sometimes drains into the superior mesenteric vein or into the angle between the splenic vein and the superior mesenteric vein.

9.1.4 Summary

The peritoneal cavity is enclosed by the visceral and parietal peritoneum, presenting as a smooth, moist, serous space containing organs associated with digestion. In males, the peritoneal cavity is closed, whereas in females, it communicates with the external environment through the reproductive tract.

The peritoneal cavity is divided into the supracolic and infracolic compartments by the transverse mesocolon. The supracolic compartment contains the stomach, the superior part of the duodenum, liver, gallbladder, and spleen, whereas the infracolic compartment contains the ascending part of the duodenum, jejunum, ileum, cecum, appendix, and colon. The supracolic and infracolic compartments communicate through a narrow gap between the anterior aspect of the greater omentum and anterior abdominal wall. Inflammations result in the adherence of the greater omentum to the peritoneum of the anterior abdominal wall, thus isolating the supracolic and infracolic compartments and limiting the spread of inflammation. The supracolic compartment is subdivided into the suprahepatic and infrahepatic spaces by the liver. The infracolic compartment, on the other hand, is subdivided into the left and right paracolic gutters and left and right mesenteric sinuses. These subdivisions are demarcated by the root of the mesentery and the ascending and descending colons. These spaces directly or indirectly communicate with each other. The pus from peritoneal inflammation freely spreads into these spaces. In cases of posterior perforation of gastric ulcers or perforation of the superior part of the duodenum, the contents spread from the omental bursa to the hepatorenal recess through the omental foramen, which further build up in the right iliac fossa and even the pelvic cavity through the right paracolic gutter. In cases of perforated appendicitis, the pus refluxes into the infrahepatic and suprahepatic spaces through the aforementioned passageways, leading to infrahepatic and subphrenic abscesses or even diffuse peritonitis.

Learning the surface projections of intraperitoneal organs, particularly those of the liver, stomach, gallbladder, spleen, and appendix, is of great significance for the clinical examinations and disease diagnosis. The liver and spleen are solid and brittle organs that can easily rupture and cause severe bleeding after being struck by an external force.

Accurately determine the position of the organ prior to surgical procedures. Precisely identify the boundaries between adjacent organs, such as that between the pylorus of the stomach and the superior part of the duodenum, and the beginning of the jejunum. Determine the incision sites of peritoneal structures (e.g., transverse mesocolon, hepatoduodenal ligament) and the sites of vascular ligation.

The peritoneum is featured by a strong regenerative ability and can either accelerate peritoneal healing or cause intestinal obstruction due to adhesion formation.

Some blood vessels in the abdominal cavity are of great clinical significance. For example, the gastroduodenal artery serves as a passageway for chemotherapy infusion or diagnosis. The left gastric artery and branches of the left gastroepiploic artery are important landmarks for subtotal gastrectomy.

9.2 Clinical Application of Key Anatomical Structures of the Abdominal Cavity

9.2.1 Laparoscopic Right Hemicolectomy

According to the scope of surgical resection of tumors or lesions, colorectal surgeries are mainly divided into the right hemicolectomy, left hemicolectomy, sigmoid colectomy, and rectal resection. Protect the superior and inferior mesenteric vessels and their branches, as well as the anatomical structures of the duodenum, ureter, pancreas, and spleen and their blood vessels, nerves, lymphatic vessels, and adjacent structures during surgery.

The dissection and surgical processing of the Toldt's fascia, ileocolic vessels, and right and middle colonic vessels are mainly concerned during the laparoscopic right hemicolectomy.

9.2.1.1 Surgical Approach

The subject is placed in a supine split-leg position and managed by general endotracheal anesthesia. A 12-mm port (12-mm trocar placement) is made at the midpoint of the line connecting the umbilicus and pubic symphysis to create pneumoperitoneum. 12- and 5-mm trocars are placed superior and inferior to the umbilicus along the left clavicle midline, respectively, and two 5-mm trocars are placed in the operating ports on the right flank (Fig. 9.28).

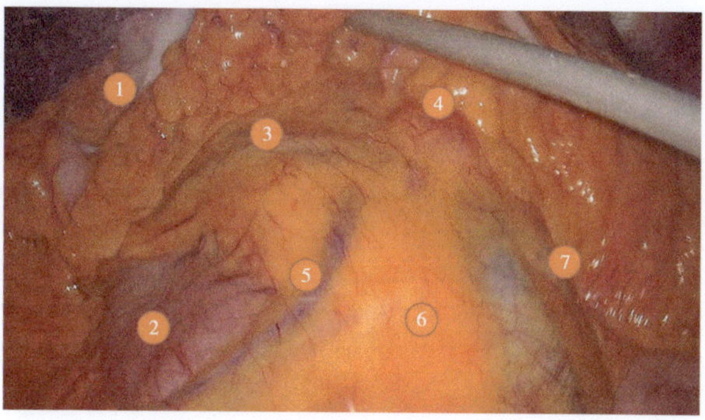

Fig. 9.28 Representative images of the laparoscopic right hemicolectomy (*1*. transverse colon; *2*. duodenum; *3*. right colic vein; *4*. middle colic artery; *5*. ileocolic vein; *6*. ileocolic artery; *7*. superior mesenteric vein)

9.2.1.2 Scope of Resection and Important Structures

A laparoscopic right hemicolectomy involves the removal of the terminal ileum, cecum, appendix, ascending colon, hepatic flexure of the colon, right half of the transverse mesocolon, and greater omentum and the resection of lymph nodes around the ileocolic artery and right and middle colic arteries. The right half of the colon and its mesentery are situated anterior to the renal capsule; posterior to the right kidney, ureter, gonadal vessels, duodenum, and head of pancreas; medially connected with the superior mesenteric vessels; and superior to the inferior margin of the liver, gallbladder, duodenal bulb, and gastric antrum. Therefore, the right ureter, duodenum, and superior mesenteric vein should be protected during the right hemicolectomy. The gastrocolic trunk of Henle is an important anatomical structure formed by the convergence of the right colic vein, right gastroepiploic vein, and anterosuperior pancreaticoduodenal vein. It is a thin, fragile venous trunk with a high risk of intraoperative bleeding that may necessitate conversion from a laparoscopic procedure to an open surgery.

Protect the body and tail of the pancreas, inferior margin of the spleen, and left ureter during laparoscopic left hemicolectomy.

Protect the left ureter during radical resection of sigmoid colon cancer.

Protect the ureters, parasympathetic nerves, and presacral vessels during radical resection of rectal cancer.

9.2.1.3 Free and Expose the Mesocolon and Its Blood Vessels

On the peripheral side of the C-shaped right half of the colon, a series of structures peripheral to the peritoneum contributes to fixing the intestine to the abdominal wall, including the peritoneal reflection lining lateral to the colon with the lateral wall of the cecum as the endpoint, phrenicocolic ligament, and gastrocolic ligament. Identifying the Toldt's fascia and performing surgical procedures in this fascial plane are key steps for freeing mesocolon. It lies anteriorly to the mesocolon, posteriorly fuses with the prerenal fascia, laterally forms the junction of the yellow and white lines by the fusion of the lateral mesocolon fat and lateral parietal peritoneum, and medially becomes the main trunk of the superior mesenteric vein. The Toldt's fascia is a natural surgical plane during human embryonic development provided for colorectal surgery.

Dissection of the Ileocolic Vessels

The ileocolic artery and vein always exist simultaneously. They are cord-like vessels that accompany each other in the ascending mesocolon. The ileocolic artery and vein slightly bulge and pulsate on the right side of the main trunk of the superior mesenteric vein. A depression sits inferomedial to the ileocolic vessels, which is the boundary that separates the inferior mesenteric vein and ileocolic vessels. It also serves as the starting point for the medial approach for right hemicolectomy, where the Toldt's fascia is observed beneath the peritoneum (Fig. 9.29). Along the Toldt's fascia, it extends laterally to the posterior aspect of the cecum and ascending colon, inferiorly to the plane of iliac vessels, superiorly to the transverse mesocolon, and medially to the surface of the duodenum and pancreas. The root of the ileocolic vessels lies near the inferior portion of the horizontal part of the duodenum. The ileocolic artery travels anteriorly to the root of the ileocolic vessels, crosses the superior mesenteric vein, and courses to the right.

Dissection of the Gastrocolic Trunk of Henle

The gastrocolic trunk of Henle, a venous trunk with the anatomic appearance rate of 69–89%, travels in the transverse retrocolic space and finally drains into the superior mesenteric vein. Its branches include the right gastroepiploic vein, right colic vein, middle colic vein, accessory right colic vein, and anterosuperior pancreaticoduodenal vein (Fig. 9.30). The gastrocolic trunk of Henle is an important anatomical structure formed by the convergence of three veins with different courses, involving the right colic vein coursing into the transverse mesocolon, the right gastroepiploic vein coursing into the mesogastrium, and the anterosuperior pancreaticoduodenal vein coursing into the Toldt's fascia. Serving as the anatomical "fingerprint" of the right half of the colon, the gastrocolic trunk of Henle is the most common site of intraoperative bleeding, often leading to conversion from laparoscopic to open right hemicolectomy. Although highly variable in morphology, the gastrocolic trunk of Henle is generally short and thick, with a mean external diameter of 5.0 (2–10) mm and a length of 14 (2.0–47.0) mm. It usually travels rightward from the ventral side to the head of the pancreas, with the root closely contacting with the inferior portion of the pancreas. The convergence of the gastrocolic trunk of Henle with the superior mesenteric vein is 22.0 mm away from the inferior portion of the pancreas. It is 10.0 mm away from the middle colic artery and 34.2 mm away from the ileocolic vein.

After dissecting the blood vessels of the gastrocolic trunk of Henle and keeping the middle colonic vessels unobstructed, free the root of the transverse mesocolon along the inferior portion of the pancreas. The middle colonic artery and vein can be seen in the caudal portion of the inferior pancreas and then ligated and dissected to complete the dissection of the gastrocolic trunk of Henle on the inner side.

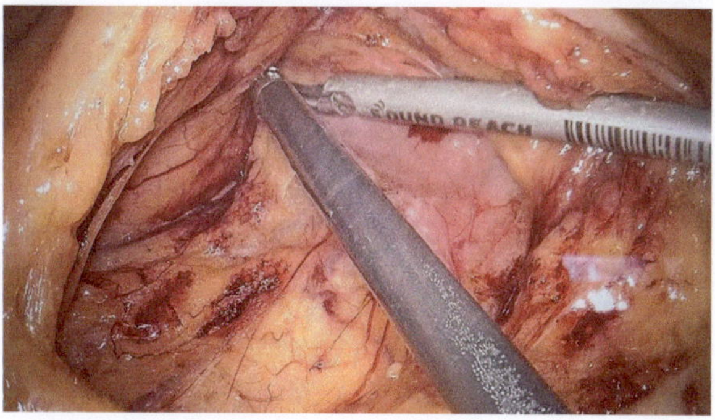

Fig. 9.29 Representative images of the laparoscopic right hemicolectomy (the Toldt's fascia)

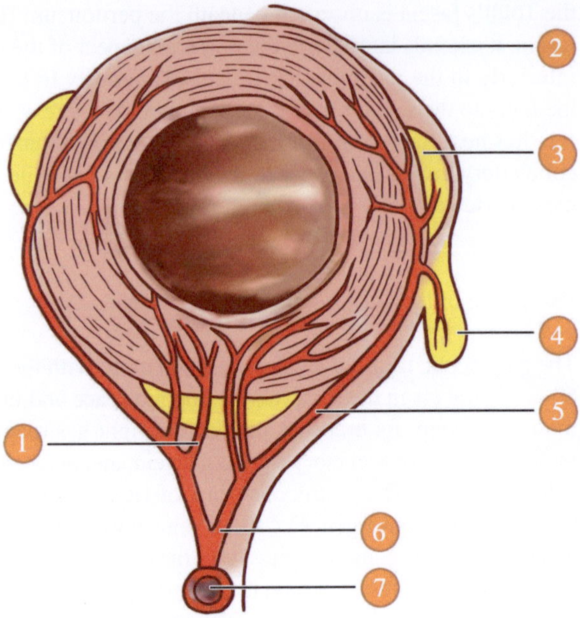

Fig. 9.30 Arteries of the colon (*1*. short branch; *2*. serosa; *3*. taeniae coli; *4*. epiploic appendages; *5*. long branch; *6*. terminal artery; *7*. marginal artery)

Dissect the gastrocolic ligament, phrenicocolic ligament, and lateral peritoneum along the head of the pancreas to completely free the right half of the transverse mesocolon.

9.2.2 *Laparoscopic Distal Subtotal Gastrectomy*

The liver, gallbladder, common bile duct, spleen, stomach, duodenum, small intestine, cecum, appendix, colon, blood vessels, nerves, and lymphatic vessels are important organs and structures in the abdominal cavity. Their position and surrounding structures should be noted in surgical procedures. The anatomical relationships among the important organs in the abdominal cavity during laparoscopic distal subtotal gastrectomy and splenectomy are thoroughly described in the following section.

9.2.2.1 Surgical Approach

The patient is placed in the supine split-leg position with a 15° abduction of both legs and managed by general endotracheal anesthesia. After creating pneumoperitoneum, an observation port and an operating port are created on the left and right flanks inferior to the umbilicus, respectively. The position of the stomach and surrounding structures are then visualized (Fig. 9.31a, b).

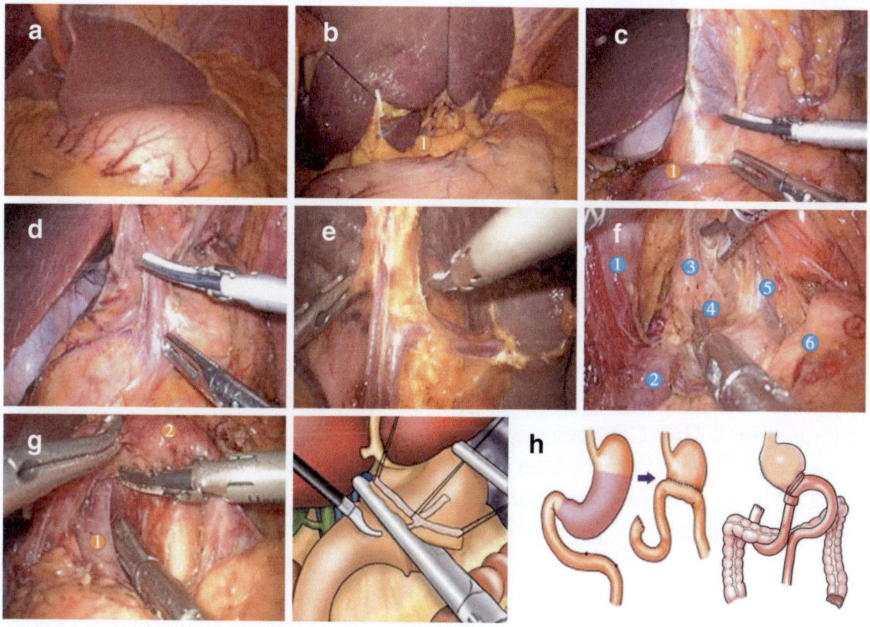

Fig. 9.31 Laparoscopic distal subtotal gastrectomy. (**a**) Stomach and its adjacent structures; (**b**) angular incisure (*1*. angular incisure); (**c**) middle colic artery (*1*. middle colic artery); (**d**) right gastroepiploic artery; (**e**) left gastroepiploic artery; (**f**) left gastric vein (*1*. duodenum; *2*. gastroduodenal artery; *3*. right gastric artery; *4*. common hepatic artery; *5*. left gastric artery; *6*. pancreas); (**g**) portal vein (*1*. portal vein; *2*. common hepatic artery); (**h**) gastrointestinal reconstruction after distal gastrectomy

The anterior wall of the stomach is located in front of the diaphragm on the left side and covered by the left lobe of the liver on the right side. On the lower left side, it directly contacts the anterior abdominal wall between the left and right costal arches inferior to the xiphoid process. Structures adjacent to the posterior wall of the stomach, including the pancreas, left adrenal gland, left kidney, and transverse mesocolon separated by the omental bursa, are known as the stomach bed. The cardia connects the esophagus and stomach, with the proximal end of the lower esophageal sphincter located 2.0–3.0 cm inferior to the esophageal hiatus. The gastrophrenic ligament is responsible for connecting the cardia and diaphragm, which should be cut off during total gastrectomy prior to freeing the cardia and esophagus. The pylorus connects the gastric antrum and duodenum. A circular groove lies on the surface of the pyloroduodenal junction, through which the prepyloric vein (of Mayo) passes and ascends to drain into the right gastric vein. It is a landmark for intraoperatively identifying the junction of the stomach and duodenum. The lesser curvature of the stomach is constantly located that attaches to the hepatogastric ligament. The angular incisure is the lowermost point of the lesser curvature of the stomach turning right and serving as a landmark for separating the antrum and body of the stomach (Fig. 9.31b). The position of the greater curvature of the stomach changes with the filling of the stomach, with the lowermost point declining to the plane of the umbilicus or lower. The inferior portion of the greater curvature of the stomach connects to the transverse colon via the gastrocolic ligament.

9.2.2.2 Dissociation of the Distal Stomach

Cut off the gastrocolic ligament that is close to the transverse colon and prevent the thermal damage to it. During the dissection of the distal stomach to the right until reaching the duodenal bulb, the gastrocolic ligament near the pylorus sometimes adheres to the transverse mesocolon posteriorly. Protect the middle colic artery lying in the transverse mesocolon when cutting the gastrocolic ligament near the pylorus (Fig. 9.31c). Cut open the gastrocolic ligament inferior to the pancreas and clean the fusion fascia space between the greater omentum and transverse mesocolon. This is an avascular space situated anterior to the middle colic artery. The superior mesenteric vein and gastrocolic trunk of Henle are further exposed during the dissection along the surface of the middle colic artery toward the root of the transverse mesocolon and inferior portion of the pancreas. Expose the right gastroepiploic vein and artery by dissecting the gastrocolic trunk of Henle that is closely contacted with the pancreas to the right side, and cut them off at the root (Fig. 9.31d). Dissect the greater omentum to the left until reaching the splenogastric ligament. Cut off the left gastroepiploic artery where it arises from the splenic artery superior to the tail of the pancreas. The origin of the left gastroepiploic artery is 2.0–3.5 cm away from the splenic hilum, and it descends after passing through the splenogastric ligament. The first gastric branch arising from the left gastroepiploic artery is an important landmark for cutting off the gastric wall at the greater curvature of the stomach during subtotal gastrectomy (Fig. 9.31e). Notably, an excessive traction of the short gastric vessels may cause splenic laceration with bleeding, especially in obese people, which is usually managed by compression, electrocauterization, or sutures to control the bleeding.

The gastroduodenal artery is the primary landmark for dissecting the anterior portion of the pancreas. Free the posterior aspect of the duodenal bulb along the ascending gastroduodenal artery. Lift the pancreatic capsule along with the anterior lobe of the transverse mesocolon to expose the superior portion of the pancreas. Radical lymph node dissection for gastric cancer is challenging in the upper part of the pancreas, where the important blood vessels, such as the posterior gastric vessels and right gastric vein, pose a high bleeding risk during the dissection. In addition, crossing over the dorsal mesogastrium and entering the superficial layer of the prerenal fascia are essential for dissecting the upper part of the pancreas. Expose the left and right crura of the diaphragm by dissecting upward until reaching the posterior aspect of the cardiac and body of the stomach. Expose the hepatic artery, gastroduodenal artery, proper hepatic artery, and splenic artery by dissecting along the upper pancreas, and protect the right gastric vein, left gastric vein, and posterior gastric vessels running perpendicular to the common hepatic artery or splenic artery

(Fig. 9.31f). They ultimately drain into the splenic vein either on the anterior or posterior aspect, which is highly risky for bleeding. The dissection of the splenic artery is necessary to reach the loose space posterior to the pancreas, and the common hepatic artery should be completely dissociated.

The common hepatic artery and the gastroduodenal artery form an arch over the superior portion of the pancreas. Dissociate the space containing loose connective tissues between the arch and superior portion of the pancreas to expose the surface of the origin of the portal vein. Bluntly dissect the surface of the portal vein into the hepatoduodenal ligament, and the tissue space anterior to the portal vein can be completely cleaned off. Generally, no vascular drainage is present anterior to the portal vein (Fig. 9.31g). Then a thorough and safe boundary is established for lymph node dissection in the superior portion of the pancreas, the superior aspect of the pylorus, and the hepatoduodenal ligament. Ligate the right gastric artery and vein, denude the superior portion of the duodenum, ligate the left gastric artery and vein upward, and free the lesser curvature of the stomach until reaching the cardia. The left gastric artery gives off five to six branches to supply the gastric wall. The space between the first two branches serves as the landmark for excising the gastric wall on the lesser curvature of the stomach during subtotal gastrectomy. The blood supply of the stomach should be preserved as much as possible during esophagogastric anastomosis. The site for anastomoses is cautiously selected to prevent anastomotic leakage.

9.2.2.3 Sample Collection

Place the resected specimens from the abdominal incisions into the retrieval bags.

9.2.2.4 Gastrointestinal Reconstruction After Distal Gastrectomy

Common gastrointestinal reconstructive procedures after distal gastrectomy include the Billroth I, Billroth II, or Billroth II with Braun anastomosis and Roux-en-Y anastomosis (Fig. 9.31).

9.2.3 Vagus Nerve-Preserving Radical Gastrectomy for Gastric Cancer

The vagus nerve to the stomach is divided into anterior and posterior trunks. The anterior trunk descends in front of the abdominal esophagus, lying deep to the serosa near the esophageal midline. The anterior trunk of the vagus nerve bifurcates into the hepatic and anterior gastric branches at the cardia. Within the lesser omentum, the anterior gastric branches accompany the left gastric artery and curve to the right at 1.0 cm away from the lesser curvature of the stomach. They give off four to six branches to the anterior gastric wall, ultimately supplying the pyloric antrum and anterior wall of the pyloric canal, like a crow's claw, near the angular incisure. The posterior trunk descends posteriorly to the abdominal esophagus and bifurcates into the celiac and posterior gastric branches at the cardia. The celiac branch follows the origin of the left gastric artery and enters the celiac plexus. The posterior gastric branches travel along the deep part of the lesser curvature of the stomach, branch off to supply the posterior gastric wall, and ultimately supply the pyloric antrum and posterior wall of the pyloric canal, resembling a crow's claw as well. Gastric branches of the vagus nerve send postganglionic fibers in the myenteric plexus of the gastric wall innervating the gastric glands and muscular layer. They are responsible for promoting the secretion of gastric acid and pepsin and enhancing gastrointestinal motility.

The common hepatic artery, left gastric artery, and celiac artery are all surrounded by the thick visceral nerves, and their surrounding lymph nodes are situated laterally to the vascular and nerve envelopes and arranged in layers. Therefore, vagus nerve-preserving lymph node dissection is theoretically feasible. Currently, the application of vagus nerve-preserving radical gastrectomy to early-stage gastric cancer has been extensively analyzed, showing its potential of the standard treatment for early-stage gastric cancer. The celiac branch of the vagus nerve is usually preserved using a two-sided approach from both the upper and lower ends. Briefly, incise the peritoneum and phrenico-esophageal membrane on the superficial layer of the abdominal esophagus anterior to the right crus of the diaphragm. Identify the posterior trunk of the vagus nerve behind the abdominal esophagus on the right side, place a traction belt, and peel off until reaching the diaphragmatic hiatus. Identify the posterior trunk and its celiac and posterior gastric branches, trace their courses to the root of the left gastric artery, and sever the posterior gastric branches. Clean off the lymph nodes from the right side of the celiac trunk on the superficial surface of the celiac ganglion to the root of the common hepatic artery and those around the celiac trunk and left gastric artery. Then the celiac trunk and left gastric artery are clearly exposed (Fig. 9.32). At the end of their junction, the left gastric artery is ligated to preserve the celiac branch. Notably, peripheral structures of the celiac trunk cannot be completely dissected; otherwise, the parasympathetic nerve fibers of the left and right celiac ganglia coursing from the root of the left gastric artery

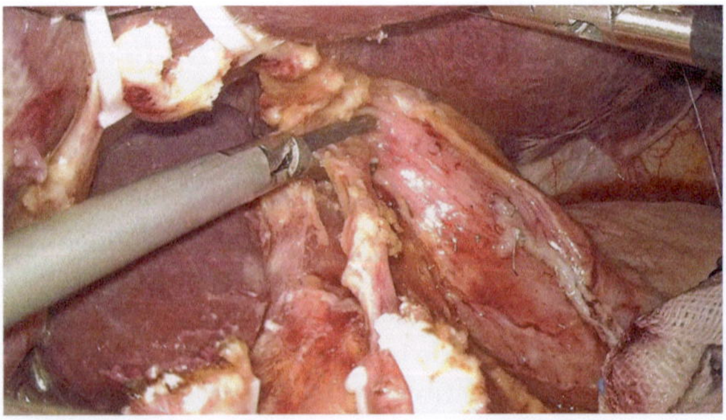

Fig. 9.32 Vagus nerve-preserving radical gastrectomy for gastric cancer

may be completely destroyed. The posterior gastric branches are sometimes close to the left gastric artery, which may be accidentally preserved.

9.2.4 *Laparoscopic Splenectomy*

9.2.4.1 Surgical Approach

The subject is placed in the supine split-leg position with a 15° abduction of both legs and managed by general endotracheal anesthesia. After creating pneumoperitoneum, an observation port and an operating port are created near the umbilicus and in the left upper quadrant of the abdomen, respectively. The position of the spleen and surrounding structures are then visualized.

The spleen is located in the deep layer of the left hypochondriac region between the fundus of the stomach and diaphragm, the long axis of which is in line with the tenth rib. Laterally, it is in contact with the diaphragm, ribs, and left abdominal wall, and medially within a depression. Near the middle of the spleen is the splenic hilum close to the tail of the pancreas, containing the splenic artery and vein, lymphatic vessels, and nerves. The splenic hilum connects to the fundus and upper portion of the greater curvature of the stomach through the gastrosplenic ligament, which is located posteroinferiorly to the left adrenal gland and left kidney and posterior to the splenic flexure. The spleen is covered by the peritoneum except at the splenic hilum and the part close to the tail of the pancreas, forming three peritoneal reflections known as the splenophrenic, splenorenal, and gastrosplenic ligaments. The splenophrenic ligament extends inferiorly to the splenocolic ligament.

9.2.4.2 Dissociation of the Ligaments of the Spleen

Dissect the gastrocolic ligament from the middle and upper portions of the greater curvature of the stomach. The omental branches of the gastroepiploic artery and vein in this area should be intraoperatively ligated and divided. Lift the omental bursa and expose the short splenogastric ligament, which contains the short gastric arteries and veins as well as the left gastroepiploic artery and vein (Fig. 9.33a). Protect the stomach and spleen during the intraoperative ligation and dissection of the splenogastric ligament.

The splenic artery and vein are then ligated and divided. First, observe the position and structure of the splenic hilum after fully mobilizing the spleen. It is located in the center of the medial side of the spleen and contains the splenic vessels and nerves that make up the splenic pedicle (Fig. 9.33d). The splenic artery branches off the left gastroepiploic artery 2.0–6.0 cm away from the splenic hilum, and the splenic artery gives off multiple branches (upper and lower branches or upper, middle, and lower branches) and then small branches that further split to enter the splenic hilum. The splenic vein is formed by the union of small venules that drain

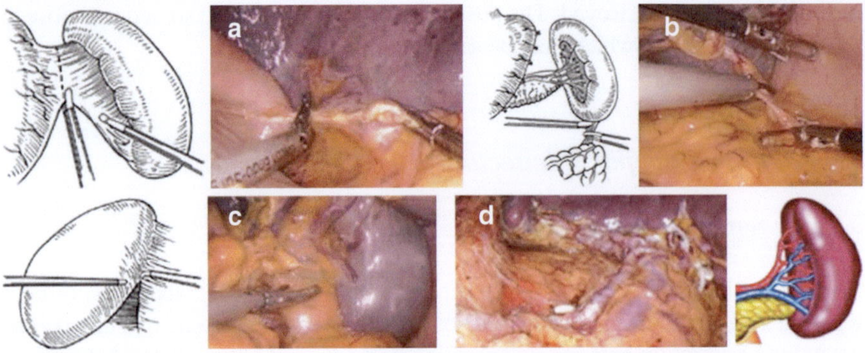

Fig. 9.33 Laparoscopic splenectomy ((**a**) cut off the splenogastric ligament; (**b**) free the lower pole of the spleen; (**c**) free the splenorenal ligament; (**d**) structures of the splenic hilum)

from the spleen posterior to the splenic hilum. It typically runs distal to the splenic artery and dorsal to the pancreas, eventually draining into the superior mesenteric vein. Intraoperative ligation and dissection of the splenic artery and vein should be performed as close as possible to the spleen to prevent damages to the tail of the pancreas and postoperative refractory pancreatic fistulas. In cases of traumatic splenic rupture and ongoing bleeding, the splenic hilum can be clamped as soon as possible to block the blood flow of the splenic artery and vein.

Chapter 10
Regional Anatomy of the Retroperitoneal Space and Its Clinical Application

Lei Li, Kuirong Jiang, Jie Yin, Chao Qin, Song Wu, and Hailiang Zhang

10.1 Regional Anatomy of the Retroperitoneal Space

10.1.1 Boundary

The retroperitoneal space is an anatomical space between the parietal peritoneum of the posterior abdominal wall and intra-abdominal fascia. It extends superiorly to the diaphragm and connects the posterior mediastinum through the lumbocostal triangles, runs inferiorly to the sacral promontory and continues with the retroperitoneal space of the pelvis, and laterally communicates with extraperitoneal areolar tissues of the anterolateral abdominal wall.

10.1.2 Retroperitoneal Structures

The main structures in the retroperitoneal space include the duodenum, pancreas, kidneys, suprarenal glands, ureters, large blood vessels in the abdomen, lymphatic vessels, and lymph nodes, which are surrounded with a large amount of loose connective tissues (Fig. 10.1). Divided by the renal fascia, the retroperitoneal space is

L. Li · K. Jiang · J. Yin · C. Qin (✉)
Nanjing Medical University, Nanjing, China
e-mail: thunderlee@njmu.edu.cn; jiangkuirong@njmu.edu.cn; qinchao@njmu.edu.cn

S. Wu
ShenZhen University South China Hospital, Shenzhen, China
e-mail: wusong@szu.edu.cn

H. Zhang
Huadong Hospital Affiliated to Fudan University, Shanghai, China

Q. Ding et al. (eds.), *Clinically Oriented Regional Anatomy*,
https://doi.org/10.1007/978-981-95-9888-5_10

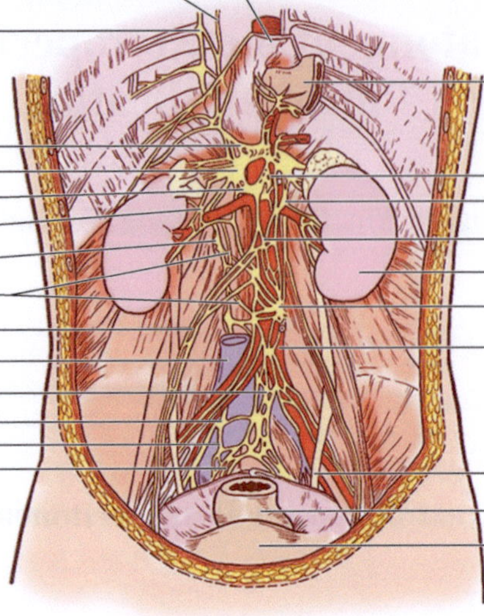

Fig. 10.1 Important organs and structures in the retroperitoneal space

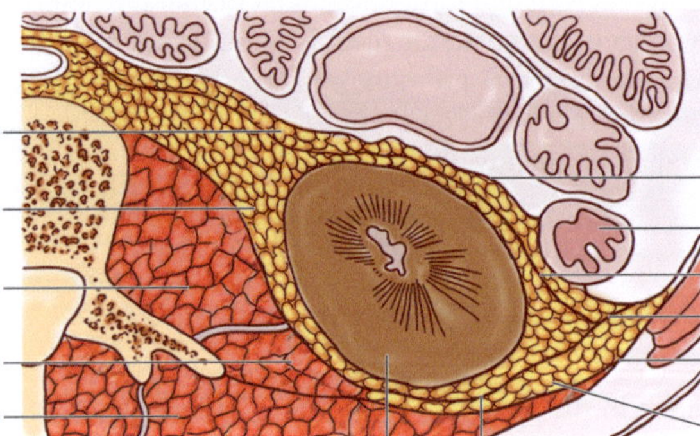

Fig. 10.2 Subdivisions of the retroperitoneal space

further subdivided into the anterior pararenal space, perirenal space, and posterior pararenal space (Fig. 10.2). The anterior pararenal space is bounded by the posterior peritoneum, the anterior leaf of the renal fascia, and lateroconal fascia and contains the ascending colon, descending colon, duodenum, and pancreas. Perirenal space is bounded by the anterior and posterior leaves of the renal fascia, which contains the kidneys, suprarenal glands, and surrounding adipose tissues. The posterior pararenal space is bounded by the posterior leaf of the renal fascia, lateroconal fascia, and transversalis fascia and just contains adipose tissues and no organs. Therefore, an oblique incision in the lumbar and abdominal regions with an extraperitoneal approach is usually made for retroperitoneal surgeries.

10.1.3 Organs and Structures in the Retroperitoneal Space

10.1.3.1 Duodenum

The descending and horizontal parts of the duodenum are situated in the retroperitoneal space. They have been described in Chap. 9.

10.1.3.2 Pancreas

Location and Surrounding Structures

The pancreas lies transversely on the posterior abdominal wall, posterior to the omental bursa and anterior to the first and second lumbar vertebrae (L1, L2). The left end of the pancreas is at a higher level than the right end. The upper border of the pancreas is projected onto the area about 10 cm above the umbilicus on the anterior abdominal wall, and the lower border onto the area about 5 cm above the umbilicus.

The pancreas is divided into the head, neck, body, and tail without a clear boundary. Except for the tail, the other parts of the pancreas are extraperitoneal (Fig. 10.3).

The head of the pancreas is surrounded by the C-shaped duodenum on the right side of the second lumbar vertebra (L2). It is anteriorly divided into the superior and inferior parts by the transverse mesocolon and posteriorly adjoins the inferior vena cava and right renal vein by the loose connective tissues. The common bile duct descends between the posterior part of the head of pancreas and the descending part of the duodenum, and sometimes, it may be partially or completely hidden by pancreatic tissue. The lower part of the head of pancreas sends out the uncinate process to the left, which hooks posteriorly to the superior mesenteric vessels. The enlarged head of the pancreas caused by chronic pancreatitis or tumor may result in duodenal

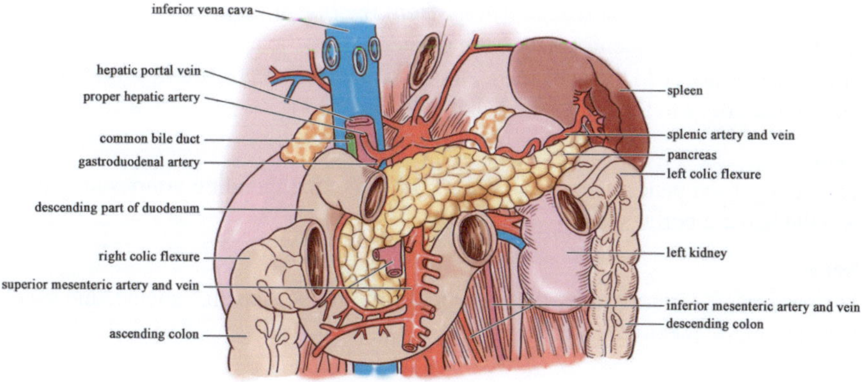

Fig. 10.3 Surrounding structures of the pancreas

obstruction, obstructive jaundice, congestion, and ascites due to its close contact with the wall of the duodenum.

The neck of the pancreas is situated posteroinferior to the pylorus of the stomach. The superior mesenteric vein passes behind it and joins with the splenic vein to form the origin of the hepatic portal vein.

The body of the pancreas lies at the level of the first lumbar vertebra (L1). It is superiorly adjacent to the celiac trunk and plexus (the splenic artery courses to the left along its upper border), inferiorly to the duodenojejunal flexure and jejunum, and posteriorly to the abdominal aorta, splenic vein, left suprarenal gland, and left kidney. Anteriorly, the body of the pancreas is adjacent to the posterior wall of the stomach, between which the omental bursa lies. As a result, perforation caused by the gastric cancer or ulcer often adheres to the pancreas.

The tail of the pancreas, a narrow part of the left end of the pancreas, is inferiorly adjacent to the left colic flexure and posteriorly to the left suprarenal gland and left kidney. The splenic artery and vein travel superiorly and posteriorly to the body of the pancreas, respectively. They further course anteriorly to the tail of the pancreas and enter the splenic hilum along with it. The tail of the pancreas should be protected during the ligation of splenic vessels and splenectomy, thus preventing the pancreatic fistulas.

The pancreas is situated deep in the abdomen, posterior to the stomach, transverse colon, and greater omentum and anterior to the left kidney. Therefore, abdominal signs are atypical in the early stage of pancreatic lesions, posing a huge challenge in the diagnosis.

Vessels, Nerves, and Lymphatics of the Pancreas

Arteries

The head of the pancreas is mainly supplied by the blood from the anterior and posterior superior pancreaticoduodenal arteries and the anterior and posterior branches of the inferior pancreaticoduodenal artery. The blood supply to the neck, body, and tail of the pancreas is mainly from the dorsal pancreatic artery (arising from the root of the splenic artery), the greater pancreatic artery (the largest branch of the splenic artery to the pancreas), and the caudal pancreatic arteries (branches of the splenic artery to the tail of the pancreas) (Fig. 10.4).

Veins

The veins of the pancreas usually accompany the corresponding arteries and drain into the hepatic portal system.

Nerves

The pancreas is innervated by the branches of the celiac, hepatic, splenic, and superior mesenteric plexuses.

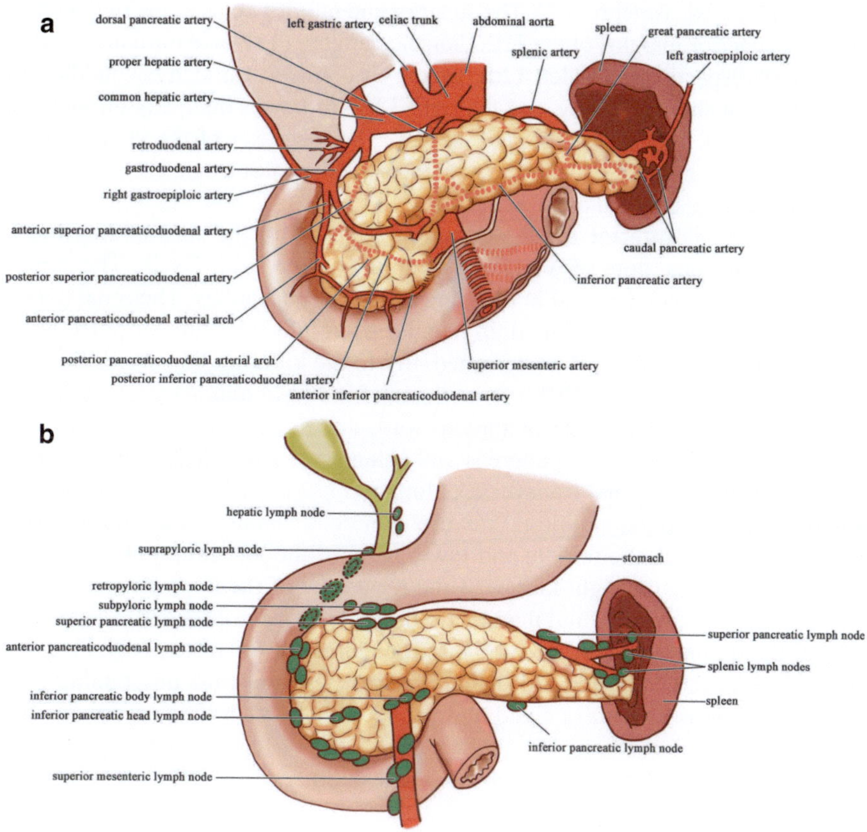

Fig. 10.4 Blood vessels and lymph nodes of the pancreas (**a**. distribution of the blood vessels; **b**. distribution of the lymph nodes)

Lymphatics

The lymphatic vessels of the head of the pancreas mainly drain into the subpyloric lymph nodes, and those of the remaining parts of the pancreas drain into the pancreatic and splenic lymph nodes. Their efferent finally drains into the celiac lymph nodes.

10.1.3.3 Kidneys

Location and Surrounding Structures

The kidneys are paired on both sides of the spine, with the posterior aspect adhering to the posterior abdominal wall. The right kidney sits 1.0–2.0 cm (half the height of a vertebra) lower than the left due to the position of the right lobe of the liver. The superior pole of the left kidney lies at the level of the inferior margin of the 11th thoracic vertebra (T11), and its inferior pole is at the level of the inferior margin of the second lumbar vertebra (L2). The superior and inferior poles of the right kidney sit at the superior margins of the 12th thoracic vertebra (T12) and third lumbar vertebra (L3), respectively. The left 12th rib courses obliquely through the middle part of the back of the left kidney, and the right 12th rib travels obliquely through the superior part of the back of the right kidney. The long axes of the kidneys point obliquely to the inferolateral aspect, with the superior poles facing each other. The two renal hila are directed opposite.

The kidney is inferior to the suprarenal gland with the surrounding loose connective tissues, both of which are wrapped by the renal fascia. The suprarenal gland does not descend in the condition of nephroptosis. The renal pelvis and ureter sit inferiorly and medially, and the left and right lumbar portions of the sympathetic trunks rest posteromedially to the kidneys. Structures that are anterior to the left kidney differ from those of the right one. Anterosuperior to the left kidney is the posterior gastric wall, and superolateral is the spleen; middle and inferior are the pancreas and splenic vessels; anterior and inferior are the jejunum, terminal transverse colon, and left colic flexure; and anterior and medial is the duodenojejunal flexure. Pancreatic and splenic vessels transversely run through the middle and lower parts of the left kidney (Fig. 10.5a). Anterosuperior to the right kidney is the right lobe of the liver, anteroinferior is the right colic flexure, and medial are the inferior vena cava and descending part of the duodenum. During surgical procedures for the left kidney, be careful to protect the body and tail of the pancreas. Besides, the descending part of the duodenum is always fixed and prone to rupture in the surgery for the right kidney.

Divided by the plane of the 12th rib, the superior part behind both kidneys is adjacent to the diaphragm and pleural cavity, and the inferior part adjoins the psoas major muscle (and the genitofemoral nerve anterior to it), quadratus lumborum muscle (and the iliohypogastric nerve and ilioinguinal nerve anterior to it), and transverse abdominal muscle from medial to lateral (Fig. 10.5b). In surgical procedures involving the 12th rib, the pleura should be carefully protected to prevent pneumothorax. Inflammation or abscess around the kidneys stimulates the psoas major muscle, and its spasm further causes the flexion of the affected lower limb.

Surface Projections of the Kidney

Two vertical lines are drawn 2.5 cm and 7.5–8.5 cm, respectively, away from the midline, and two horizontal lines are drawn at the levels of the 11th thoracic vertebra (T11) and third lumbar vertebra (L3). The kidney is projected on the quadrangle formed by the four lines. The renal hilum is projected anterior to the ninth rib on the anterior abdominal wall and in the angle (known as the costovertebral angle or renal angle) formed by the lateral side of the erector spinae muscle and the 12th rib on the posterior wall. Tenderness or percussion pain in the quadrangle and costovertebral angle is the clinical sign of kidney diseases.

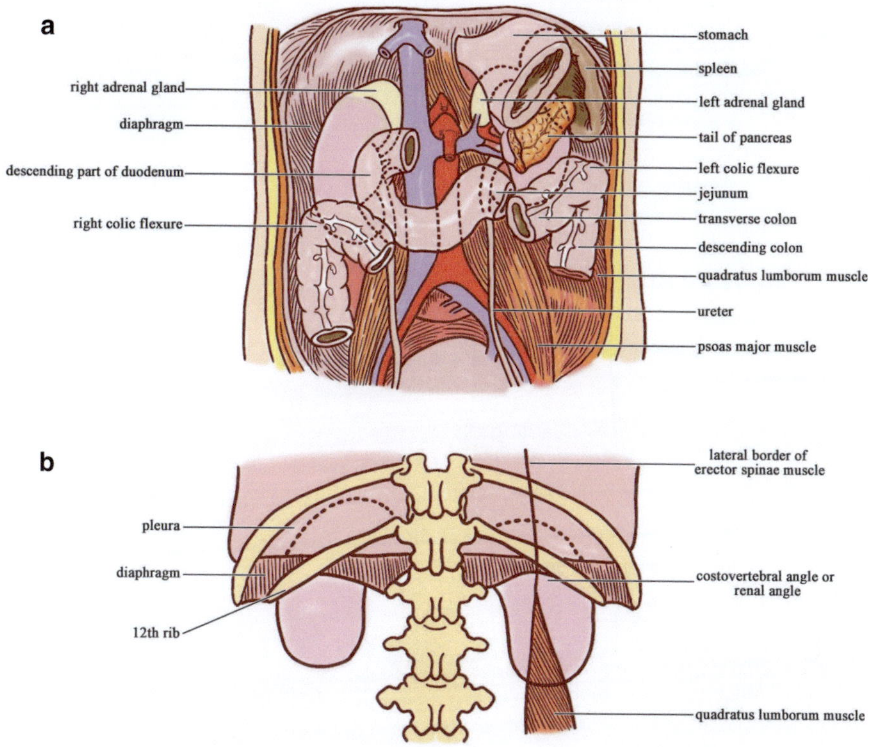

Fig. 10.5 Location and surrounding structures of the kidney (**a**. anterior view; **b**. posterior view)

Renal Capsule

The renal capsule is divided into three layers: renal fascia, adipose capsule, and fibrous capsule from outside to inside (Fig. 10.6).

The renal fascia is a dense, elastic connective tissue enveloping the kidney and suprarenal gland and divided into the anterior and posterior renal fascia. In the medial side of the kidney, the anterior renal fascia passes through the abdominal aorta, travels anterior to the inferior vena cava, and combines with that on the other side. The posterior renal fascia fuses with the fasciae of the quadratus lumborum and psoas major muscles and attaches to the vertebrae and intervertebral discs medially. The anterior and posterior renal fasciae fuse laterally to the kidney to form the lateroconal fascia, which extends to the transversalis fascia superior to the suprarenal gland and combines into the subdiaphragmatic fascia. Inferior to the kidney, the anterior renal fascia joins with the extraperitoneal fascia, and the posterior renal fascia extends downward to fuse with the iliac fascia. The anterior and posterior renal fasciae do not merge below the kidney but extend inferiorly to communicate with the retrorectal space.

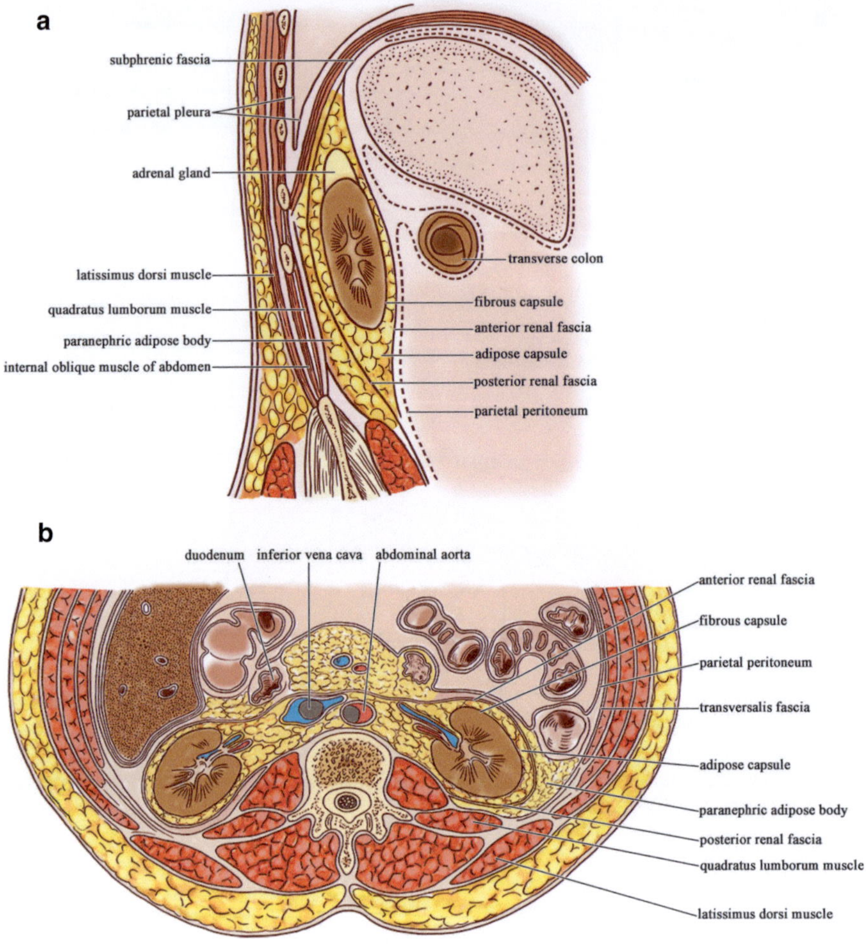

Fig. 10.6 Renal capsule (**a**. a sagittal section; **b**. a transverse section)

Many fiber bundles, composed of connective tissues derived from the renal fascia, pass through the adipose capsule and connect the fibrous capsule, serving to fix the kidney. The inferior end of the renal fascia is completely open. As a result, the increase of renal mobility, due to the weakening of the abdominal wall muscles, decrease in the perirenal adipose tissues, and visceroptosis, further causes nephroptosis (or floating kidney). The pus can spread downward along the renal fascia in cases of pyonephrosis or perirenal inflammation.

The adipose capsule, or renal fat pad, is a layer of adipose tissue with a thickness of 2.0 cm in adults (thicker on the posterior side and at the margin). It is responsible for supporting and protecting the kidney. X-rays easily pass through adipose tissues, and therefore, the morphology of the kidney can be clarified as the layer of the adipose capsule, thus favoring the diagnosis of kidney diseases. Solutions are injected into the adipose capsule to seal the renal capsule for performing kidney surgeries via an extraperitoneal approach.

The fibrous capsule, also known as the fibrous membrane, is the lamina propria of the kidney composed of dense, thin, and tough connective tissues. It covers the outer surface of the kidney and protects it. It can be easily peeled off from the surface of the kidney in vivo. Using the fibrous capsule, the floating kidney can be fixed on the 12th rib or psoas major muscle. The fibrous capsule should be sutured during the partial nephrectomy or surgical procedures for renal trauma. However, the fibrous capsule adheres to the kidney in cases of kidney diseases.

Collectively, layers located at the lumbar region to the renal capsule include the skin, subcutaneous tissue, deep fascia, latissimus dorsi muscle or external oblique abdominis, serratus posterior inferior muscle or internal oblique abdominis, aponeurosis of transverse abdominis, quadratus lumborum muscle, transversalis fascia, retroperitoneal structures, posterior layer of the renal fascia, and adipose capsule.

Vessels, Nerves, and Lymphatics of the Kidney

Arteries

The renal arteries, with one mostly, two occasionally, and three to five rarely on each side, arise from the abdominal aorta at the level of the second lumbar vertebra (L2). They travel transversely and superiorly behind the renal veins and enter the kidney through the renal hilum (Fig. 10.7). The abdominal aorta lies

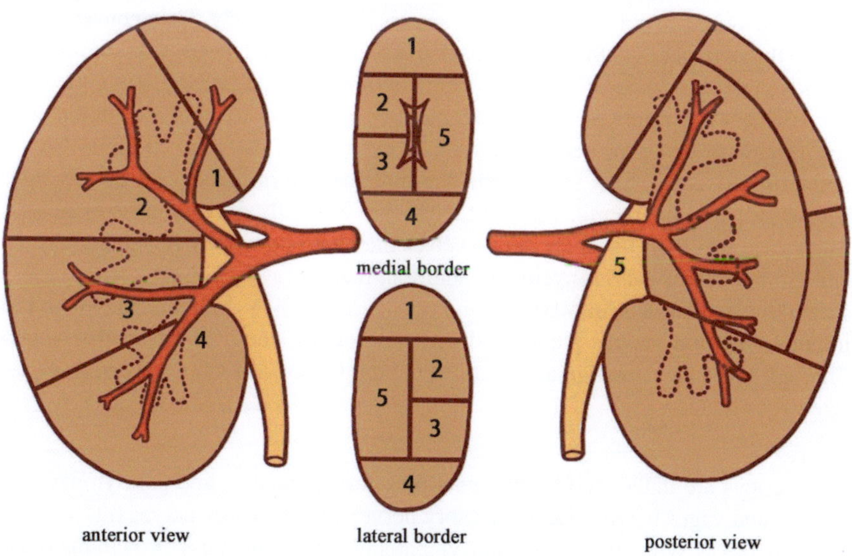

Fig. 10.7 Renal segmental arteries (1. superior segmental artery; 2. anterior superior segmental artery; 3. anterior inferior segmental artery; 4. inferior segmental artery; 5. posterior renal segmental artery)

on the left front of the lumbar spine; therefore, the right renal artery is longer than the left one and turns to the right and passes posteriorly through the inferior vena cava, till entering the kidney. Before entering the renal hilum, the renal artery (primary branch) splits into the anterior and posterior trunks (secondary branches), which further give off segmental arteries (tertiary branches). The area of renal parenchyma, which is supplied by a segmental artery, is known as renal segment. The anterior branch travels anteriorly to the renal pelvis and divides into the superior, anterosuperior, anteroinferior, and inferior segmental arteries. The posterior branch travels posterior to the renal pelvis and continues with the posterior segmental artery. Each kidney is therefore divided into the superior, superior anterosuperior, anteroinferior, inferior, and posterior segments. Blockage of a segmental artery causes ischemic necrosis in the renal parenchyma it supplies, due to the lack of the anastomosis between renal segmental arteries.

The renal arteries demonstrate anatomical variations. Superior polar renal arteries are the accessory branches that enter the superior pole of the kidney without passing through the renal hilum, and inferior polar renal arteries are those entering the inferior pole without passing through the hilum. The incidence of superior and inferior polar renal arteries is about 28.0%, and the superior polar renal arteries are more commonly detected. They mainly arise from the renal arteries and sometimes from the abdominal aorta or superior mesenteric artery. Accessory renal arteries should be highly concerned during kidney surgery to prevent ischemia or necrosis of the areas supplied by them.

Veins

The renal veins are non-segmental and anastomose extensively. They converge into two to three branches in the renal sinus and fuse into one renal vein after running out of the renal hilum. They course anterior to the renal arteries and drain into the inferior vena cava at a right angle. The left renal vein is relatively long, due to the inferior vena cava being located anterior and to the right of the spine. It arises from a point slightly lower than start of the superior mesenteric artery and travels right across the abdominal aorta. The right renal vein generally does not have extrarenal tributaries, while the left renal vein receives the blood flow from the left suprarenal and left testicular (ovarian) veins. In addition, the left renal vein joins with the left ascending lumbar vein in 50.0% of the population, which communicates with the internal vertebral venous plexus and cerebral venous sinus via the lumbar veins. Through this course, malignant tumors of the left kidney and left testis can metastasize to the brain.

Nerves

The kidneys are innervated by the renal plexus (sympathetic and parasympathetic nerves) and vagus nerve (visceral sensory nerve). Most sensory nerves travel along the branches of sympathetic and parasympathetic nerves and pass through the renal plexus. Therefore, resection or sealing of the renal plexus contributes to alleviating the pain induced by kidney diseases.

Lymphatics

The lymphatic vessels of the kidney are divided into the superficial and the deep sets. The superficial lymphatic vessels are situated on the deep side of the fibrous capsule that drain lymphatic vessels of the renal capsule, and the deep ones are situated around the intrarenal network of blood vessels that drain lymphatic vessels of the renal parenchyma. Both of superficial and deep lymphatic vessels of the kidney drain into the renal hilum lymph nodes posterior to the renal pelvis, and their efferent drains into the lumbar lymph nodes. The collecting lymphatic vessels in the anterior part of the left kidney drain into the preaortic lymph nodes and lateral aortic lymph nodes at the origin of the left renal artery, and those in the posterior part drain into the lateral aortic lymph nodes. The collecting lymphatic vessels in the anterior part of the right kidney drain into the precaval, para-aortic, and preaortic lymph nodes, and those in the posterior part drain into the postcaval lymph nodes. Malignant tumors of the kidney may involve the abovementioned lymph nodes.

10.1.3.4 Suprarenal Gland

Location and Surrounding Structures

The suprarenal glands are paired on both sides of the spine at the level of the 11th thoracic vertebra (T11), attached to the kidneys superiorly and medially, and covered by the renal capsule. The left suprarenal gland is semilunar and the right one is triangular. The surrounding structures of the left suprarenal gland differ from those of the right one. Anteroinferior to the left suprarenal gland is the stomach separated by the omental bursa, inferior are the tail of the pancreas and splenic vessels, and medial is the abdominal aorta. Anterior to the right suprarenal gland is the liver, lateral and anterosuperior is the bare area of the liver, and medial is the inferior vena cava. They are both adjacent to the diaphragm, and between them is the celiac plexus.

Blood Vessels, Nerves, and Lymphatic Vessels

Arteries

The suprarenal glands, although small in size, have a rich arterial supply (Fig. 10.8). The superior suprarenal artery arising from the inferior phrenic artery, the middle suprarenal artery arising from the abdominal aorta, and the inferior suprarenal artery arising from the renal artery all supply to the suprarenal glands. They form rich anastomoses in the renal capsule before entering the suprarenal glands, and their branches finally supply the adrenal cortex and medulla.

Veins

The suprarenal veins are usually one on each side and two on the left side occasionally. The left adrenal vein, with the mean length of 2.0 cm, drains into the left renal vein. The right adrenal vein, with the mean length of 1.0 cm,

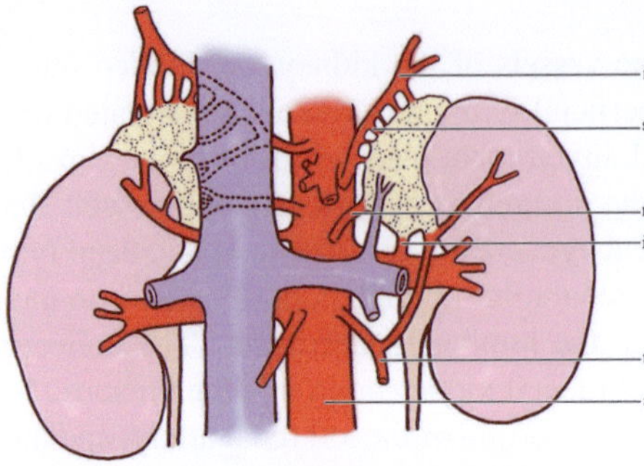

Fig. 10.8 Blood supply to the suprarenal glands

drains into the right posterior wall of the inferior vena cava, and occasionally into the right inferior phrenic vein, right renal vein, or right accessory hepatic vein, and rarely into the right hepatic vein. Therefore, care should be taken to protect the inferior vena cava when ligating the right adrenal vein during right adrenalectomy.

Nerves
The preganglionic fibers of the greater and lesser splanchnic nerves via the celiac plexus innervate the suprarenal glands, and they mainly provide innervation to the adrenal medulla.

Lymphatics
The lymphatic vessels of the suprarenal glands mostly run obliquely inward and downward and drain into the lateral aortic, lateral caval, and intermediate lumbar lymph nodes. Some lymphatic vessels of the superior part of the suprarenal glands travel along the superior suprarenal artery and drain into the inferior phrenic lymph nodes.

10.1.3.5 Abdominal Ureter

Location and Surrounding Structures

The ureters are slender and elastic tubes made of smooth muscles and paired on both sides of the spine. The abdominal ureter is about 13.0–14.0 cm long. Its superior end continues with the renal pelvis. Close to the anterior surface of the psoas major muscle, the abdominal ureter travels obliquely inward and downward, crosses the testicular (ovarian) artery posteriorly just below the midpoint of the psoas major muscle, then descends to cross over the iliac blood vessels, and continues with the pelvic ureter. The abdominal ureter is projected on the semilunar line of the anterior abdominal wall and the line connecting the tip of the lumbar transverse processes on the back. Anterior to the left abdominal ureter are the duodenojejunal flexure, testicular (ovarian) vessels, and blood vessels of the descending colon; anterior to the right abdominal ureter are the descending part of the duodenum, testicular (ovarian) vessels, blood vessels of the ascending colon and ileocolon, and terminal ileum. Inflammation of the retroileal appendix usually causes ureteritis. Most of the abdominal ureter is adjacent to blood vessels of the ascending and descending colon, and it should therefore be protected during colon surgeries.

Variations are rare in the ureter. The ureter that lies posterior to the iliac artery or inferior vena cava is prone to obstruction, and the obstructed ureter needs to be cut away and sewn back to allow to perform ureteroureterostomy. Malformations of both renal pelvises and ureters with normal courses and openings (e.g., ureters open into the urinary bladder) generally do not cause functional abnormalities; otherwise, the opening of ureters into the external urethra or vagina causes urinary incontinence due to the damage to the sphincter control that needs surgical interventions.

Blood Vessels, Nerves, and Lymphatics

Arteries

The abdominal ureter receives a rich arterial supply (Fig. 10.9). The branches of the renal arteries and inferior polar renal arteries provide blood supply to the upper part of the abdominal ureter. Its lower part is supplied by the branches of abdominal aorta, testicular (ovarian) artery, first lumbar artery, and common iliac artery. These branches mainly enter the ureter from the medial side and form an arterial network through anastomoses. Therefore, the ureter is usually dissociated laterally, and the damage to one branch may not significantly influence the blood flow. Because of the small anastomoses, it is not recommended to free the ureter in a large scale to prevent local ischemic necrosis.

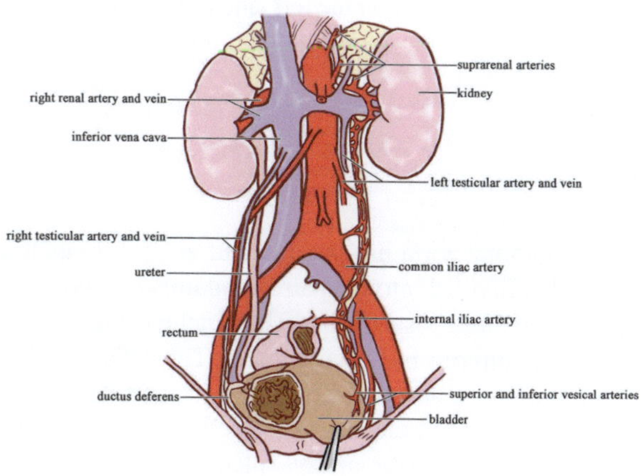

Fig. 10.9 Arteries of the ureter

Veins

The veins of the abdominal ureter accompany the arteries and drain into the renal vein, testicular (ovarian) vein, the common iliac vein, and finally the inferior vena cava.

Nerves

The ureter is innervated by the autonomic nervous system from the renal plexus and hypogastric plexus. Distributed in a network, the nerves that innervate the ureter lie in the connective tissue and finally enter the muscular layer. The abdominal ureter only contains a few ganglion cells.

Lymphatics

The lymphatic vessels of the abdominal ureter drain into the lumbar lymph nodes and common iliac lymph nodes that are arranged along the common iliac artery.

10.1.3.6 Abdominal Aorta

Location and Surrounding Structures

The abdominal aorta is about 14.0 cm long and continues with the thoracic aorta at the aortic hiatus anterior to the 12th thoracic vertebra (T12), which descends along the spine on the left front and splits into the left and right common iliac arteries at the level of the fourth lumbar vertebra (L4). The surface projection of the abdominal aorta starts from 2.5 cm above the midpoint of the line connecting the jugular notch and superior margin of pubic symphysis and extends to 2.0 cm below the left side of the umbilicus, forming a band-shaped area with 2.0 cm in width. Anterior to the abdominal aorta are the pancreas, splenic vein, left renal vein, horizontal part of the duodenum, and root of the mesentery, and posterior to the abdominal aorta are the first to fourth lumbar vertebrae (L1–L4) and intervertebral discs. It adjoins with the left sympathetic trunk on the left, and the inferior vena cava on the right. The lumbar lymph nodes, celiac lymph nodes, and nerve plexuses are arranged around the abdominal aorta.

Vascular Branches

The abdominal aorta has parietal and visceral branches, and the visceral branches are further divided into the paired and unpaired branches (Fig. 10.10).

The unpaired visceral branches include the celiac trunk, superior mesenteric artery, and inferior mesenteric artery. The celiac trunk arises from the anterior wall of the abdominal aorta slightly below the aortic hiatus at the level of the first lumbar vertebra (L1). The branches of the celiac trunk are variable, and most of them serve as the common hepatic artery, splenic artery, and left gastric artery. The superior

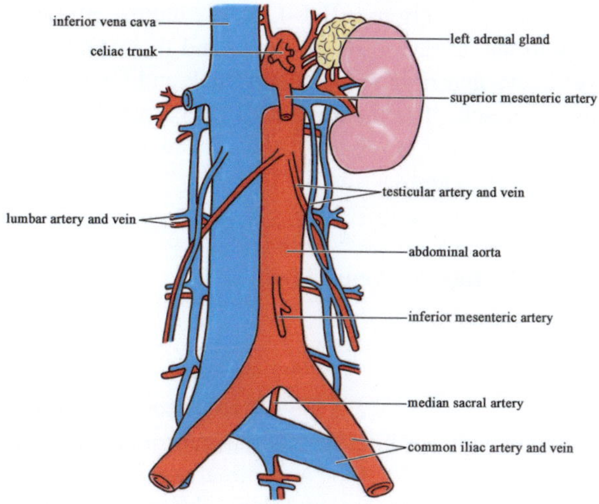

Fig. 10.10 Abdominal aorta and its branches

mesenteric artery arises from the anterior wall of the abdominal aorta slightly below the celiac trunk, travels to the root of the mesentery between the neck of the pancreas and horizontal part of the duodenum, and curves into the right iliac fossa. The inferior mesenteric artery arises from the anterior wall of the abdominal aorta 3.0–4.0 cm above the bifurcation of the abdominal aorta at the level of the third lumbar vertebra (L3), descends deep to the peritoneum on the posterior abdominal wall to the left, and enters the pelvic cavity after passing through the sigmoid mesocolon. It gives off the terminal branch of the superior rectal artery.

Paired visceral branches include the middle suprarenal artery, renal arteries, and testicular (ovarian) artery. The middle suprarenal artery arises from the lateral wall of the abdominal aorta at the level of the first lumbar vertebra (L1) and travels laterally from the medial crus of the diaphragm to the middle part of the suprarenal gland. The renal arteries usually originate from the lateral wall of the abdominal wall at the level of the second lumbar vertebra (L2), slightly below the origin of the superior mesenteric artery, and course into the kidney. The testicular (ovarian) artery starts from the anterolateral wall of the abdominal aorta slightly below the origin of the renal arteries. Descending for a short distance, it accompanies the corresponding vein, crosses anteriorly to the ureter, and travels downward anteriorly to the psoas major muscle. The testicular artery enters the inguinal canal through the deep inguinal ring and descends within the spermatic cord to the testis and epididymis. The ovarian artery descends within the suspensory ligament of the ovary and distributes across the ovary and fallopian tube.

The parietal branches include the inferior phrenic arteries, lumbar arteries, and median sacral artery. The inferior phrenic arteries, usually paired, arise from the origin of the abdominal aorta at the abdominal hiatus, travel superolaterally to the diaphragm, and give off the superior suprarenal artery to the suprarenal gland. The lumbar arteries, usually in four pairs, spring from both sides of the posterior wall of the abdominal aorta and travel laterally through the anterior aspect of the first to fourth lumbar vertebrae (L1–L4). The lumbar arteries lie on the left course posteriorly to the left sympathetic trunk, and those on the right pass behind the inferior vena cava and right sympathetic trunk and finally enter the deep side of the psoas major muscle. The median sacral artery, usually with one branch, arises from the posterior wall of the abdominal aorta and descends anteriorly along the fifth lumbar vertebra (L5) and sacrum.

10.1.3.7 Inferior Vena Cava

Location and Surrounding Structures

The inferior vena cava is the largest venous trunk formed by the joining of the left and right common iliac veins at the level of the fifth lumbar vertebra (L5). It ascends along the right side of the abdominal aorta, passes into the thoracic cavity through the vena caval foramen, and drains into the right atrium. Anterior to the inferior vena cava exist the liver, head of the pancreas, horizontal part of the duodenum, right testicular (ovarian) artery, and the root of mesentery; posterior to it lie the right crus of the diaphragm, first to fourth lumbar vertebrae (L1–L4), right lumbar sympathetic trunk, and parietal branches of the abdominal aorta. The psoas major muscle, right kidney, and right suprarenal gland are situated on the right side of the inferior vena cava, and the abdominal aorta sits on the left side.

Variations of the inferior vena cava include the double inferior vena cava, left-sided inferior vena cava, and absence of the hepatic segment of the inferior vena cava. Due to the different origins, courses, sites of drainage, and adjacent structures of variated inferior vena cava, it should be carefully protected during surgical procedures in the retroperitoneal space.

Tributaries

The tributaries of the inferior vena cava include the common iliac vein, right testicular (ovarian) vein, renal vein, right adrenal vein, hepatic vein, inferior phrenic vein, and lumbar veins, which usually accompany the corresponding arteries (Fig. 10.11).

Visceral Tributaries

The testicular vein, usually with two branches on each side, arises from the pampiniform plexus. It travels to the posterior peritoneum on the posterior abdominal wall through the deep inguinal ring, accompanies the corresponding artery, ascends on the anterior aspect of the psoas major muscle and ureter, and finally merges into one branch. The right-sided testicular vein drains obliquely into the inferior vena cava, and the left-sided one almost vertically ascends and drains into the left renal vein. The paired ovarian vein ascends along the lateral pelvic wall, with the same course and site of drainage as those of the testicular vein after passing through the external iliac vessels.

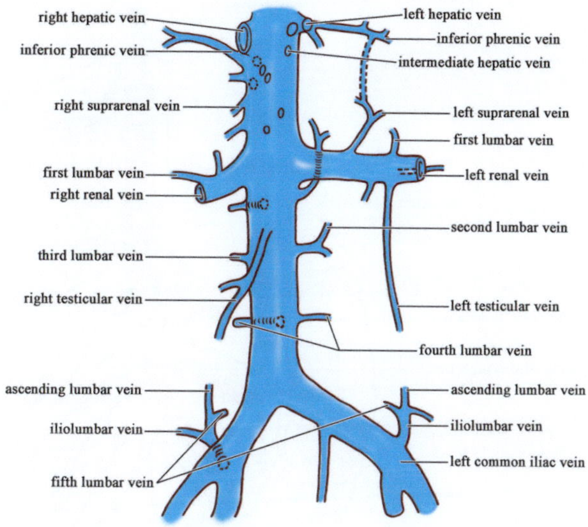

Fig. 10.11 Inferior vena cava and its tributaries

Parietal Tributaries

The parietal tributaries of the inferior vena cava include the inferior phrenic veins and lumbar veins. The inferior phrenic veins receive the venous blood flow from the diaphragm and left suprarenal gland and accompany the corresponding arteries. The lumbar veins, in four pairs, receive the venous blood flow from the lumbar tissues and drain into the inferior vena cava. The communicating branches of the left and right lumbar veins are interconnected upward and downward to form the ascending lumbar vein, which then courses superiorly, passes through the diaphragm, and enters the thoracic cavity. The right-sided ascending lumbar vein is continuous with the azygos vein, and the left-sided one continues with the hemiazygos vein. Therefore, the ascending lumbar vein is a significant collateral anastomosis between the superior and inferior vena cava.

10.1.3.8 Cisterna Chyli and Its Lymphatic Trunks

The cisterna chyli is dilated or reticular in shape and situated anterior to the first to second lumbar vertebrae (L1–L2), right rear of the abdominal aorta. Its superior end continues with the thoracic duct and enters the thoracic cavity through the aortic hiatus (Fig. 10.12). The cisterna chyli drains the lymphatic vessels from the lumbar trunk and intestinal trunk. The lumbar trunk is paired on both sides, formed by the union of the efferent vessels from the lumbar lymph nodes around the abdominal aorta and inferior vena cava. The intestinal trunk, with one branch, is formed by the union of the efferent vessels from the celiac, superior, and inferior mesenteric lymph nodes. The cisterna chyli is invisible in 14% of the population and usually presents as the anastomoses of multiple lymphatic vessels.

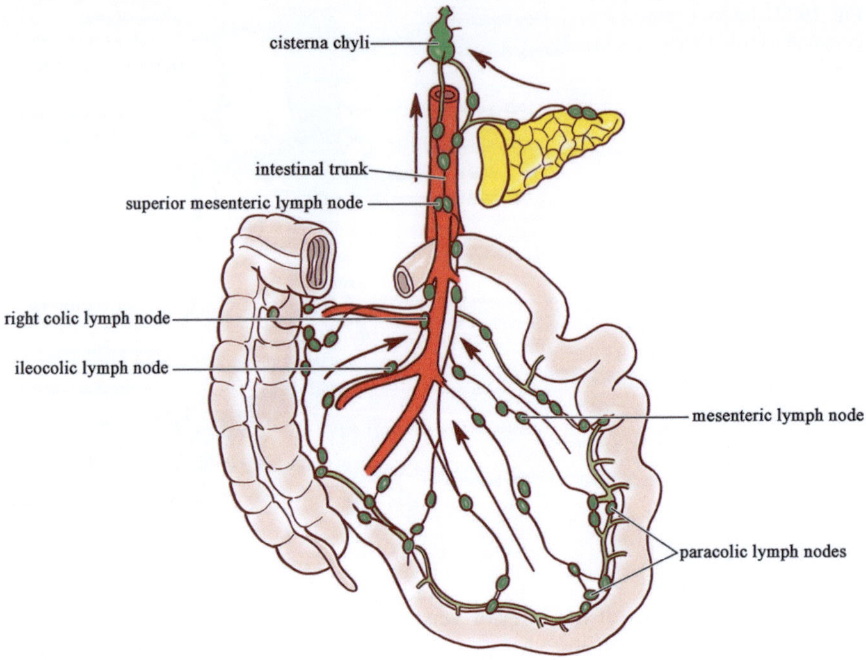

Fig. 10.12 Cisterna chyli

10.1.3.9 Lumbar Plexus

The lumbar plexus is situated deep to the psoas major muscle, anterior to the transverse process of the lumbar vertebrae. It is composed of the anterior branches of the 12th thoracic nerve to the fourth lumbar nerve (T12–L4) (Fig. 10.13). The main branches of the lumbar plexus include the iliohypogastric, ilioinguinal, lateral femoral cutaneous, femoral, obturator, and genitofemoral nerves, which supply the iliopsoas muscle, quadratus lumborum muscle, inferior part of the anterior abdominal wall, muscles and skins on the anterointernal part of the thigh, and skin on the lateral side of the thigh, medial side of the leg and foot, and external genitalia.

10.1.3.10 Lumbar Sympathetic Trunk and Autonomic Plexus

The lumbar sympathetic trunk is situated on both sides of the spine and internal to the psoas major muscle, giving off the lumbar splanchnic nerves and coursing to the abdominal aorta. It is composed of three to four lumbar ganglia and interganglionic branches on each side. The lumbar sympathetic trunk is continuous superiorly with the thoracic sympathetic trunk and inferiorly with the sacral sympathetic trunk. Communicating branches transversely travel between the left and right lumbar sympathetic trunks (Fig. 10.14), which need to be resected as well during the resection of the lumbar sympathetic ganglia.

Nerve fibers of the sympathetic and parasympathetic nervous systems are interconnected around the abdominal aorta and the root of its thick branches to form nerve plexuses, mainly including the celiac plexus and abdominal aortic plexus. The celiac plexus is situated around the celiac trunk and root of the superior mesenteric artery, containing the paired celiac, aorticorenal, and unpaired superior mesenteric ganglia. Along the branches of the celiac trunk, superior mesenteric artery, and renal arteries, the celiac ganglia help form the accessory nerve plexuses (e.g., hepatic plexus, gastric plexus, splenic plexus, pancreatic plexus, renal plexus, and superior mesenteric plexus) that distribute in the organs. The abdominal aortic plexus is superiorly continuous with the celiac plexus and gives off the branches that accompany the inferior mesenteric artery to form the inferior mesenteric plexus. The inferior mesenteric ganglion lies at the root of the inferior mesenteric artery (Fig. 10.14). The greater and lesser splanchnic nerves and preganglionic sympathetic fibers of the lumbar splanchnic nerves change the neurons in the inferior mesenteric ganglion, and the postganglionic fibers climb around the arteries and accompany the arterial branches to distribute in the organs. The parasympathetic preganglionic fibers of the vagus nerve and pelvic splanchnic nerve also enter the abovementioned nerve plexuses and change neurons in the intramural ganglia within the organs they innervate. In addition, nerve plexuses also contain the visceral afferent fibers.

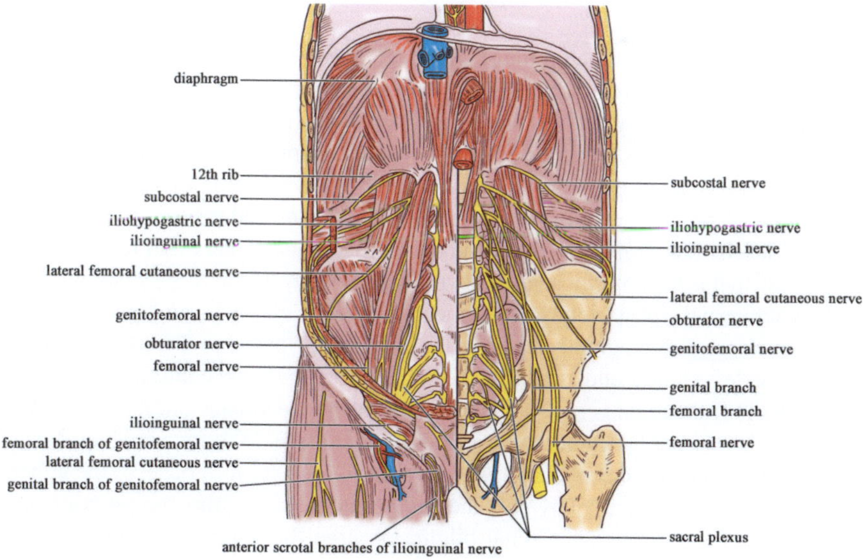

Fig. 10.13 Lumbar plexus

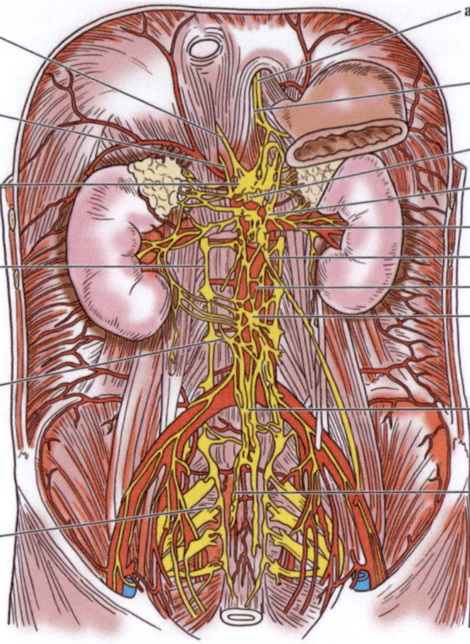

Fig. 10.14 Lumbar sympathetic trunk and autonomic plexus

10.1.4 Dissection of the Retroperitoneal Space

10.1.4.1 Dissect the Kidney, Suprarenal Gland, Renal Hilum, and Ureter

Step 1. Peel off the peritoneum lining in the renal area and observe the position and surrounding structures of the kidney. Cut open the renal fascia anterior to the kidney longitudinally and turn it outward to expose a thick layer of adipose tissues (adipose capsule) or a thin layer in slim people. Explore the suprarenal gland in the superior pole of the kidney that is contained in the renal fascia. Lift the lateral margin of the kidney and observe the adipose tissues and posterior layer of the renal fascia that wrap the kidney and suprarenal gland. Then observe the fibrous capsule that is the innermost layer covering the kidney. Identify the anatomic relation between the posterior aspect of the kidney and 12th rib. Insert your right hand into the costodiaphragmatic recess in the left thoracic cavity to identify its relation with the left kidney, and similarly check their relation in the contralateral side.

Step 2. Cut off the renal vessels and ureter inferior to the kidney and remove it. The kidney is covered by a smooth layer of fibrous capsule. Make an arc-shaped incision on the fibrous capsule and peel off a small piece of it to observe the adherence to the renal parenchyma. The kidney is then cut into the anterior and posterior parts through the renal hilum. Observe the internal structures of the renal parenchyma on the coronal section of the kidney, followed by the renal sinus and inner structures after cleaning off the adipose tissues in the renal sinus.

Step 3. Identify the suprarenal gland on the top of the kidney, which is occasionally similar to the connective tissues in color and texture. Observe the morphology and surrounding structures of the left and right suprarenal glands. Remove the three arteries of the suprarenal gland and identify the anterior veins. Trace the suprarenal veins to the site where they drain into the inferior vena cava or left renal vein.

Step 4. Remove the adipose tissues at the renal hilum and dissect the renal hilum. Observe the renal vein, renal artery, and renal pelvis within the renal pedicle from anterior to posterior. Observe the presence of accessory renal arteries, which usually arise from the main trunk of the renal arteries or abdominal aorta. Dissect the ureter and observe its course, strictures, and surrounding structures. The right-sided ureter passes anteriorly to the origin of the right external iliac artery at the pelvic inlet, and the left-sided one crosses in front of the left common iliac artery to enter the pelvic cavity. The ureter within the pelvic cavity is later dissected.

10.1.4.2 Dissect the Blood Vessels and Nerves

Step 1. Peel off the lymph nodes and connective tissues around the celiac trunk and roots of the superior and inferior mesenteric arteries to expose the thick abdominal aorta surrounded by nerve plexuses. Trace the abdominal aorta downward at the level of the fourth lumbar vertebra (L4), where it gives off the left and right common iliac arteries. The nerve plexus extends downward to the pelvis to form the hypogastric plexus. Peel off the peritoneum on the right side of the abdominal aorta, and observe the inferior vena cava lying parallel to it. Identify the origin of the inferior vena cava formed by the union of the left and right common iliac veins posterior to the right common iliac artery. The left common iliac vein is situated between the left and right common iliac arteries, and the right common iliac vein lies deep to the artery.

Step 2. Remove the left renal vein that arises from the renal hilum, travels posterior to the roots of the superior mesenteric artery and vein, and drains the blood from the left testicular (ovarian) vein. Dissect the left suprarenal vein anterior to the left suprarenal gland, and trace its drainage into the left renal vein. The right renal vein is shorter than the left one in length.

Step 3. Observe the testicular (ovarian) vein anterior to the lower part of the psoas major muscle. Peel off the peritoneum and trace upward along the left testicular vein, which is observed to drain into the left renal vein at a right angle. The right testicular vein, however, directly drains into the inferior vena cava. The testicular (ovarian) artery is accompanied by the corresponding vein medially. Trace it upward and observe its origin of the abdominal aorta slightly inferior to the renal artery.

Step 4. Observe the left renal artery that arises from the left portion of the abdominal aorta slightly inferior to the origin of the superior mesenteric artery and travels transversely to the left to enter the left renal hilum. The right renal artery arises from the right portion of the abdominal aorta at the level of the origin of the left renal artery and travels transversely to the right to enter the right renal hilum.

Step 5. Remove the psoas major and quadratus lumborum muscles. Then observe the subcostal, iliohypogastric, ilioinguinal, and lateral femoral cutaneous nerves and the genitofemoral nerve that perforates the psoas major muscle, as well as their anatomic relationship with the psoas major muscle. Cut open the peritoneum covering the iliac fossa, and remove the testicular artery and vein and the vas deferens that turns from the abdominal ring to the pelvic cavity. In the female cadaver, remove the ovarian artery and vein and round ligament of the uterus. Cut open the fascia lining between the lateral portion of the psoas major muscle and the iliacus muscle to explore the femoral nerve.

Step 6. Dissect along the medial margin of the psoas major muscle, and observe the lumbar sympathetic trunks running longitudinally on both sides of the spine. The lumbar sympathetic trunk on each side contains three to four enlarged sympathetic ganglia that give off lumbar splanchnic nerves coursing to the abdominal aortic plexus. The lumbar sympathetic trunk continues with the thoracic portion and descends to the pelvic cavity after passing through the deep side of the common iliac artery and vein. The left lumbar sympathetic trunk is adjacent to the left margin of the abdominal aorta, and the right-sided one is anteriorly covered by the inferior vena cava.

Step 7. Lift up the left margin of the inferior vena cava and remove the connective tissue. Expose the last three pairs of the lumbar arteries on the right side by lifting up the abdominal aorta, which arise from the posterior wall of the abdominal aorta and travel posterior to the lumbar sympathetic trunk to the deep side of the psoas major muscle. Similarly, expose the last three pairs of the lumbar arteries on the left side by lifting up the left margin of the abdominal aorta. The lumbar veins accompany with the corresponding arteries.

10.2 Clinical Application of Key Anatomical Structures of the Retroperitoneal Space

10.2.1 Anatomy of the Pancreas and Its Clinical Application

The pancreas is a retroperitoneal organ situated anteriorly to the abdominal aorta and the inferior vena cava, between the celiac trunk and superior mesenteric artery. It is adjacent to the stomach, duodenum, spleen, and transverse colon. The head of the pancreas is surrounded by the C-shaped curve of the duodenum. The ampulla of Vater is formed by the common bile duct running within the head of the pancreas that fuses with the pancreatic duct, and opens at the major duodenal papilla. The pancreas receives a rich blood supply. Briefly, the anterior and posterior arterial arcades formed by the gastroduodenal artery (branch of the common hepatic artery) and inferior pancreaticoduodenal artery (branch of the superior mesenteric artery) provide the arterial supply to the head of the pancreas. The dorsal pancreatic artery, greater pancreatic artery, and anastomoses formed by the transverse pancreatic artery (or the inferior pancreatic artery) that arises from the splenic artery supply the body and tail of the pancreas (Fig. 10.4a). A precise dissection of the abovementioned blood vessels is of great significance in pancreatic surgeries. The application of anatomical structures of the pancreas in common pancreas surgeries is thoroughly described in the following section.

10.2.1.1 Pancreaticoduodenectomy

The Whipple procedure, or pancreaticoduodenectomy, is a common surgical procedure to remove tumors around the ampulla and reconstruct the digestive tract. Typically, it involves the removal of the distal stomach, gallbladder, common bile duct, duodenum, head of the pancreas, and part of the proximal jejunum, followed by the pancreaticojejunostomy, cholangioenterostomy, and gastrointestinal anastomosis (Fig. 10.15).

A skin incision is made on the left side of the upper abdomen below the xiphoid process, bypassing the umbilicus to its inferior aspect. The Kocher maneuver is performed to dissociate the descending and horizontal parts of the duodenum and head of the pancreas and to expose the inferior vena cava and abdominal aorta. The position, size, and texture of the tumors in the head of the pancreas are then palpable, as well as its anatomic relation with surrounding blood vessels. Dissociate the greater omentum close to the avascular area of the transverse mesocolon to expose the omental bursa and pancreas (Fig. 10.16).

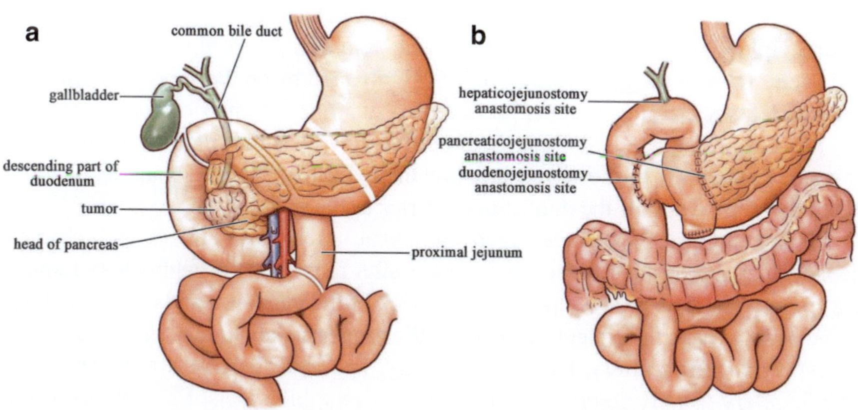

Fig. 10.15 Representative images of the pancreaticoduodenectomy and digestive tract reconstruction (**a**. standard Whipple procedure with the resection of a portion of the stomach and preservation of the pylorus; pancreaticoduodenectomy involves the resection of the duodenum inferior to the pylorus; **b**. Child-type reconstruction of the digestive tract)

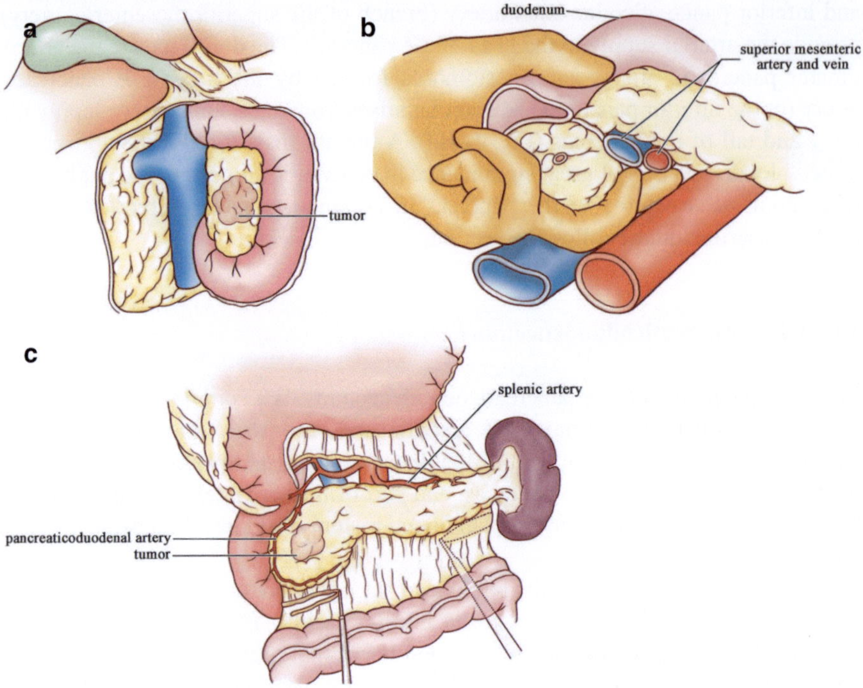

Fig. 10.16 Representative images to expose the pancreas (**a**. dissociation of the duodenum and head of the pancreas via the Kocher maneuver; **b**. palpation of the head of the pancreas; **c**. exposure of the body and tail of the pancreas)

Dissect the inferior portion of the neck of the pancreas to expose the superior mesenteric vein. The gastrocolic trunk of Henle formed by the union of the right gastroepiploic vein and accessory right colic vein drains into the superior mesenteric vein. Dissect the gastrocolic trunk of Henle, and reach the superior portion of the pancreas by creating a tunnel between the superior mesenteric vein and head of the pancreas. The standard Whipple procedure involves the removal of the distal stomach at the body of the stomach, while the pylorus-preserving pancreatoduodenectomy aims to cut off the duodenum inferior to the pylorus.

Dissect the Calot's triangle, ligate the cystic artery, and cut off the common hepatic duct approaching to the porta hepatis after removing the gallbladder. Expose the common hepatic artery superior to the neck of the pancreas, and dissect it along to the porta hepatis to sequentially expose the proper hepatic artery, gastroduodenal artery, right gastric artery, left hepatic artery, and right hepatic artery. The right hepatic artery usually enters the liver anterior to the bile ducts. Be cautious to the alternative or variation of the right hepatic artery on the right side or posterior to the bile ducts, the potential damage to which may cause liver ischemia, biliary tumors, liver abscesses, or even liver failure. Posterior to the common bile duct is the portal vein formed by the union of the superior mesenteric vein and splenic vein inferior to the neck of the pancreas. Dissect along the common hepatic artery to the left to expose the celiac trunk and the left gastric and splenic arteries arising from it. The gastroduodenal artery is the main blood vessel supplying the head of the pancreas and duodenum. Its ligation needs to be carefully performed due to a high risk of corrosive effects of pancreatic fistulas after pancreaticoduodenectomy. A gradient ligation procedure is clinically adopted to first make a ligature (not too tight) of the root of the gastroduodenal artery, followed by a tight figure-of-eight suture at the distal end and disconnection. Finally, dissect the pancreas at the neck, identify the position of the pancreatic duct, and determine its diameter, and suture bleeding wounds (Fig. 10.17).

Dissociate the duodenojejunal flexure inferior to the ligament of Treitz, and cut off the proximal jejunum after freeing the mesojejunum. Pull the proximal jejunum from the posterior aspect of mesenteric vessels to the right side, as well as the portal and superior mesenteric veins to the left to fully expose the uncinate process. Remove the nerves and connective tissues on the right half of the superior mesenteric artery, ligate the inferior pancreaticoduodenal artery that arises from the superior mesenteric artery, and completely resect the uncinate process (Fig. 10.18).

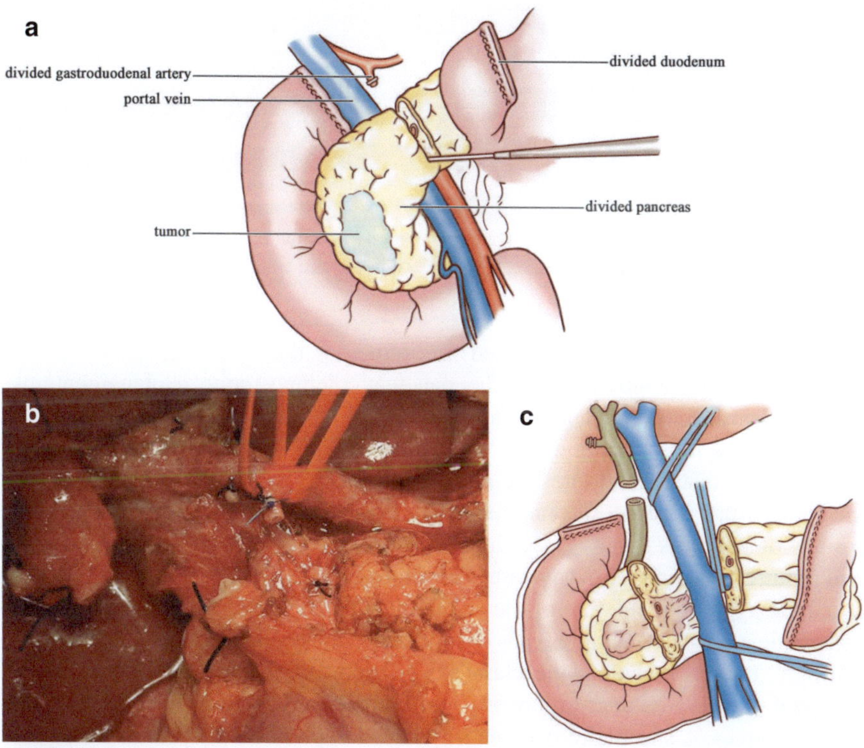

Fig. 10.17 Representative images before and after dissecting the pancreas (**a**. before dissecting the pancreas; **b**. regional anatomy of the porta hepatis after dissecting the common hepatic artery and gastroduodenal artery; **c**. exposure of the portal vein system after dissecting the pancreas)

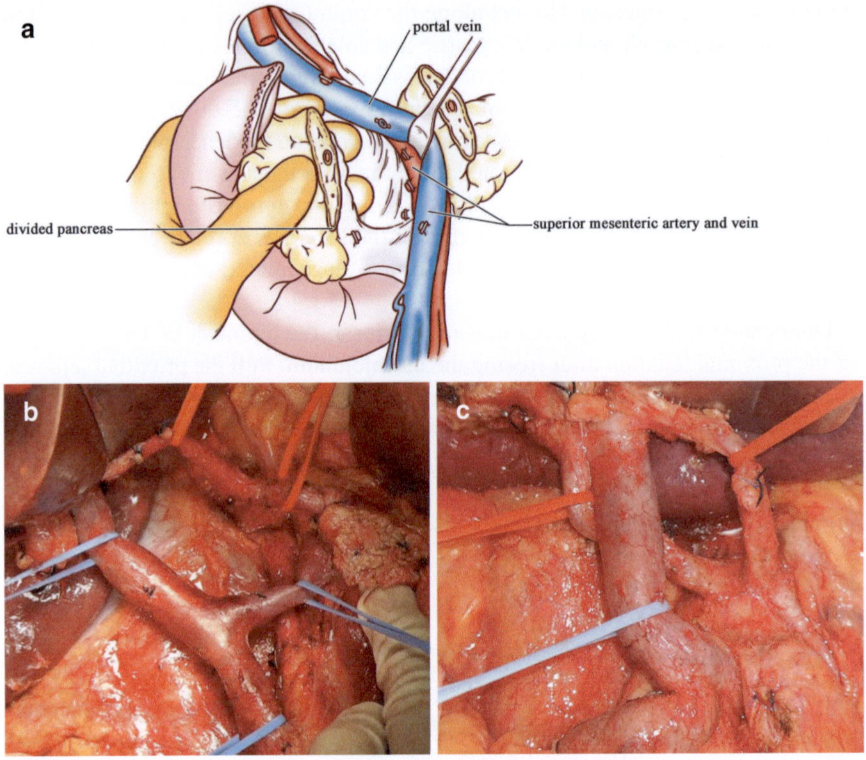

Fig. 10.18 Representative images of removing the uncinate process (**a**. removal of the uncinate process; **b**. a representative image after pancreaticoduodenectomy; **c**. a representative image after pancreaticoduodenectomy with the presence of the right hepatic artery with an ectopic position)

The digestive tract is reconstructed after removing the head of the pancreas, and the common procedure involves the pancreaticojejunostomy, cholangioenterostomy, and gastrointestinal anastomosis. The Child-type reconstruction of the digestive tract is the most common procedure, involving the pancreaticojejunostomy by lifting up the distal small intestine at first, followed by cholangioenterostomy and gastrointestinal anastomosis. Pancreatic fistulas are one of the most serious complications of pancreas surgeries, leading to abdominal infection, vascular corrosion and rupture, bleeding, or even death. The Child-type reconstruction can effectively avoid the aggressive mixture of the acidic bile and the pancreatic juice to activate pancreatic enzymes. Multiple types of procedures are available for pancreaticojejunostomy, mainly including the classic two-layered duct-to-mucosa anastomosis, modified one-layered duct-to-mucosa anastomosis, and invaginating and telescoping techniques. A successful pancreaticojejunostomy effectively prevents the postoperative pancreatic fistulas. The one-layered duct-to-mucosa anastomosis is a simple procedure that effectively lowers the incidence of postoperative pancreatic fistulas and features a wider spacing between sutures to close more pancreatic

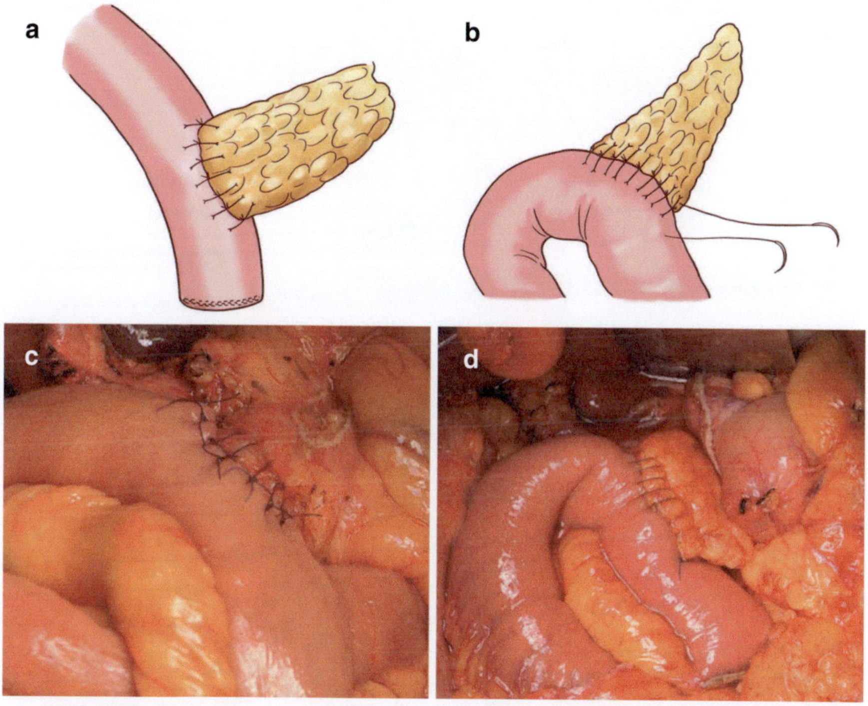

Fig. 10.19 Representative images of the modified duct-to-mucosa anastomosis for pancreaticojejunostomy (**a**, **c**. one-layered duct-to-mucosa anastomosis with interrupted sutures; **b**, **d**. one-layered duct-to-mucosa anastomosis with continuous sutures)

tissues, sparser needle spacing to ensure the normal blood supply without influences by too dense sutures, and loose sutures to prevent from tissue edema and cutting pancreatic tissues by sutures in this condition. The continuous suture technique is also available for pancreaticojejunostomy (Fig. 10.19).

10.2.2 Distal Pancreatectomy

The distal pancreatectomy is the classic surgical treatment of tumors of the body and tail of the pancreas, which removes the body and tail of the pancreas and spleen. Spleen-preserving distal pancreatectomy is an option for benign lesions, involving the Kimura technique with the preservation of the splenic vessels and the Warshaw technique without preserving splenic artery and vein (Fig. 10.20).

Cut open the gastrocolic ligament close to the transverse colon, and enter the omental bursa to expose the pancreas and visualize the lesions in the body and tail of the pancreas. Dissect the gastrosplenic ligament and dissociate the short gastric veins from the greater curvature of the stomach proximal to the left side of the

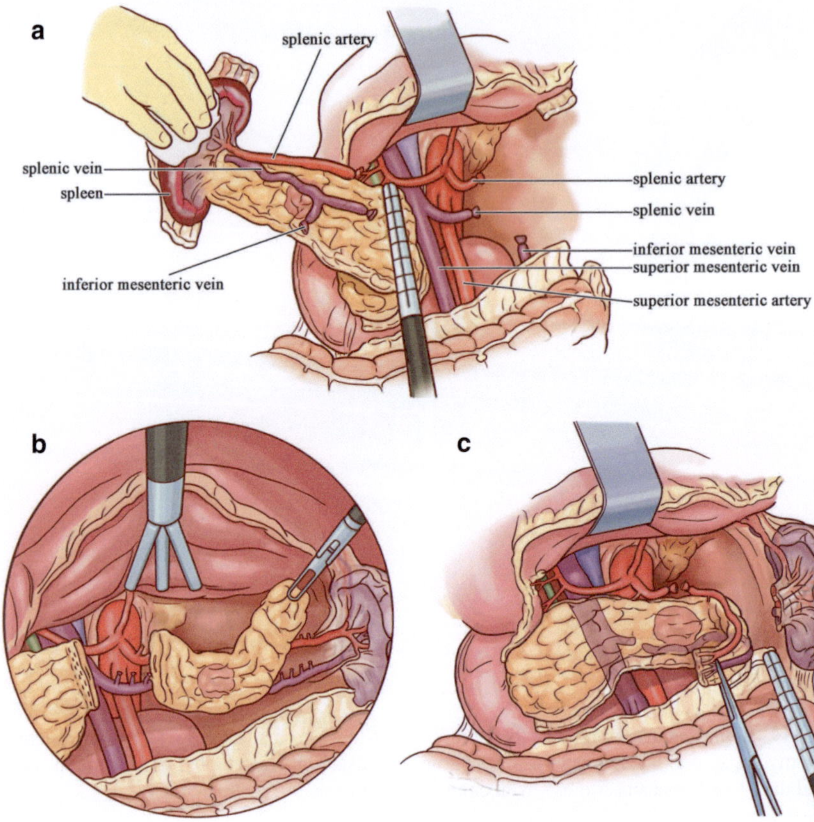

Fig. 10.20 Representative images of distal pancreatectomy (**a**. classic distal pancreatectomy with the removal of the spleen; **b**. laparoscopic distal pancreatectomy with the Kimura technique to preserve splenic vessels; **c**. laparoscopic distal pancreatectomy with the Warshaw technique to dissect splenic vessels)

cardia. Expose the superior mesenteric vein inferior to the neck of the pancreas, and create a tunnel to separate it upward. Then expose the common hepatic artery superior to the pancreas and dissect it to the left to further expose the splenic and left gastric arteries. They are ligated and disconnected at the root of the splenic artery. Dissociate the pancreas at the tail and the splenic vein inferior to the pancreas. After lifting up the pancreas and dissociating it toward the body and tail until reaching the hilus, the splenophrenic, splenocolic, and splenorenal ligaments are dissociated to completely remove the body and tail of the pancreas and spleen. A margin-negative resection (R0) at the retroperitoneum after cutting off the Gerota's fascia is essential for the surgical treatment of malignant lesions. The left suprarenal gland and adipose capsule are also required to be resected on the surface of the left renal vein (Fig. 10.21).

A modified Appleby procedure involving the resection of the body and tail of the pancreas and celiac trunk is feasible for patients with pancreatic tumors invading the

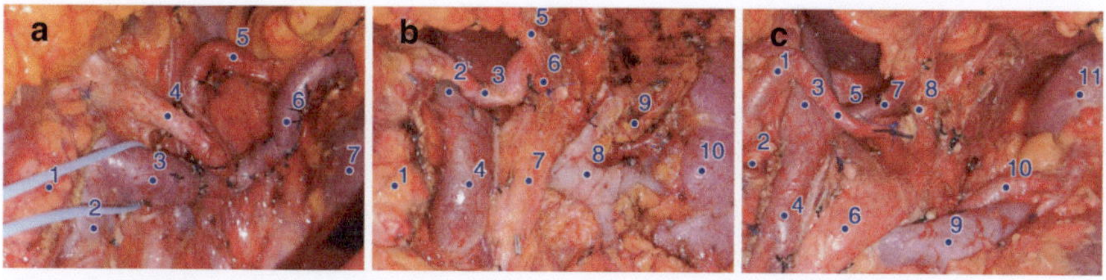

Fig. 10.21 Representative images after distal pancreatectomy. (**a**) Distal pancreatectomy with the Kimura technique (1. pancreas; 2. superior mesenteric vein; 3. splenic vein; 4. splenic artery; 5. splenic artery; 6. splenic vein; 7. spleen). (**b**) Anterior radical antegrade modular pancreatosplenectomy (RAMPS) with the preservation of the left suprarenal gland (1. pancreas; 2. portal vein; 3. common hepatic artery; 4. superior mesenteric vein; 5. left gastric artery; 6. splenic artery stump; 7. superior mesenteric artery; 8. left renal vein; 9. suprarenal gland; 10. kidney). (**c**) Posterior RAMPS with the removal of the left suprarenal gland (1. gastroduodenal artery; 2. pancreas; 3. portal vein; 4. superior mesenteric vein; 5. common hepatic artery; 6. superior mesenteric artery; 7. left gastric vein; 8. left gastric artery; 9. left renal vein; 10. left renal artery; 11. kidney)

celiac trunk. It allows to dissociate blood vessels at the root of the celiac trunk, resects the common hepatic and left gastric arteries, but preserves the gastroduodenal artery. The arterial arcades, formed by the inferior pancreaticoduodenal artery arising from the superior mesenteric artery at the head of the pancreas, provide the blood to the liver through the gastroduodenal and proper hepatic arteries (Fig. 10.22). Considering the potential risk of liver and gastric ischemia due to the reduced hepatic blood flow, indications for the modified Appleby procedure should be strictly concerned.

10.2.3 Anatomy of the Kidney and Its Clinical Application

The main structures in the retroperitoneal space include the duodenum, pancreas, kidneys, suprarenal glands, ureters, large blood vessels in the abdomen, lymphatic vessels, and lymph nodes. Their anatomical structures and adjacent tissues should be intraoperatively concerned. The regional anatomy of important structures in the retroperitoneal space during kidney surgeries is thoroughly described in the following section.

10.2.3.1 Surgical Approach

Open Surgery

A skin incision for an open surgery of the kidney is made about 1.0 cm below the inferior border of the 12th rib, lateral to the erector spinae muscle, obliquely extending forward and downward to the internal side of the anterior superior iliac spine (Fig. 10.23a–c).

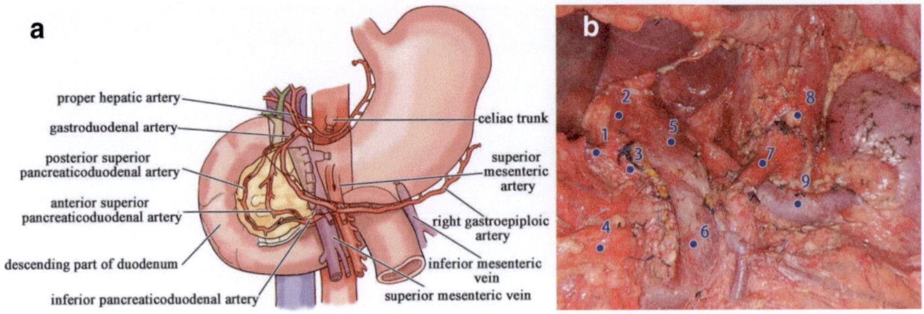

Fig. 10.22 Modified Appleby procedure. (**a**) Arterial supply to the liver during the modified Appleby procedure. (**b**) Intraoperative images of the modified Appleby procedure (1. right gastric artery; 2. proper hepatic artery; 3. gastroduodenal artery; 4. pancreas; 5. portal vein; 6. superior mesenteric vein; 7. superior mesenteric artery; 8. tumor residue; 9. left renal vein)

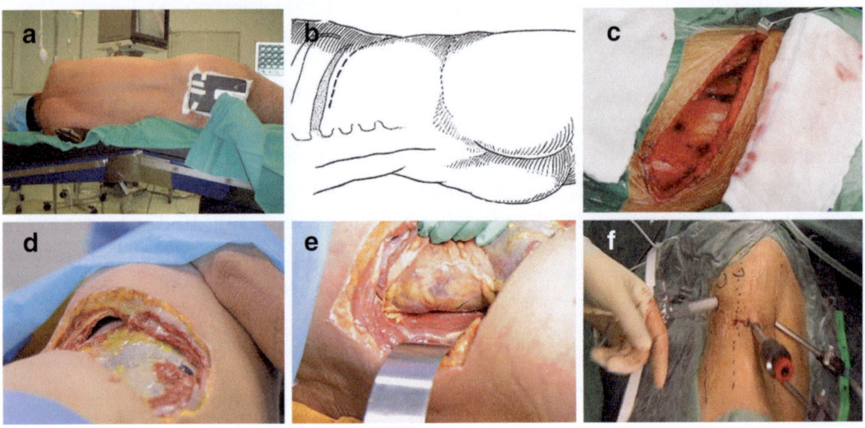

Fig. 10.23 Skin incisions for the kidney surgery (**a**. intraoperative position; **b**. a position for exposing the incision; **c**. an intraoperative incision; **d**. layers at the skin incision; **e**. anatomy under the skin incision; **f**. trocar placement for minimally invasive laparoscopy)

Laparoscopic Retroperitoneal Approach

Similar to the open surgery, the patient is placed in a lateral position on the uninjured side with the lumbar extension. Trocars A and B are inserted at 2.0 cm superior to the anterior superior iliac spine and inferior to the rib margin along the posterior axillary line, respectively. Trocars C and D are inserted subcostal in the anterior axillary line (Fig. 10.23d–f).

10.2.3.2 Major Structures in the Regional Anatomy of the Kidney

Location and Surrounding Structures

The kidneys are paired on both sides of the spine, with the posterior aspect approaching to the posterior abdominal wall. The long axes of the kidneys obliquely point to the inferolateral aspect, with the superior poles orienting to each other. The kidney is inferior to the suprarenal gland with the surrounding loose connective tissues, both of which are wrapped by the renal fascia. Inferior and internal to the kidney are the renal pelvis and ureter, posterointernal is the lumbar sympathetic trunk, lateral is the quadratus lumborum muscle, and posterointernal is the psoas major muscle backward. Anterosuperior to the kidney is the right lobe of the liver and a cover of the visceral peritoneum, anteroinferior is the right colic flexure, and internal is the inferior vena cava. The descending part of the duodenum lies on the inner side of the right-sided renal hilum, which is constantly located and prone to rupture in the surgery. The inferior vena cava should be intraoperatively protected to prevent uncontrollable bleeding. Internal to the left kidney is the abdominal aorta, anterosuperior is the posterior gastric wall, superior and lateral is the spleen, and inferior are the jejunal loops and splenic flexure. The pancreas transversely lies in front of the middle part of the left kidney, and the tail of the pancreas and splenic vessels closely approach to the renal hilum. The body and tail and the pancreas and abdominal aorta should be protected during the left kidney surgery (Fig. 10.24).

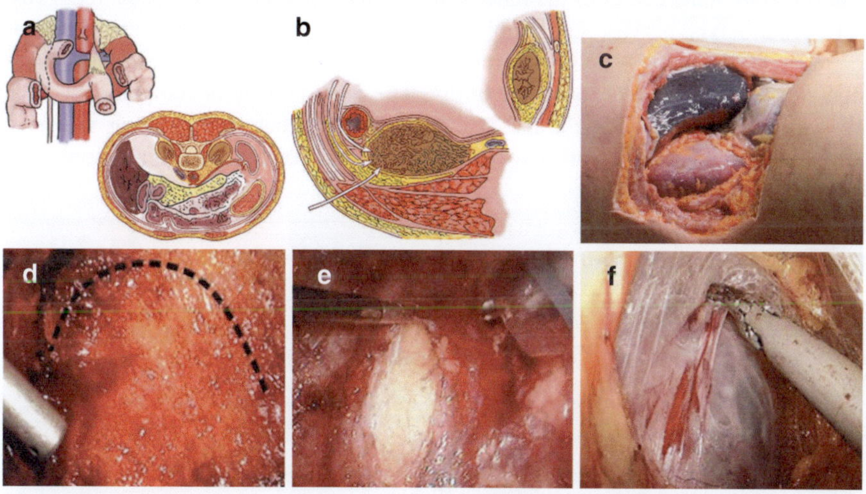

Fig. 10.24 Anatomical structures of the kidney (**a**, **c**. adjacent structures of the kidney; **b**. renal capsule and adjacent muscles; **d**, **e**. removal of extraperitoneal fat and perinephric fascia; **f**. removal of perinephric adipose to expose the renal cysts)

Key Points to Expose the Kidney

The kidneys in the retroperitoneal space are often squeezed forward due to body position and pneumoperitoneum pressure and can be visualized only after removing the extraperitoneal fat, cutting open the perinephric fascia and cleaning off the perinephric fat. Three layers of renal capsule are exposed during the dissection of perirenal tissues, namely, the renal fascia (Gerota's fascia), adipose capsule, and fibrous capsule from outside to inside. The renal fascia is a dense, elastic connective tissue envelop that encloses the kidney and suprarenal gland. The adipose capsule is a layer of adipose tissue with a thickness of 2.0 cm in adults, thicker on the posterior side and at the margin. It is responsible for supporting and protecting the kidney. The fibrous capsule, also known as the fibrous membrane, is the lamina propria of the kidney composed of dense, thin, and tough connective tissue that covers the outer surface and protects the kidney. It should be sutured during the partial nephrectomy or surgical procedures for renal trauma.

For radical nephrectomy, it is necessary to separate the kidney from perirenal fat as much as possible. Dissection of the perirenal fat to expose renal lesions is essential for partial nephrectomy and renal cyst deroofing and decompression.

Key Points in Processing the Renal Hilum

The renal hilum is usually processed during kidney surgeries (Fig. 10.25), which is a depression in the center of the inner side of the kidney that contains the renal vessels, renal pelvis, nerves, and lymphatic vessels. The margin of the renal hilum is bounded by the anterior and posterior hilar lips, which are elastic that can be intraoperatively retracted to expand the hilum. The renal pedicle is composed of renal vessels, renal pelvis, nerves, and lymphatic vessels that pass through the renal hilum. The renal arteries arise from the lateral side of the abdominal aorta, run

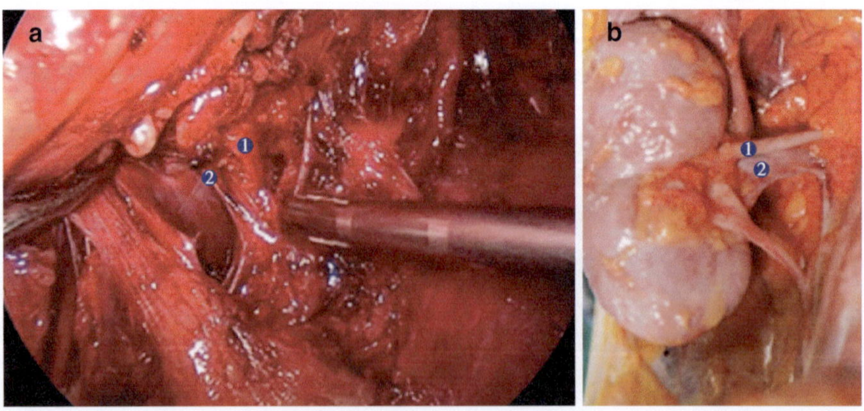

Fig. 10.25 Anatomy of the renal hilum. (**a**) Representative intraoperative images (1. renal arteries; 2. renal veins). (**b**) Gross specimen (1. renal arteries; 2. renal veins)

transversely and outward from the posterior and superior part of the renal vein, and enter the kidney via the renal hilum. Accessory renal arteries are considered as the variations of the renal arteries that arise from the abdominal aorta. Ignorance of accessory renal arteries poses a high risk of intraoperative bleeding. The right renal artery is longer than the left one in length due to the left-sided position of the abdominal aorta and enters the right kidney posterior to the inferior vena cava. The right renal vein is shorter than the left one because of the inferior vena cava situated in the right side. Cautions should be made to protect the inferior vena cava during the surgery for the right kidney, thus preventing massive bleeding. A retroperitoneal approach is usually adopted to expose and dissociate the renal pedicle. From posterior to anterior, the renal pelvis, renal artery, and renal vein lie within the renal pedicle. From superior to posterior are the renal artery, renal vein, and renal pelvis. Renal artery can be intraoperatively identified by arterial pulsation because of the low position of the renal pelvis.

10.2.3.3 Anatomy of the Branches of Renal Arteries and Veins

The main trunk of the renal arteries gives off multiple segmental arteries before and after entering the renal hilum, which has been described in the previous section. In partial nephrectomy, the anatomy of renal segmental arteries could be kept clear in mind to prevent renal dysfunction due to ischemia-reperfusion injury following the complete blockage of renal blood flow. The renal segmental arteries are highly variable and can be preoperatively visualized by computed tomography angiography (CTA) to favor the precise blockage of renal arteries (Fig. 10.26).

The left suprarenal vein and left gonadal (testicular or ovarian) vein drain into the left renal vein and should be carefully identified and protected intraoperatively (Fig. 10.27).

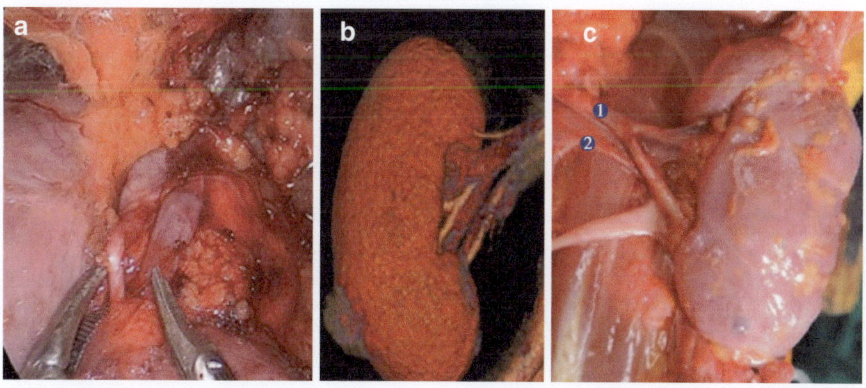

Fig. 10.26 Branches of the renal arteries. (**a**) Representative intraoperative images. (**b**) Representative radiological images. (**c**) Gross specimen (1. renal arteries; 2. renal veins)

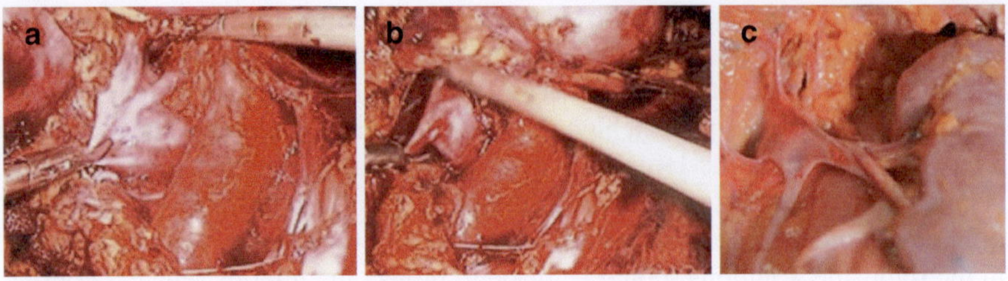

Fig. 10.27 Branches of the renal veins. (**a**) Intraoperative dissociation of the suprarenal veins. (**b**) Intraoperative dissociation of the gonadal vein. (**c**) Gross specimen

Chapter 11
Regional Anatomy of the Pelvic Cavity and Its Clinical Application

Yongjie Zhang, Weiwei Sun, Kun Xiong, Pengfei Shao, and Jian Qian

11.1 Regional Anatomy of Pelvic Cavity

11.1.1 Boundary

Pelvic cavity is the lacuna bounded by the pelvic wall and diaphragm. The pelvic wall, comprising lesser pelvis, parietal pelvic muscles, and parietal pelvic fascia, surrounds the pelvic cavity. The lower bound of the pelvic cavity is the pelvic diaphragm, also called the pelvic floor. The upper bound is the inlet of the lesser pelvis, serving as the junction of the abdominal and pelvic cavities.

11.1.2 Structural Characteristics

As part of the body cavity, pelvic cavity is composed of the pelvic peritoneal cavity and the inferior pelvic peritoneal cavity.

Y. Zhang · W. Sun (✉) · P. Shao · J. Qian
Nanjing Medical University, Nanjing, China
e-mail: zhangyongjie@njmu.edu.cn; sunweiwei@njmu.edu.cn

K. Xiong
Central South University Xiangya School of Medicine, Changsha, China

Q. Ding et al. (eds.), *Clinically Oriented Regional Anatomy*,
https://doi.org/10.1007/978-981-95-9888-5_11

11.1.2.1 Pelvic Peritoneal Cavity

Pelvic peritoneal cavity is a part of the peritoneal cavity (Fig. 11.1). At the junction of the middle and lower third of the rectum, the peritoneum covers the anterior wall of the rectum and folds forward. In males, the peritoneum continues to migrate to the surface of the bladder, forming a rectovesical pouch between the rectum and the bladder, the bottom of which is about 7.5 cm away from the anus; in females, the peritoneum extends downward and forward to the posterosuperior fornix of the vaginal fornix, stretches upward to cover the cervix and posterior wall of the uterus and wrap the fundus of uterus, then descends along the anterior uterus, and reflects forward near the uterine isthmus to the bladder, forming rectouterine pouch (between rectum and uterus) and vesicouterine pouch (between bladder and uterus). The rectouterine pouch (also known as Douglas pouch) is deeper, with its bottom about 5.5 cm from the anus. In sitting and semirecumbent positions, rectovesical and rectouterine pouches are the lowest parts of the peritoneal cavity in males and females, respectively, where fluid accumulates in case of peritoneal effusion. Accordingly, in clinical practice, paracentesis can be performed via the anterior rectal wall or posterior fornix of vagina for effusion drainage. Semirecumbent position can also be applied in patients with acute abdominal disease or after abdominal or pelvic cavity surgeries.

Lying on the two flanks of rectovesical and rectouterine pouches are rectovesical and rectouterine folds, respectively. In males, the ureter and vas deferens extend toward the base of the bladder in front of the deep surface of the rectovesical fold. In females, the deep surface of the rectouterine fold is the sacrouterine ligament.

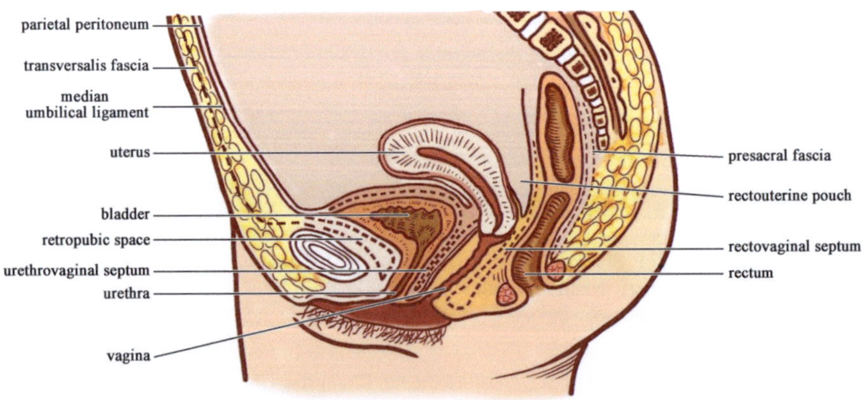

Fig. 11.1 Medial sagittal section of the pelvic cavity in females

11.1.2.2 Pelvic Subperitoneal Cavity

Between the pelvic peritoneum and pelvic floor surrounded by pelvic wall is the pelvic subperitoneal cavity, which extends into the extraperitoneal space through the pelvic inlet. Inside the cavity are several organs of the digestive, urinary, and reproductive systems, some vital blood vessels, nerves, lymph nodes, as well as a large amount of loose connective tissues, pelvic fasciae, and their formations.

Pelvic Fascia

As the immediate extension of intra-abdominal fascia, the pelvic fascia consists of parietal and visceral components: parietal pelvic fascia and visceral pelvic fascia.

Parietal pelvic fascia (Fig. 11.2), also known as the parietal layer of pelvic fascia, covers the inner side of the pelvic wall. The parts that cover the piriformis and internal obturator muscle are called piriformis fascia and obturator fascia, respectively. At top of the obturator fascia, the incrassated section between the posterior symphysis pubis and the ischial spine is the tendinous arch of levator ani, one origin of the levator ani muscle. The fascia covering the musculus levator ani is the superior fascia of pelvic diaphragm, a component of the pelvic diaphragm. It connects to the obturator fascia at the tendinous arch of the levator ani. Another part of parietal pelvic fascia is in front of the sacrum, called presacral fascia. Between the presacral fascia and the sacrum is a large quantity of venous plexus. Therefore, the damage of the presacral fascia during intrapelvic surgery may lead to massive hemorrhage.

Visceral pelvic fascia, also known as the visceral layer of pelvic fascia or intrapelvic fascia, surrounds the intrapelvic organs, blood vessels, and nerves and forms vascular and neural sheaths, visceral fascia, fascia septum, and some ligaments.

Visceral fascia, such as rectus sheath, vesicle pouch, and prostatic capsule, wraps the intrapelvic organs. Near the pelvic floor, the visceral fascia migrates with the superior fascia of pelvic diaphragm and presacral fascia. The fascia of pelvic organs

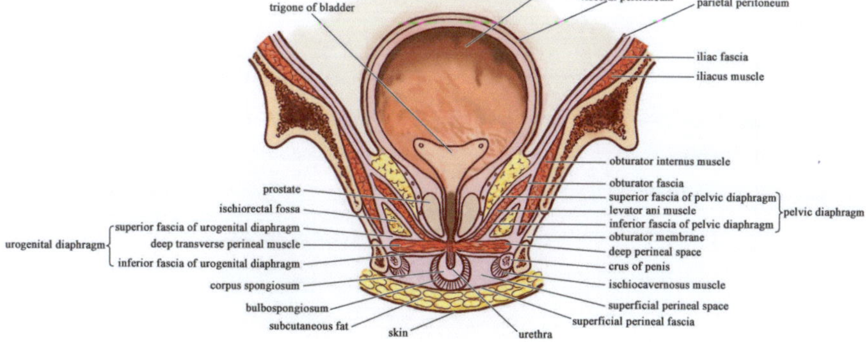

Fig. 11.2 Frontal section of male pelvic cavity (via urinary bladder)

presents varying patterns of development, which is associated with the changes in the volume of organs. The fascia surrounding the organ with a large extent of volume change (e.g., vesicle pouch) does not develop to a perfect level, but with a better adapt ability, while the organ with a small extent of volume change (e.g., prostatic capsule) tends to have a fascia well developed.

Vascular and neural sheaths are composed of pelvic fascia wrapping the intrapelvic vessels and nerves, including internal iliac arteries, veins, and their branches (or tributaries), together with pelvic plexus and their branches. The vascular and neural sheaths link the ischial spine and the cervix uteri (in females) or bladder base (in males) and extend to the areas surrounding the bladder, uterus, and vagina. The fascial sheaths at both lateral sides of the cervix uteri are called the cardinal ligaments of uterus, and those at both sides of the rectum are called the lateral ligaments of the rectum.

Fascia septum is the structure between the adjacent organs in frontal position. One example is the fascia peritoneoperinealis, which starts from the bottom of rectovesical pouch (in males) or rectouterine pouch (in females) and extends downward to the central tendon of the perineum. In males, the fascia septum is located between the rectum and bladder, the prostate and seminal vesicle, called rectovesical septum. In females, the fascia septum is located between the rectum and vagina, called the rectovaginal septum. Besides, the septum between the bladder and vagina is called the vesicovaginal septum and that between the urethra and vagina is the urethrovaginal septum.

Ligaments are incrassated pelvic fascia around the pelvic organs. They connect the organ and the bones to support and fixate the organs. Males have pubicoprostatic ligaments, while females have pubovesical and uterosacral ligaments (Fig. 11.3).

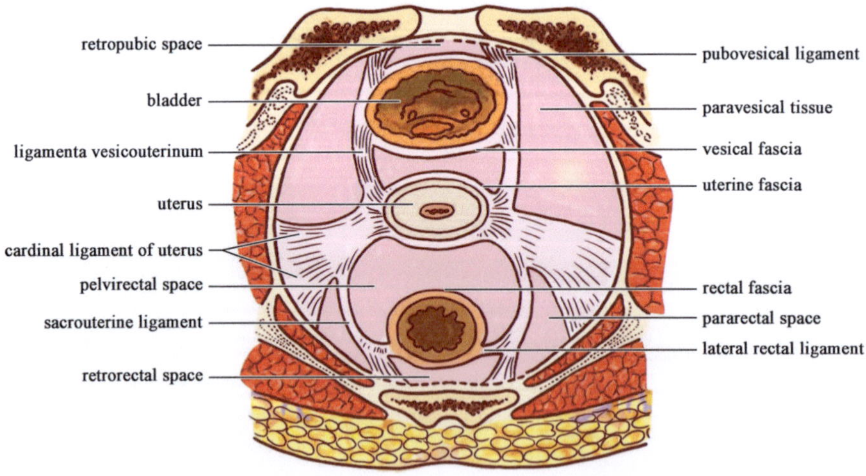

Fig. 11.3 Uterine ligaments and pelvic fascial spaces

Pelvic fascial spaces refer to the spaces between the parietal and visceral layers of the pelvic fascia, containing a large quantity of loose tissues. The retropubic and retrorectal spaces are of great clinical significance.

Retropubic space, also known as the prevesical or Retzius space, lies between the symphysis pubis and bladder. It is bilaterally lined by pubicoprostatic (in males) or pubovesical (in females) ligaments. The lower bound of retropubic space is the urogenital diaphragm, and the upper bound is connected to the extraperitoneal space of the anterior abdominal wall. In clinical practice, extraperitoneal surgeries on bladder, prostate, or uterus can be performed via this space.

Retrorectal space, also known as the presacral space, lies between the rectal and presacral fascia, with its top adjacent to the retroperitoneal space through the pelvic inlet and its two sides lined by the rectal lateral ligaments. The important structures inside the retrorectal space include the middle sacral artery, hypogastric plexus, sacral lymph nodes, sacral plexus, and lumbosacral trunk.

Vessels, Lymphatics, and Nerves in the Pelvic Cavity

Internal iliac artery, a short trunk about 4 cm long, travels downward against the pelvic posterior lateral wall and divides into the anterior and posterior trunks at the superior border of the piriformis (Fig. 11.4). The anterior trunk branches into the umbilical artery, obturator artery, inferior vesical artery, uterine artery (deferential artery in males), inferior rectal artery, internal pudendal artery, and inferior gluteal

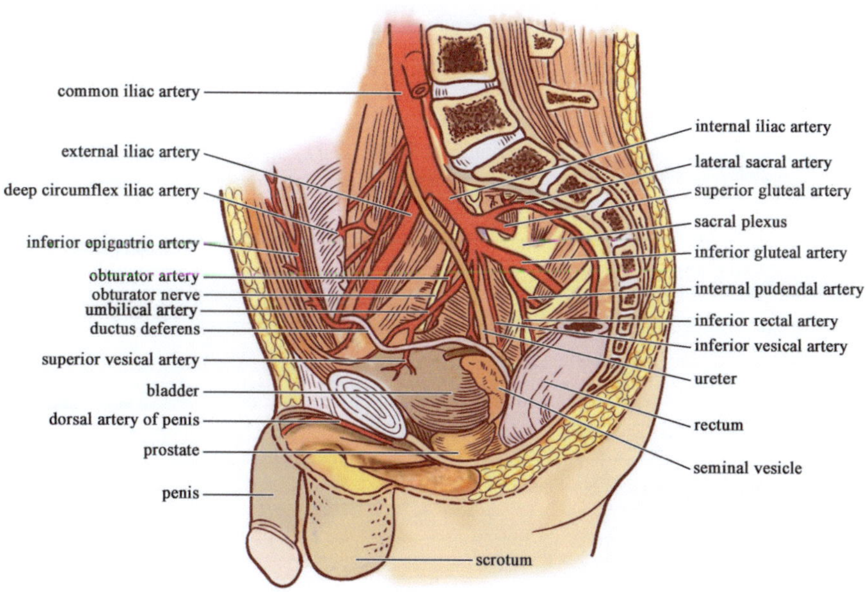

Fig. 11.4 Arteries in pelvic cavity

artery. The posterior trunk branches into the iliolumbar artery, lateral sacral artery, and superior gluteal artery.

The obturator artery is mostly the parietal branch of anterior trunk of the internal iliac artery. It courses anteriorly along the lateral pelvic wall and through the obturator canal to the inner thigh. The obturator artery sends out the pubic branch that anastomoses to the pubic branch of the inferior epigastric artery behind the superior ramus of pubis. In some cases, the anastomotic branch is thick, the obturator artery is thin or even absent, and the anastomotic branch takes the place of the obturator artery. Thus, this abnormal obturator mainly derives from the inferior epigastric artery. It can also stem from the external iliac or femoral arteries either directly or indirectly. The abnormal obturator artery usually travels along the lateral margin of the femoral ring (some along the internal margin or the central part), then goes downward, and enters the obturator canal. In femoral herniorrhaphy, damage to the obturator artery may result in hemorrhage.

Apart from the internal iliac artery and its branches, there are superior rectal artery and median sacral artery in the pelvic cavity. The former is the branch of the inferior mesenteric artery, and the latter originates from the posterior wall of the abdominal aorta bifurcation, runs across anterior to fourth and fifth lumbar vertebrae and descends into the pelvic cavity, and then goes down between the sacrum and presacral fascia.

The internal iliac vein travels along the posteromedial side of the internal iliac artery. All venous branches corresponding to eponymous internal iliac arterial branches, except the umbilical vein, are subordinate to the internal iliac vein (Fig. 11.5). The veins of pelvic visceral organs form venous plexuses (e.g., rectal,

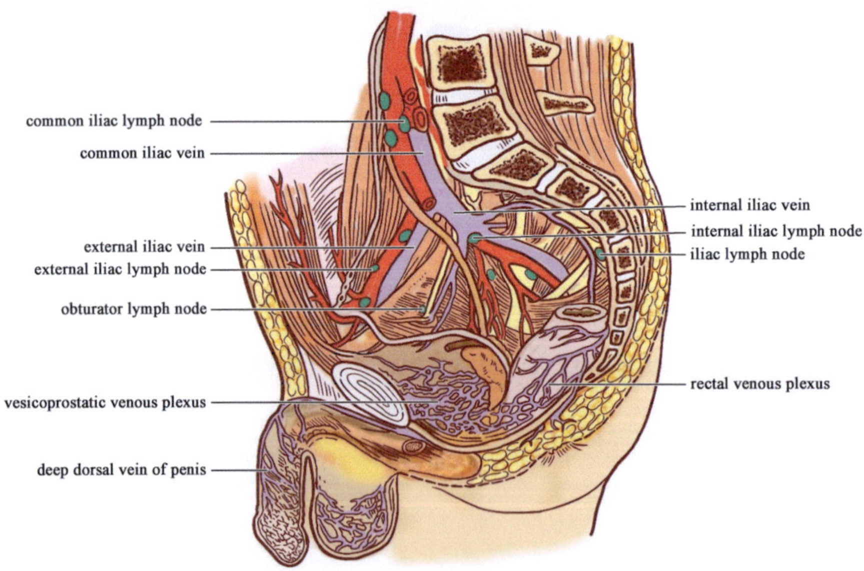

Fig. 11.5 Veins and lymph nodes in the pelvic cavity

vesical, prostatic, and uterine venous plexuses) at the proximal pelvic diaphragm and then congregate as accompanying veins of the corresponding arteries. Among these venous plexuses, the presacral venous plexus is located between the sacrum and presacral fascia; the rectal venous plexus is divided into internal venous plexus (located in the rectal submucosa and subcutaneous tissue) and external venous plexus (located outside the muscular layer); the vesical venous plexus is located around the lower part of the bladder; the male prostatic venous plexus is located in the anterior and lateral parts of the prostatic sheath; the female uterine and vaginal venous plexuses are located bilaterally along the uterus and vagina, and the ovarian venous plexus is located around the ovary and inside the uterine broad ligament near the fallopian tube.

The venous plexuses in the pelvic cavity have no valves. The anastomoses among the plexuses are abundant, thus benefiting venous drainage. The presacral venous plexus is connected to the intracranial vein via the internal and external vertebral venous plexuses and serves as an intracranial metastatic pathway of the pelvic tumor.

Lymph nodes in the pelvic cavity include the internal iliac lymph nodes and sacral lymph nodes. The internal iliac lymph nodes, distributing along the internal iliac artery and its branches, collect the lymph in the blood supply areas of the internal iliac artery. The sacral lymph nodes, distributing along the middle sacral artery, collect partial lymph from the posterior pelvic wall and intrapelvic visceral organs. The external iliac lymph nodes, distributing along the external iliac artery (Fig. 11.5), also collect some lymph from the intrapelvic visceral organs.

Nerves in the pelvic cavity are categorized as somatic nerves and visceral nerves (Fig. 11.6).

Somatic nerves in the pelvic cavity include obturator nerves, sacral plexus, and its branches. Obturator nerves, as branches of lumbar plexus, thread through the obturator canal with the obturator vessels in the pelvic cavity and then run out of the cavity. The sacral plexus is located anterior to the piriformis. Its branches exit the pelvic cavity via the suprapiriform and infrapiriform foramens.

The visceral nerves in the pelvic cavity include the sacral segment of the sympathetic trunk, hypogastric plexus, and pelvic visceral nerves. The sacral segment of the sympathetic trunk, also called the sacral sympathetic trunk, descends along the internal side of the anterior sacral foramen. The left and right sacral segments of the sympathetic trunk join at the front of the coccyx. The hypogastric plexus is composed of superior and inferior hypogastric plexuses. The superior hypogastric plexus descends from anterior fifth lumbar to the pelvic cavity and branches into the left and right hypogastric nerves near the sacral promontory. At the level of the third sacral vertebra, the left and right hypogastric nerves congregate with the lateral postganglionic fibers from the sacral ganglia and the pelvic splanchnic nerves to form the inferior hypogastric plexus, which is also known as pelvic plexus. The fibers of inferior hypogastric plexus run along the branches of internal iliac artery and reach the pelvic visceral organs. The pelvic splanchnic nerves are preganglionic parasympathetic fibers arising from the anterior branches of S2–S4 nerves; their postganglionic fibers innervate the descending and sigmoid colon, apart from the pelvic visceral organs.

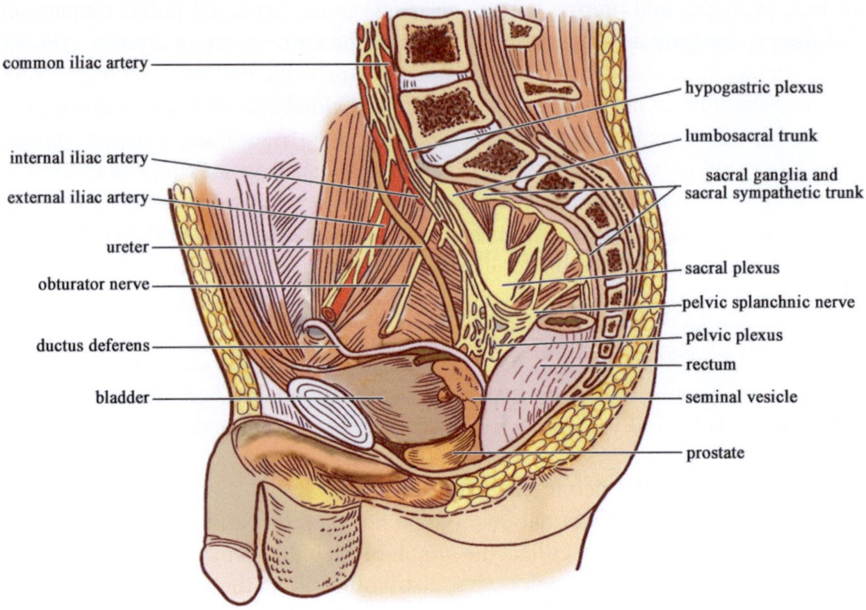

Fig. 11.6 Nerves in the pelvic cavity

11.1.3 Pelvic Viscera

Pelvic viscera include the digestive, urinary, and reproductive organs in the pelvic cavity. In the front of the pelvic cavity are bladder and urethra, and at the back are the inferior segment of the sigmoid colon and rectum. Between these viscera are the pelvic part of vas deferens, seminal vesicle, and prostate (in males) or ovaries, ductus deferens, uterus, and superior part of vagina (in female). Besides, the pelvic part of ureter runs along the lateral pelvic wall from the back forward to the internal part (Figs. 11.7 and 11.8). The present section focuses on bladder, prostate, and rectum.

11.1.3.1 Bladder

Location and Adjacencies of the Bladder

The bladder, an organ in the anterior pelvic cavity that stores urine, can be divided into an apex, a body, a fundus, and a neck. When empty, the bladder is an extraperitoneal organ, with its front and both sides adjacent to the pubic symphysis and lateral pelvic wall and its upper part next to the intestinal loop. In males, the inferior bladder neck is adjacent to the prostate, the lower part of the bladder fundus is adjacent to the seminal vesicles and ampulla of vas deferens, and the upper part of the base is next to the rectum. In females, the inferior bladder neck is adjacent to the

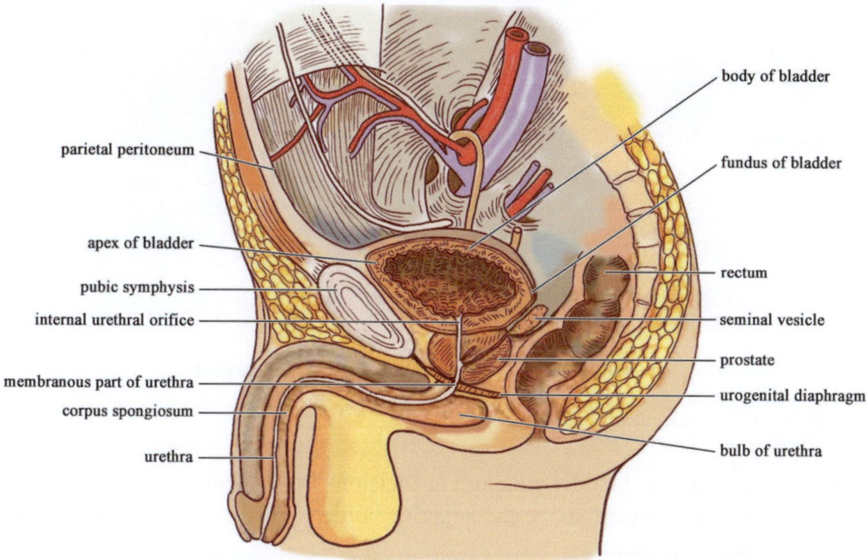

Fig. 11.7 Median sagittal section of male pelvic cavity

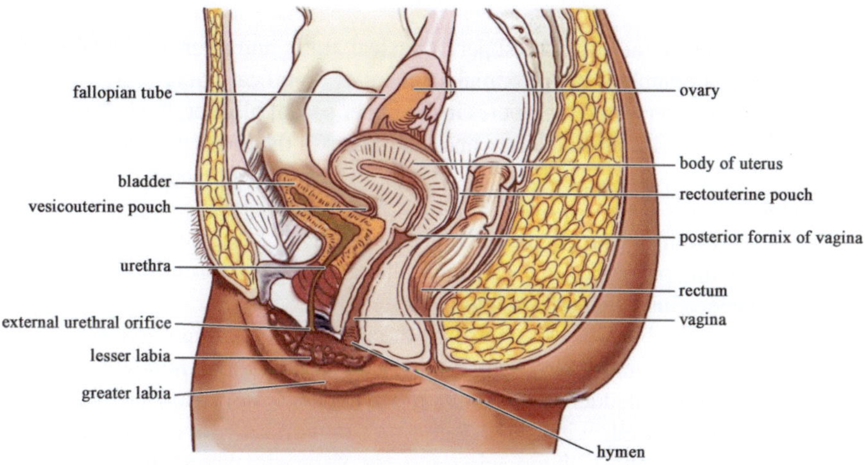

Fig. 11.8 Median sagittal section of female pelvic cavity

urogenital diaphragm, and the bladder fundus is next to the anterior wall of uterus and superior vaginal segment. In children, the bladder is located higher with part of it lodged in the abdominal cavity. In adults, the empty bladder is entirely situated in the pelvic cavity. But when it is full, the bladder apex and body can rise above the superior border of the pubic symphysis (Fig. 11.9); meanwhile, the peritoneal reflection between the anterior abdominal wall and upper bladder moves upward, making the anterior bladder wall adjacent to the anterior abdominal wall. Therefore,

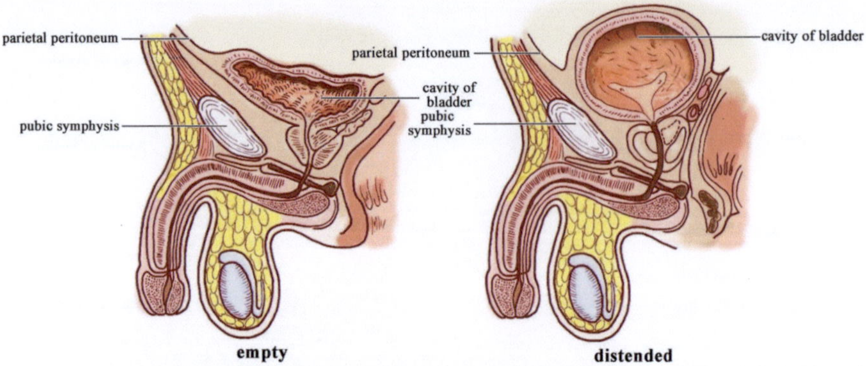

Fig. 11.9 Location change of bladder

during bladder filling, bladder puncture or incisions for bladder, prostate, or uterus surgeries should be made above the superior border of pubic symphysis to avoid damage to the peritoneum.

Vessels, Lymphatics, and Nerves of the Bladder

The vesical arteries comprise the superior vesical artery and inferior vesical artery. The former is a branch of the proximal segment of umbilical artery (deriving from the internal iliac artery) and distributes in the upper part of bladder; the latter springs directly from the internal iliac artery and distributes in the lower part of bladder. In addition, the inferior rectal and uterine arteries also have subbranches distributed in the bladder.

The vesicle veins first form the vesicle venous plexus at the neck of the bladder and on either side of the prostate gland and then converge to form the superior and inferior vesicle veins, which drain into the internal iliac vein.

Lymph from the bladder can drain into the internal iliac lymph nodes, external iliac lymph nodes, common iliac lymph nodes, and sacral lymph nodes.

The nerves of the bladder come from the pelvic plexus and follow the blood vessels to the bladder wall, with sympathetic preganglionic fibers coming from the lateral horns of 11th and 12th thoracic segments of the spinal cord and the first and second lumbar segments, and parasympathetic preganglionic fibers from the second to fourth sacral medullary segments.

11.1.3.2 Prostate

The prostate is located between the bladder neck and the urogenital diaphragm (Fig. 11.10). The base of the prostate faces up adjoining the neck of the bladder; the tip of the prostate faces down adjoining the urogenital diaphragm; the front of the

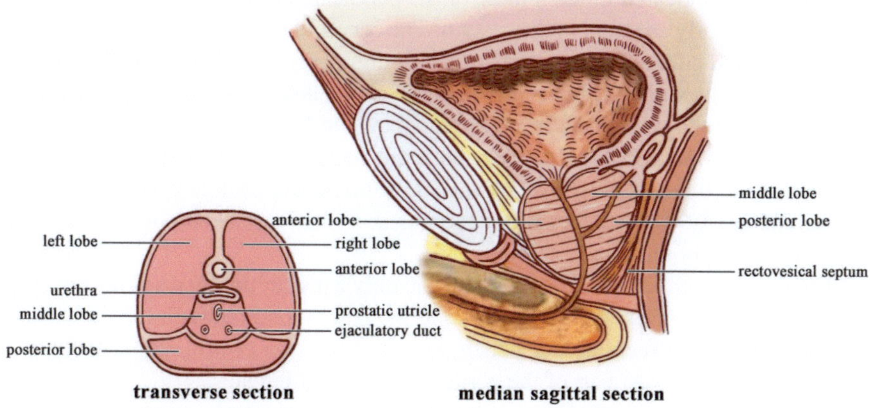

Fig. 11.10 Location and lobes of prostate

prostate is connected to the back of pubic bone by the puboprostatic ligament; the back is adjacent to the rectum with the rectovesical septum in between, and therefore, the digital rectum examination or prostatic massage can be performed through the anterior rectal wall. The prostate consists of anterior, median, posterior, left, and right lobes. The prostatic urethra is in front of the median lobe and between the left and right lobes. Prostate enlargement is a common disease in elderly men. The enlargement of the median lobe or the left or right lobe can compress the urethra and result in dysuria.

The prostate is wrapped in a prostatic capsule, and between the capsule and the prostate is the prostatic venous plexus, which converges with the vesical venous plexus to form the vesical vein and then injects into the internal iliac vein.

11.1.3.3 Uterus

Morphology, Location, Proximity, and Support of the Uterus

The uterus is an inverted pear-shaped organ that slightly flattens from anterior to posterior. It can be divided into four parts: the fundus, the body, the isthmus, and the cervix. The uterine isthmus is only 1 cm long in non-pregnancy and can be gradually prolonged during pregnancy, reaching 7–11 cm long at the time of labor. The obstetrician often performs a caesarean section at the uterine isthmus to remove the fetus from the uterus. The upper lateral edge of the uterus, where it meets the fallopian tube, is called the uterine horn. In this area, the round ligament of the uterus and the proper ligament of ovary are located on the anterior and posterior aspects of the fallopian tubes, respectively. These structures need to be carefully identified when performing tubal ligation.

The uterus is located in the middle of the pelvis, anteriorly adjacent to the bladder and posteriorly adjacent to the rectum. The cervix and the lower part of the body can be palpated clinically during an intranasal digital rectal examination. The uterus is attached to the vagina below. On both sides of the uterus are the broad ligaments of uterus and fallopian tubes. In non-pregnancy, the fundus of the uterus does not extend beyond the pelvic inlet when both the rectum and bladder are empty; in pregnancy, the fundus, body, and isthmus of the uterus are enlarged and rise into the abdominal cavity. The cervix of the uterus is in a relatively fixed position, usually above the plane of the sciatic spine.

The uterus is an interperitoneal organ, and only a part of the cervix is not covered by the peritoneum. Between the uterus and the rectum and between the uterus and the bladder are the rectouterine pouch and vesicouterine pouch, respectively, the former being the lowest part of the peritoneal cavity in females.

The uterus needs mostly the support of the pelvic floor and perineum to stay in position, but the ligaments of uterus also play a very important role in maintaining its position and posture. The ligaments of uterus are of the following four types:

The broad ligament of uterus: a double-layered peritoneal fold in a frontal position connected between the lateral margin of the uterus and the lateral pelvic wall, which restricts the movement of the uterus from side to side.

The uterosacral ligament travels posteriorly from the back of the supravaginal part of the cervix and ends at the front of the sacrum, where it can pull the cervix backward and upward. In concert with the round uterine ligament, it maintains the uterus in an anteflexed and anteverted position.

The cardinal ligament of uterus is a paired, fan-shaped fibrous band at the base of the broad ligament of uterus. It extends from the cervix to the lateral pelvic wall and provides primary lateral support of the uterus.

Vessels, Lymphatics, and Nerves of the Uterus

The uterine artery provides nutrients to the uterus. As a larger branch of the internal iliac artery, it courses medially and anteriorly in the base of the broad ligament to reach about 2 cm lateral to the cervix, then crosses the anterior superior ureter, and travels inward. The uterine artery divides into two branches on the lateral side of the cervix, with the lower branch traveling downward and branching to the cervix and vaginal wall, while the upper branch ascending along the lateral margin of the uterus, branching to the isthmus, body, and fundus of the uterus (with some branches to the uterine tubes and the ovaries). Its ovarian branch anastomoses with the ovarian artery. When managing the uterine artery in the uterine surgery, care should be taken to avoid injury to the ureter (Fig. 11.11).

Veins of the uterus: The uterine venous plexus is formed on either side of the uterus and then joins the vaginal venous plexus near the cervix to form the uterine vein, which is then injected into the internal iliac vein.

Lymphatic return of the uterus: Most lymphatic vessels of the uterine fundus and upper part of the uterine body follow the ovarian artery upward and inject into the

Fig. 11.11 Relationship of the uterine artery to the ureter

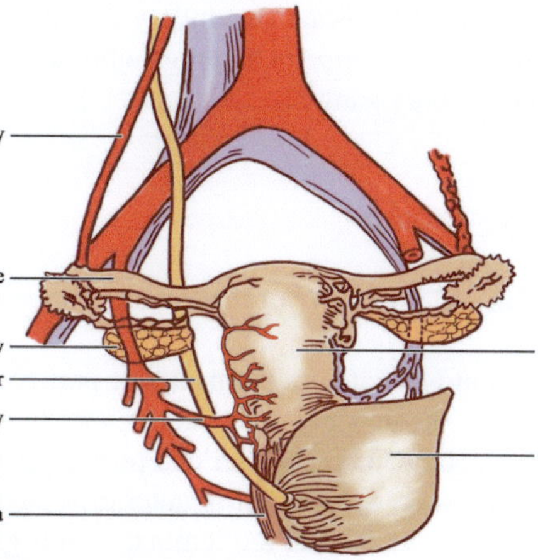

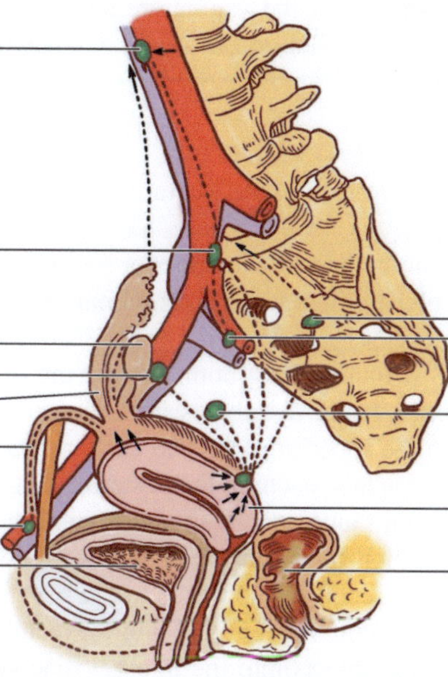

Fig. 11.12 Lymphatic return of the uterus

lumbar lymph nodes; some follow the round ligament of the uterus to the superficial inguinal lymph nodes; and those of the lower part of the uterine body and cervix are injected into the internal and external iliac lymph nodes with the uterine arteries; some are also injected into the sacral lymph nodes (Fig. 11.12). There are anastomoses between the lymphatic vessels of all the pelvic visceral organs, so cervical cancer can metastasize extensively via the lymph.

The nerves of the uterus are derived from the uterovaginal plexus springing from the pelvic plexus, with sympathetic preganglionic fibers arising from the lateral horns of the 12th thoracic medullary ganglia and first and second lumbar medullary ganglia and parasympathetic preganglionic fibers arising from the second to fourth sacral medullary ganglia.

11.1.3.4 Rectum

Location and Proximity of the Rectum

The rectum is located in the posterior part of the pelvis and anterior to the sacrum and coccyx. Its upper end is connected to the sigmoid colon at the level of the third sacral vertebrae, and its lower end penetrates the pelvic diaphragm to join the anal canal. In males, the rectum is anteriorly adjacent to the bladder, seminal vesicle glands, and prostate, and the seminal vesicle glands and prostate can be touched via the anterior rectal wall during digital rectal examination; in females, the cervix of the uterus and the upper part of the vagina are anterior to the rectum, and in the process of labor, the cervical dilation status can be known through digital anterior rectal wall examination.

Vessels, Lymphatics, and Nerves of the Rectum

The rectum is mainly nourished by the superior and inferior rectal arteries, which are derived from the inferior mesenteric and internal iliac arteries, respectively. The superior rectal artery divides into left and right branches at the level of the third lumbar vertebra and distributes along both sides of the upper rectum. The inferior rectal artery, on the other hand, distributes in the lower part of the rectum, and it anastomoses with both the superior rectal and anal arteries. In addition, the median sacral artery has also branches reaching the posterior rectal wall (Fig. 11.13).

The veins of the rectum anastomose in and around the rectal wall to form the rectal venous plexus, which then converges to form the superior and the inferior rectal veins. The superior rectal vein belongs to the hepatic portal vein system and injects into the inferior mesenteric vein; the inferior rectal vein belongs to the inferior vena cava system and injects into the internal iliac vein. When hepatic portal hypertension is present, the veins of the rectum are one of the collateral circulation routes of the hepatic portal vein.

Lymphatics from the upper rectum are injected into the inferior mesenteric lymph nodes, while those from the lower rectum are injected into the internal iliac and sacral lymph nodes.

The nerves of the rectum are derived from the inferior mesenteric plexus and the pelvic plexus, with sympathetic preganglionic fibers from the lateral horns of the lumbar medullary ganglia and parasympathetic preganglionic fibers from the pelvic visceral nerves.

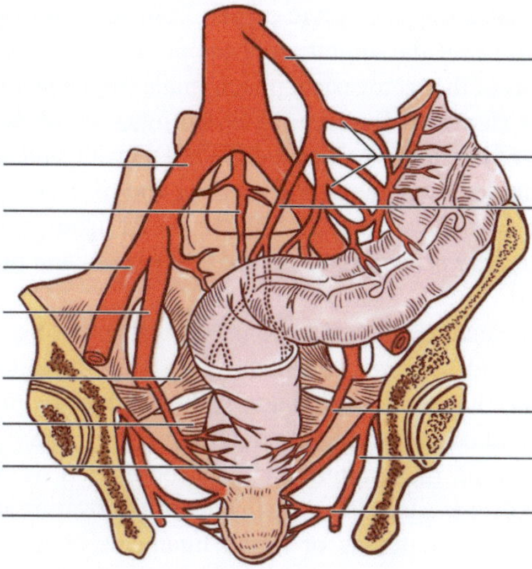

Fig. 11.13 Arteries of the rectum and anal canal

11.1.4 Anatomy of the Pelvic Cavity

11.1.4.1 Objectives

The following objectives should be achieved after dissection of the pelvic cavity.

(a) To understand the boundary and structure of the pelvic cavity
(b) To understand the distribution and migration of the pelvic peritoneum, the names of the pouches in the pelvic peritoneal cavity in both sexes, and their clinical significance
(c) To understand the distribution of the pelvic fascia and the formations of its visceral layers, and master the important pelvic fascial spaces
(d) To master the blood vessels, lymph nodes, and nerves in the pelvic cavity
(e) To master the location, proximity, and vascularity of important organs in the pelvis and understand their lymphatic return and innervation
(f) To know the structures that pass through the pelvic inlet

11.1.4.2 Dissection and Observation

Step 1: Push the sigmoid colon and small bowel collaterals in the pelvic cavity into the abdominal cavity to fully expose the pelvic peritoneal cavity and observe the locations of the bladder, uterus, and rectum. Find the uterine tubes and ovaries on either side of the uterine fundus. With the help of the pelvic median sagittal section specimen, observe the locations and adjacencies of the prostate (male) and vagina (female), the normal position of the uterus, and the curvature of the rectum.

Step 2: Slide the fingers along the pelvic organs from back to front and then from center to sides to observe the migration of the peritoneum; pay particular attention to the locations of the rectovesical pouch (male) or the rectouterine and vesicouterine pouches (female). Observe the broad ligament of the uterus between the lateral margin of the uterus and the pelvic lateral wall, and locate the suspensory ligament of the ovary between the superior end of the ovary and the pelvic lateral wall. Near the uterine horns, locate the round ligament of the uterus, the fallopian tubes, and the proper ligaments of the ovaries, and observe their positional relationships.

Step 3: Peel the peritoneum from the lateral pelvic wall toward the pelvic cavity to the pelvic organs, and observe the structures passing through the pelvic inlet: (from back to front) the median sacral artery, the hypogastric plexus, the sympathetic trunk, the lumbosacral trunk, the obturator nerves, the sigmoid colon and mesocolon, the superior rectal artery and vein (on the left side), the ureters, the internal iliac vessels, the suspensory ligaments of the ovaries and ovarian blood vessels, and the ductus deferens or round ligaments of the uterus, and note their course.

Step 4: Insert the fingers into the space between the bladder and the pubic symphysis, where lies the retropubic space. This space contains a large amount of loose tissue. Here, the pubovesical ligament between the inferior border of the pubic symphysis and the neck of the bladder (in females), or the puboprostatic ligament between the inferior border of the pubic symphysis and the prostate (in males), can be touched. Insert the fingers into the space between the rectum and the sacrum, where the retrorectal space is called and its floor is the pelvic diaphragm. Observe the pelvic fascial septum with the help of the pelvic sagittal section specimens and illustrations, and further observe the locations and understand the clinical significance of the retropubic space and the retrorectal space.

Step 5: Identify the ureter and ductus deferens at the male pelvic inlet, and trace them inward the pelvis to the base of the bladder. The ureter can be seen traveling in front of the internal iliac artery inferiorly and inwardly; then cross anteriorly over the obturator vessels and nerves, until reaching near the base of the bladder; and then runs posteriorly below the ductus deferens to the base of the bladder. The ductus deferens expands posteriorly to the bladder base and medially to the seminal vesicle glands to form the vas deferens jugularis. In the female pelvic cavity, identify the ureter, which travels from the front of the obturator to the base of the broad ligament of the uterus, and then from about 2 cm lateral to the cervix, posteriorly below the uterine artery, to the base of the bladder.

Step 6: Identify the internal iliac artery and internal iliac vein (which is posterior and medial to the internal iliac artery) in the posterior lateral wall of the pelvis, and search for lymph nodes around them. Identify the important branches of the internal iliac artery. The one that exits the pelvis between the lumbosacral trunk and the first sacral nerve is the superior gluteal artery. The arteries that exit the pelvis between the first and second (or the second and third) sacral nerves are the inferior gluteal artery and the internal pubic artery. The artery exiting the pelvis via the obturator canal is the obturator artery; observe the pubic branch and its anastomoses with the homonymous branch of the other artery, and note if there exists any anomalous obturator artery. In the case of anomalous obturator artery, observe its origin and location in relation to the femoral ring. The superior and inferior bladder arteries and the inferior rectal artery are thinner and may be identified according to their distribution. On the lateral side of the cervix, look for the uterine artery and note its position in relation to the ureter.

Step 7: Identify the superior rectal artery at the root of the sigmoid mesocolon and trace it to the rectum.

Step 8: Use the specimens and illustrations and observe the important venous plexuses in the pelvis, such as the rectal venous plexus and bladder venous plexus.

Step 9: Clean the posterior pelvic wall and locate the median sacral artery; locate the superior hypogastric plexus anterior to the sacral promontory, and from there, explore for the left and right hypogastric nerves and the inferior hypogastric plexus, and locate the pelvic visceral nerves.

11.1.5 Summary

The pelvic cavity can be divided into two parts: the pelvic peritoneal cavity and the pelvic subperitoneal cavity. The pelvic peritoneal cavity is part of the peritoneal cavity, and the rectovesical pouch and rectouterine pouch are the lowest part of the peritoneal cavity in males and females in the semirecumbent position, respectively, which has certain significance in clinical practice. The pelvic subperitoneal cavity, which is located between the pelvic peritoneum and the pelvic wall, contains the pelvic fascia and important blood vessels, lymph nodes, nerves, and pelvic organs. The pelvic fascia can be divided into visceral and parietal layers, with the latter migrating with the intra-abdominal fascia. The retropubic space and the retrorectal space are important pelvic fascial spaces, both of which are superiorly connected to the extraperitoneal space of the abdominal cavity. Clinically, extraperitoneal surgeries of the bladder, prostate, or uterus can be performed through the retropubic space; gas contrast radiography of the retroperitoneal space is feasible through the retrorectal space.

The major arteries of the pelvic cavity include the internal iliac artery and its branches. In addition, there are the superior rectal artery and the median sacral artery, both of which have branches to the rectum; the former is a branch of the inferior mesenteric artery, and the latter is from the abdominal aorta. The veins of the pelvic organs first form venous plexuses in or around the walls of the organs before draining into the internal iliac or inferior mesenteric veins. There are anastomoses between the pelvic venous plexuses or between the pelvic venous plexuses and the vertebral venous plexus. The rectal venous plexus is also one of the anastomoses between the hepatic portal venous system and the inferior vena cava system.

The major lymph nodes in the pelvis include the internal iliac lymph nodes and the sacral lymph nodes. Apart from the above lymph nodes, the lymph from the pelvic organs is injected into the external iliac and common iliac lymph nodes. In addition, the lymph from the upper rectum and the uterine fundus and upper body may also be injected into the inferior mesenteric lymph nodes, lumbar lymph nodes, and superficial inguinal lymph nodes, respectively.

Somatic and visceral nerves distribute in the pelvic cavity. The somatic nerves include the sacral plexus and the obturator nerves, and the visceral nerves include the sympathetic trunk sacral, pelvic splanchnic nerve, and the hypogastric plexus. The inferior hypogastric plexus, also known as the pelvic plexus, contains sympathetic and parasympathetic fibers that follow blood vessels to the pelvic viscera.

The pelvic organs include the intrapelvic portions of the urinary system, reproductive organs, and digestive tract, the former two being in the anterior middle of the pelvis and the latter in the posterior part of the pelvis. Since the pelvic organs are close to each other, organs such as the prostate or uterus can be examined through the anterior rectal wall.

11.2 Clinical Application of Key Anatomical Structures of the Pelvis

Pelvic organs mainly involve the urinary system, reproductive system, and part of the digestive system, which are highly concerned in urological surgeries (such as prostate surgery and bladder surgery), gynecological surgeries (such as uterine and adnexal surgery), and general surgeries (such as colon or rectal surgery). Because of the uniqueness of the surgery in these specialties, it is impossible to list them one by one. Hence, we take radical cystectomy, which involves more organs and is more complicated, as an example to describe the important anatomical structures in the pelvis and the related clinical significance.

1. Establish a surgical approach

After general anesthesia, the patient is placed in the supine position with legs slightly apart, head down and feet high. A subumbilical or supraumbilical incision is made, and the pneumoperitoneum is established by using pneumoperitoneum needling or incision, and the pneumoperitoneum pressure is maintained at 15 mm Hg. Using either the pneumoperitoneum needling or the incision method, the parietal peritoneum should be penetrated, and the pneumoperitoneum is established only after entering the abdominal cavity to avoid damaging the intestinal tubes. Generally, for patients without a history of abdominal surgery, pneumoperitoneum needling is adopted to establish the pneumoperitoneum, while for patients with a history of abdominal surgery or trauma, the incision method is often applied for the entry of the abdominal cavity in order to avoid the adherence of the intestinal tubes to the abdominal wall and the resulting damage to the intestines (Fig. 11.14a). Before entering the abdominal cavity, a finger is usually used to probe deeply into the abdominal cavity at the incision site to search for the presence of surrounding adhesions. After establishing the pneumoperitoneum, the surgical trocars are

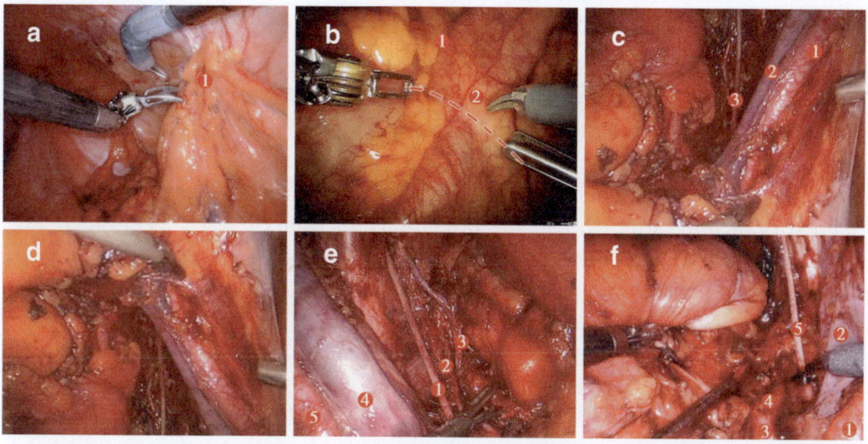

Fig. 11.14 A surgical approach for freeing the lower and middle ureter and clearing the pelvic lymph nodes. (**a**) Adherent omentum and bowel (1. large omentum and bowel adherent to the abdominal wall). (**b**) Ureter and external iliac arteries (1. right external iliac artery; 2. right ureter). (**c**) Iliac vessels and obturator nerve (1. right external iliac artery; 2. right external iliac vein; 3. obturator nerve). (**d**) Pelvic lymph node dissection is completed. (**e**) Obturator nerve (1. left obturator nerve; 2. left obturator artery; 3. left obturator vein; 4. left external iliac vein; 5. left external iliac artery). (**f**) Obturator nerve and iliac vessels (1. right external iliac artery; 2. right external iliac vein; 3. right internal iliac artery; 4. right umbilical artery; 5. right obturator nerve)

usually inserted by puncturing beside the right and left rectus abdominis muscles, 2–3 cm below the umbilicus, and 2–3 cm inboard above the right and left anterior superior iliac spines under the direct vision of the observation mirror.

2. Free the lower and middle ureter

The abdominal cavity is explored under laparoscopy, and the intestinal and other organs were examined for injury and intra-abdominal metastasis. Visualize the pulsatile right external iliac artery by pulling the ileum cephalad from the right pelvic inlet. The ureter is often seen above the bifurcation of the internal and external iliac arteries, which is the second physiologic narrowing of the ureter and is superficial enough to be easily accessible through the peritoneum (Fig. 11.14b). Therefore, the ureter is often detected here and freed down to the bladder wall. Since the left ureter is often covered by the sigmoid colon, it requires pulling the sigmoid colon down inward and freeing the lateral adhesions to the sigmoid colon to expose the left ureter (Fig. 11.14c).

In female patients, the ureter often runs below the uterine artery, and extra care is needed to avoid injury to the ovarian and uterine arteries, which may cause hemorrhage. Similarly, when resecting the uterus and adnexa, protect the ureter when disconnecting the uterine artery in order to avoid ureteral injury.

3. Remove pelvic lymph nodes

Open the posterior peritoneum along the surface of the external iliac artery and cut the ductus deferens above the external iliac artery. Dissect the iliac artery sheath along the lymph nodes on the surface of the external iliac artery, distal to the point where the artery passes the abdominal wall and proximal to the bifurcation of the common iliac artery (Fig. 11.14d). The external iliac artery generally has no well-defined branching arteries, and the probability of injury-caused bleeding is low. However, because the external iliac artery is an important vessel supplying the lower extremities and injury can have serious consequences, extra care should be taken when clearing the external iliac lymph nodes.

Find the accompanying external iliac vein medially inferior to external iliac artery. Free the external iliac vein along its inner and lower edge and find the inner wall of the pelvic cavity. Then in the adipose lymph node tissues here, find the obturator nerve, and the obturator artery and vein (Fig. 11.14e), and clear the surrounding adipose lymphoid tissues along the obturator nerve. Since the obturator nerve is located deep in the adipose lymphoid tissues, the obturator nerve should be found first, and it is important not to blindly use ultrasonic scalpel or other thermal injury instruments, like electrocoagulation hooks, to cut the tissue without identifying the location of the nerve, so as not to cause injury to the obturator nerve. Unilateral injury to the obturator nerve often decreases the power of internal thigh contraction, and thus the affected limb cannot be rested on the healthy thigh, and the skin sensation of the medial femur is impaired. Simultaneous bilateral injury to the obturator nerve leads to postoperative walking disorders. If the nerve is found to be severed, it should be repaired in one stage.

Explore the internal iliac artery from the bifurcation of the common iliac artery and free it medially and inferiorly to locate the umbilical artery, which is then clamped and severed (Fig. 11.14f). The superior segment of the umbilical artery occludes into the medial umbilical ligament, and the inferior segment gives off the superior vesical artery, which is an important source of blood supply to the bladder. Internal iliac lymph nodes can be cleared along the surface of the internal iliac artery. Upward along the bifurcation of the common iliac artery, the common iliac lymph nodes on the surface of the vessel can be cleared up to the bifurcation of the right and left common iliac arteries at the abdominal aorta (Fig. 11.15a). Internal iliac lymph nodes can be cleared along the surface of the internal iliac arteries. In addition, presacral lymph nodes can be cleared medial posteriorly to the internal iliac artery. The left pelvic lymph nodes can be cleared in the same way.

4. Free the ductus deferens, seminal vesicles, and posterior prostate wall

Push the posterior wall of the bladder upward and tract the sigmoid colon cephalad to reveal the rectovesical pouch (Fig. 11.15b). Observe the rectovesical pouch and identify two transverse peritoneal reflex arches, with the ureter under the shallower arcuate eminence and the ductus deferens and seminal vesicles under the deeper arcuate eminence (Fig. 11.15b). Incise the deeper arcuate eminence to free the ductus deferens and seminal vesicles to the junction with the prostate, and then

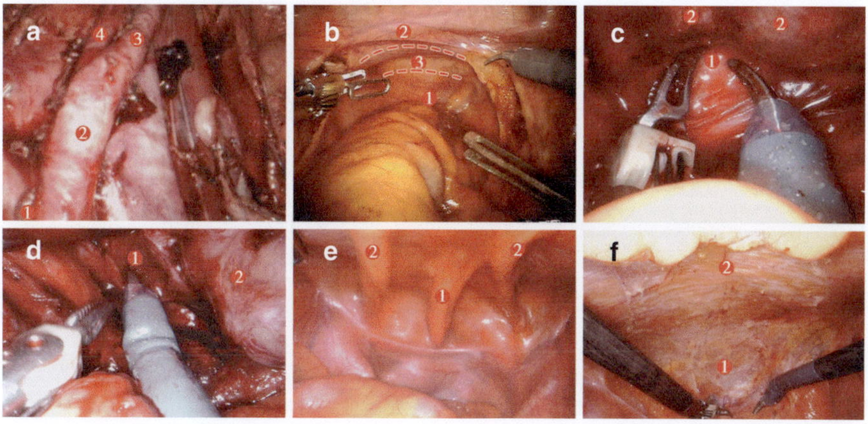

Fig. 11.15 Free the ductus deferens, seminal vesicles, and posterior prostate wall. (**a**) Complete lymph node dissection (1. iliac artery branches; 2. right common iliac artery; 3. right external iliac artery; 4. right internal iliac artery). (**b**) Rectovesical pouch and two arcuate eminences (1. recto-vesical pouch; 2. superficial arcuate eminence; 3. deep arcuate eminence). (**c**) Peritoneal perineal fascia (1. peritoneal perineal fascia; 2. spermatic vesicle). (**d**) Peritoneal perineal space (1. peritoneal perineal space; 2. seminal vesicles). (**e**) Median umbilical and lateral umbilical ligaments (1. median umbilical ligament; 2. paramedian umbilical ligament). (**f**) Retzius space (1. Retzius space; 2. abdominal wall)

sever the ductus deferens. The seminal vesicle artery is present at the base of the seminal vesicle on the lateral side, which is prone to hemorrhage in case of injury, and therefore, it needs to be severed by electrocoagulation or ultrasonic coagulation.

Tract the ductus deferens and seminal vesicles upward and press downward the sigmoid colon and rectum to reveal the peritoneal perineal fascia (Denonvilliers' fascia) (Fig. 11.15c). Incise the peritoneal perineal fascia transversely above the junction of the prostate and seminal vesicles to expose the peritoneal perineal space (Fig. 11.15d), which is then separated to the tip of the prostate. When freeing the peritoneal perineal space, it is necessary to free it closely along the side of the prostate to avoid injury to the rectum. Clinically, it is generally recommended to separate the space with scissors or blunt dissection, and the use of thermoinvasive instruments such as ultrasonic scalpels or electrocoagulation hooks is not recommended, to enable one-stage repair in case of injury.

5. Free the anterior bladder wall

Open the parietal peritoneum to the incised peritoneum from the umbilical median ligament to its sides, during which the paramedian median ligament and peritoneal reflex are severed (Fig. 11.15e). Continue to separate the anterior bladder space (Retzius space) downward (Fig. 11.15f) to reveal the pubicoprostatic ligament and the endopelvic fascia (Fig. 11.16a).

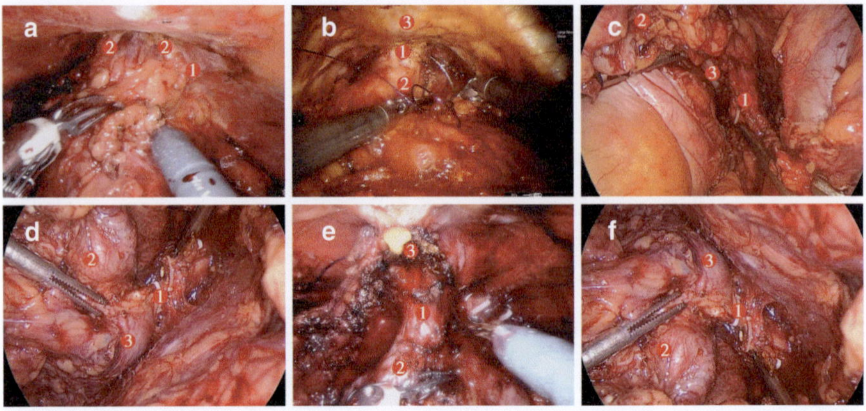

Fig. 11.16 Free the bladder, ligate blood vessels, and remove the bladder and prostate. (**a**) Puboprostatic ligament and endopelvic fascia (1. endopelvic fascia; 2. puboprostatic ligament). (**b**) Dorsal penile vascular complex (1. dorsal penile vascular complex; 2. prostate; 3. pubic symphysis). (**c**) Lateral bladder ligaments (1. lateral bladder ligaments; 2. bladder; 3. seminal vesicles). (**d**) Lateral prostatic ligaments (1. lateral prostatic ligaments; 2. bladder; 3. prostate). (**e**) Urethra (1. urethra; 2. prostate; 3. sutured dorsal vascular complex). (**f**) Urethrorectal muscle (1. urethrorectal muscle; 2. proximal urethra; 3. distal urethra)

6. Suture the deep dorsal penile vein complex

Incise the endopelvic fascia and pubicoprostatic ligament on both sides to expose the two sides of the tip of the prostate, and then suture the dorsal vascular complex (DVC) of the penis (Fig. 11.16b). During radical cystectomy and radical prostatectomy for prostate cancer, suturing of the venous complex before incision is clinically recommended to avoid hemorrhage caused by vein complex incision.

7. Free the lateral bladder ligament and the lateral prostate ligament

Lift the lower part of the ureter and cut it off after clamping it on the lateral side of the bladder wall. Lift the top of the bladder and free the lateral ligament of the bladder (Fig. 11.16c), clamping it and then severing it if necessary. When freeing downward to the base of the prostate, separate the lateral prostatic ligament closely against the lateral side of the prostate (Fig. 11.16d). The lateral bladder and prostatic ligaments contain neurovascular bundles and should be associated with postoperative urinary control and male sexual function. Clinical recommendations for early-stage, low-risk prostate cancer include intrafascial prostatectomy with preservation of the neurovascular bundles to reduce the possibility of postoperative urinary leakage and to protect sexual function.

8. Dissect the urethra and remove the bladder and prostate gland

Dissect the sutured deep dorsal penile vein complex, separate it downward to the tip of the prostate, and cut the urethra closely against the tip (Fig. 11.16e). When cutting the posterior part of the urethra, turn up the tip of the prostate cephalad to reveal the posterior urethrorectal muscle, and sever the urethrorectal muscle closely against the capsule of prostate (Fig. 11.16f) to avoid rectal injury.

Chapter 12
Regional Anatomy of the Perineum and Its Clinical Application

Wei Zhang, Pu Li, Shangqian Wang, and Yao Zhu

12.1 Regional Anatomy of the Perineum

The perineum can be defined broadly and narrowly. In a broad sense, the perineum refers to all the soft tissue below the pelvic diaphragm that encloses the outlet of the lesser pelvis. In a narrow sense, the perineum refers only to the soft tissue between the anus and the external genitalia. In women, the perineum in the narrow sense in also known as the obstetric perineum, which needs to be protected from tearing during natural childbirth.

12.1.1 Boundary

The perineum in the broad sense is diamond shaped, with its boundary consistent with the outlet of the lesser pelvis. The anterior border is the lower edge of the pubic symphysis, the posterior border is the tip of the coccyx, and the sides are the inferior ramus of pubis, the ramus of ischium, the ischial tuberosity, and the sacrotuberous ligament. A line passing through the ischial tuberosity on both sides can divide the perineum into two triangles, anterior and posterior. The former is the urogenital triangle, containing the urethra and external genitalia. The latter is the anal triangle, containing the anal canal and the ischioanal fossa.

W. Zhang · P. Li (✉) · S. Wang
Nanjing Medical University, Nanjing, China
e-mail: wangshangqian@njmu.edu.cn

Y. Zhu
Fudan University Shanghai Cancer Center, Shanghai, China
e-mail: zhuyao@fudan.edu.cn

Q. Ding et al. (eds.), *Clinically Oriented Regional Anatomy*,
https://doi.org/10.1007/978-981-95-9888-5_12

12.1.2 Anatomical Landmarks

The main markers of the perineum on the body surface include pubic symphysis, pubic arch, ischial tuberosity, ischial spine, and coccygeal tip. In obstetrics and gynecology, these bony landmarks are commonly used in the measurement of pelvic diameter. For example, the distance between the medial edges of the two sides of the ischial tuberosity is the intertuberous diameter, that is, the transverse diameter of the pelvic outlet, which is about 9 cm on average, and the distance between the lower edge of the pubic symphysis and the sacrococcygeal joint is the anterior-posterior diameter of the pelvic outlet, about 11.5 cm on average.

12.1.3 Characteristics of Layers and Structures

12.1.3.1 Skin

The perineal skin is rich in sweat and sebaceous glands. The skin around the anus forms radial folds and may present sparse hair in males. In the urogenital triangle, the skin of the penis and scrotum can move in phase in males, while in females, the skin here forms into the labia majora and labia minora.

12.1.3.2 Superficial Fascia and Superficial Muscles

The superficial fascia of the perineum is divided into two layers: a superficial fatty layer and a deep membranous layer. The superficial layer of superficial fascia at the anal triangle is rich in adipose tissue, forming a fat pad that fills the ischioanal fossa. The deeper layer of superficial fascia is thin and inconspicuous and not easy to be peeled off completely.

The superficial layer of the superficial fascia at the urogenital triangle migrates with the superficial layer of the superficial fascia of the lower part of the anterior lateral abdominal wall (i.e., Camper's fascia); the deeper membranous layer of the superficial fascia is called the superficial perineal fascia or Colles' fascia, which is thinner and covers the surface of the superficial muscles of the perineum. It extends anteriorly into the dartos of the scrotum and the superficial penile fascia; expands upward with the deep layer of the superficial fascia of the lower part of the anterior lateral abdominal wall (i.e., Scarpa's fascia); attaches bilaterally to the inferior ramus of pubis, the ramus of ischium, and the ischial tuberosity; and unites posteriorly with the inferior fascia of urogenital diaphragm at the posterior edge of the urogenital triangle, till to the central tendon of the perineum on the median line.

The superficial muscles in the urogenital triangle are located on the deep side of the superficial perineal fascia and include the superficial transverse perineal muscle, bulbospongiosus, and ischiocavernosus (Fig. 12.1).

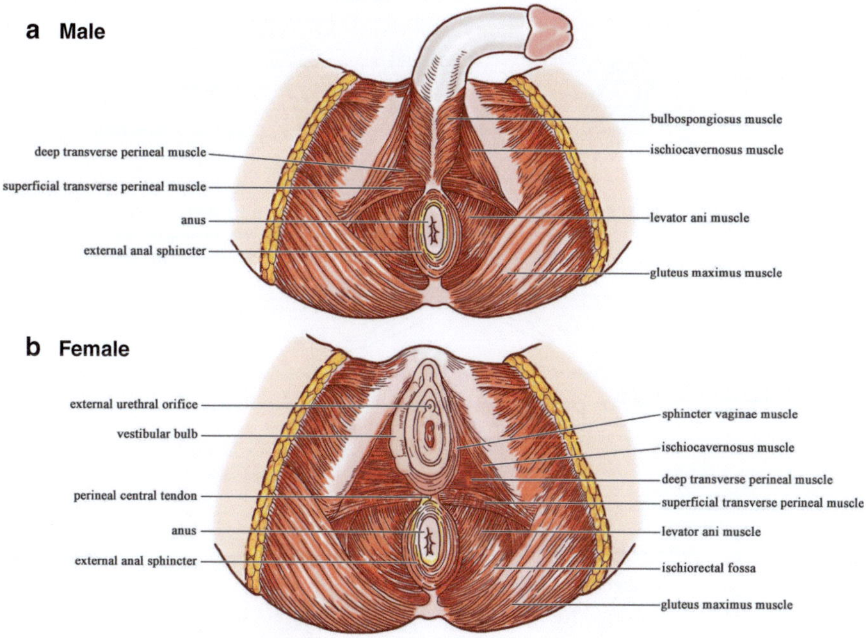

Fig. 12.1 Superficial muscles in the urogenital triangle

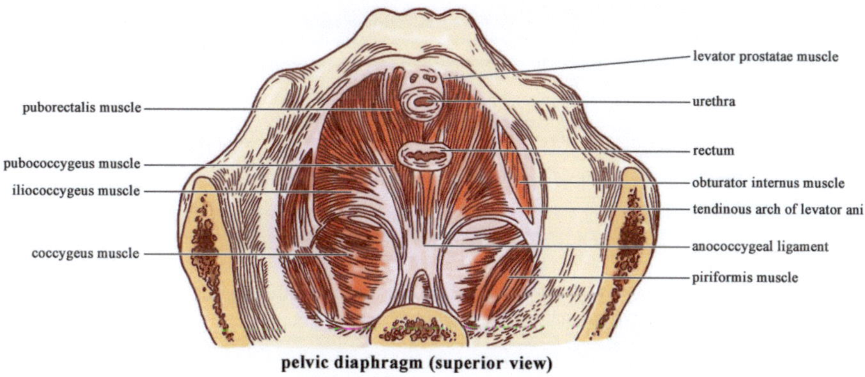

Fig. 12.2 Deep muscles at the anal triangle

12.1.3.3 Deep Fascia and Deep Muscles

The deep muscles at the anal triangle include the levator ani, coccygeus, and sphincter ani externus (Fig. 12.2). The superficial and deep surfaces of the levator ani and coccygeus muscle are covered by the inferior fascia of the pelvic diaphragm and the superior fascia of the pelvic diaphragm, respectively, and these three layers together form the pelvic diaphragm (Fig. 12.3). After passing through the center of the pelvic

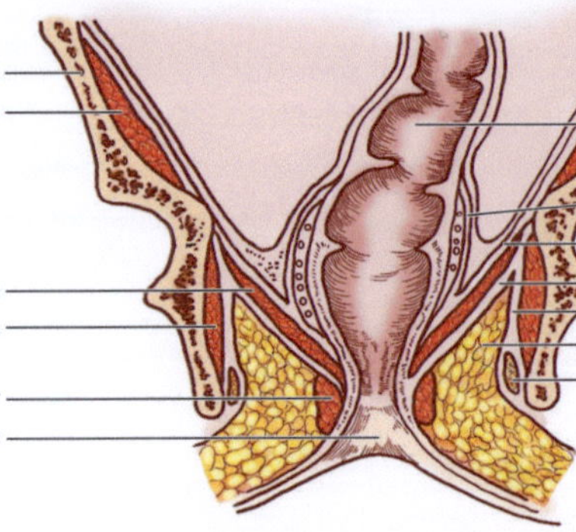

Fig. 12.3 Pelvic diaphragm

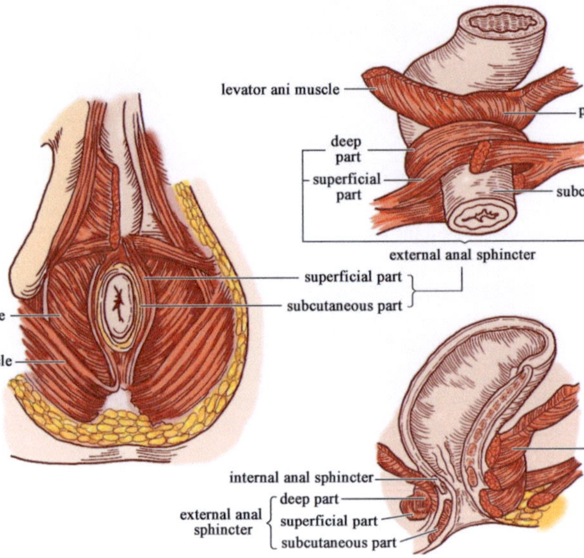

Fig. 12.4 Internal and external anal sphincter and anorectal ring

diaphragm, the rectum transits into the anal canal. The superficial and deep portions of the external anal sphincter, together with the internal anal sphincter, the longitudinal muscles of the lower rectum, and a portion of the levator ani muscle (puborectalis), surround the junction of the anal canal and the rectum, making up a powerful muscular ring called the anorectal ring (Fig. 12.4). This ring functions to open and close the anus, and if severed during surgery due to carelessness, fecal incontinence may appear.

At the urogenital triangle, the deep fascia is divided into two layers, superficial and deep. The superficial layer is called the inferior fascia of urogenital diaphragm, also known as the perineal membrane, which is triangular in shape and covers the superficial surface of the deep perineal muscles. It is bilaterally attached to the periosteum of the inferior ramus of pubis and ramus of ischium and posteriorly fused with the superficial fascia of the perineum. The deep layer is the superior fascia of urogenital diaphragm, which covers the deep surface of the deep muscles and extends to the obturator fascia. This fascia is also bilaterally attached to the inferior ramus of pubis and ramus of ischium, and its anterior and posterior margins fuse with the superior fascia of urogenital diaphragm.

The deep muscles of the urogenital triangle include the deep transverse perineal muscle and the sphincter of urethra (urethrovaginal sphincter in females). The deep transverse perineal muscle and the sphincter of urethra, along with the superior and inferior fasciae of the urogenital diaphragm located on their deep and superficial surfaces, form the urogenital diaphragm (Fig. 12.5).

The perineal central tendon, also known as the perineal body, is a fibrous septum located between the anus and the root of the penis in males and between the anus and the posterior end of the vaginal vestibule in females. It is about 3–4 cm deep and wedge shaped in the sagittal position, with the tip facing upward and the bottom facing downward. The external anal sphincter, bulbospongiosus muscle, and pairs of superficial transverse perineal muscles, deep transverse perineal muscles, and levator ani muscle are attached to the perineal central tendon, all contributing to strengthening the pelvic floor and supporting pelvic visceral organs.

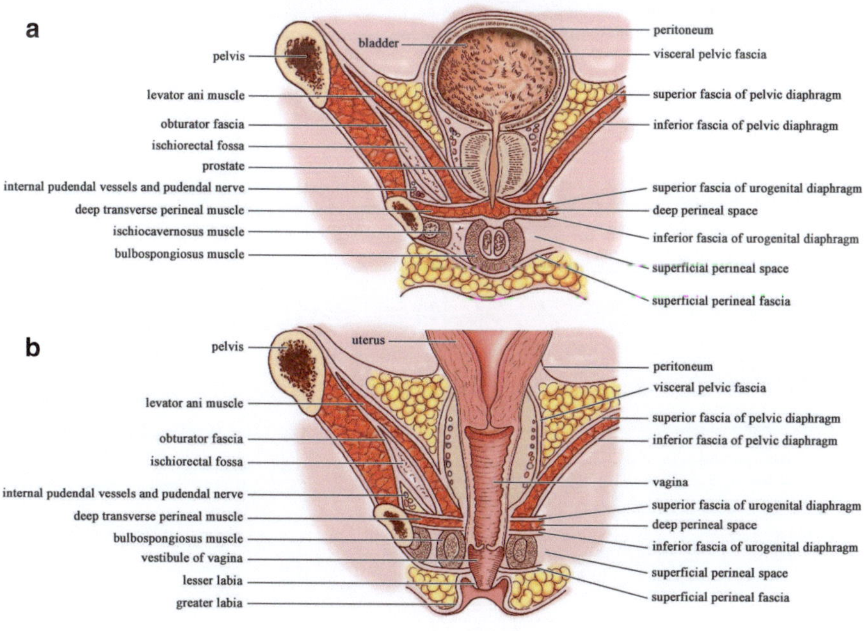

Fig. 12.5 Male and female urogenital diaphragm

12.1.3.4 Perineal Spaces

The superficial perineal space, also known as the superficial perineal pouch, is a triangular space located between the superficial perineal fascia and the inferior fascia of urogenital diaphragm. The superficial perineal space opens anteriorly and superiorly to the scrotum, penis, and abdominal wall. Within it are the superficial transverse perineal muscles, bulbospongiosus muscles, ischiocavernosus muscles, branches of the pudendal nerve and internal pudendal blood vessels, as well as the crus of penis, bulb of urethra, and the part of urethra in it (in males) and the urethra, the lower part of the vagina, crus of clitoris, the vestibular bulb, and the greater vestibular gland in females (Fig. 12.6). In males with straddle injuries, if the bulb of urethra ruptures, urine may extravasate into the superficial perineal space, leak

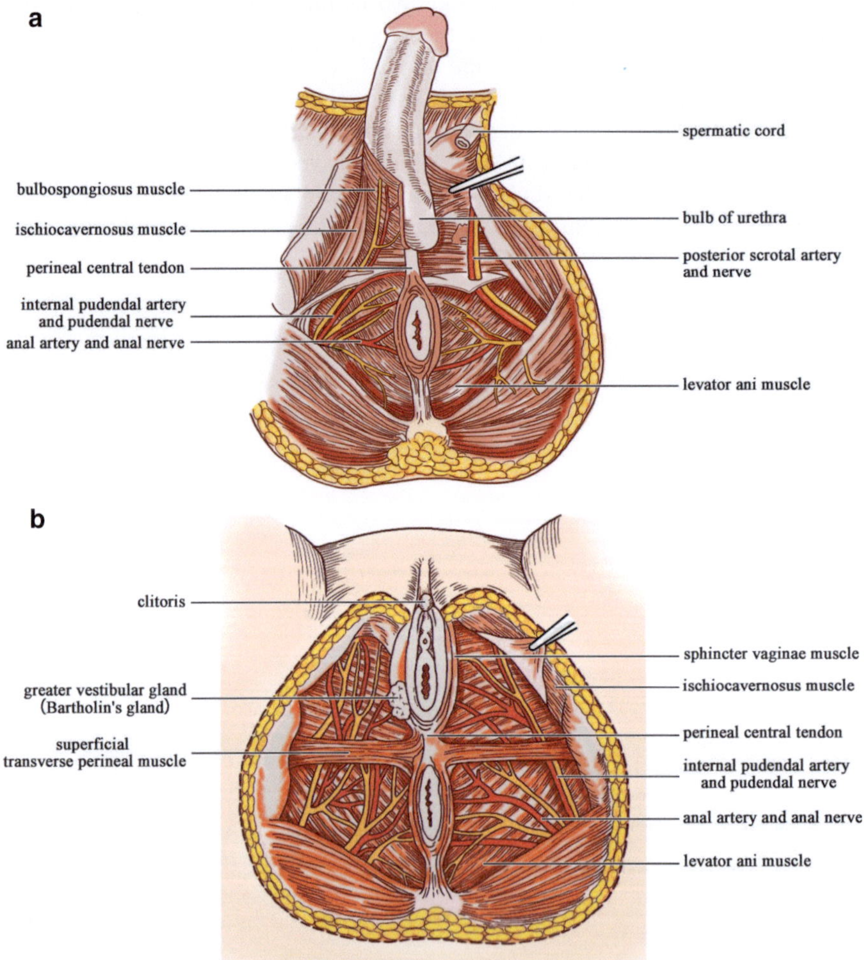

Fig. 12.6 Male and female superficial perineal space

through the anterior superior opening into the scrotum and penis, and then spread to the deeper surface of Scarpa's fascia in the lower part of the anterior lateral wall of the abdomen, causing swelling in the affected area (Fig. 12.7).

The deep perineal space, also known as the deep perineal pouch, is located between the superior and inferior fascia of the urogenital diaphragm. In this space, apart from the deep transverse perineal muscles, urethral sphincter, terminal branches of pudendal nerves, and internal pudendal vessels, the membranous part of urethra and bulbourethral glands are present in males (Fig. 12.8), and the urethra and lower part of the vagina are present in females.

The ischioanal fossa, also known as the ischiorectal fossa, is located on both sides of the anal canal, providing a pyramid-shaped space with the tip facing upward and the bottom facing downward. The tip of the fossa is formed by the confluence of the inferior fascia of pelvic diaphragm and the obturator fascia; the bottom of the fossa is the skin and superficial fascia on both sides of the anus. The anterior wall is the urogenital diaphragm; the posterior wall is the inferior border of the gluteus maximus muscle and the sacrotuberous ligament on its deep surface; the lower part of the medial wall is the external anal sphincter, and the upper part is the levator ani muscle and coccygeus muscle; and the lateral wall is the ischial tuberosity, obturator internus, and its fascia. In the lateral wall of the fossa, there is a pudendal canal formed by the obturator fascia, also known as Alcock's canal, into which the internal pudendal vessels and pudendal nerves enter after passing through the lesser sciatic foramen. Within the canal, the internal pudendal artery gives off two or three anal arteries, which are distributed around the anus. Its trunk travels forward and divides into the perineal

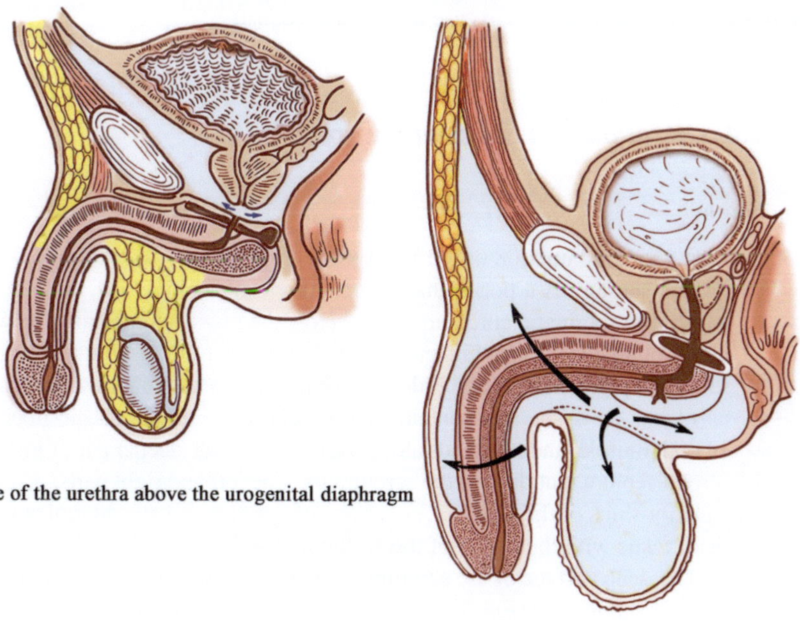

Fig. 12.7 Rupture of bulb of urethra

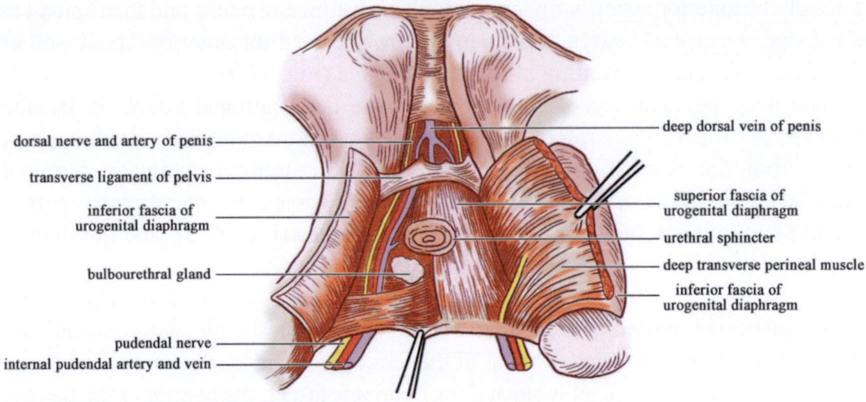

Fig. 12.8 Male deep perineal space

artery and dorsal artery of penis (clitoris) as it reaches the posterior border of the urogenital diaphragm. The pudendal nerve divides into three branches within the pudendal canal and the anal, perineal, and dorsal penile (clitoral) nerves, each of which accompanies the corresponding artery in its course and distribution. The large amount of adipose tissue that fills the fossa is called the adipose body of ischioanal fossa and serves as an elastic cushion and facilitates adequate dilation of the anal canal during defecation. When perianal infection is present, abscesses and fistulas in the ischioanal fossa are likely to occur, and they can spread upward through the pelvic diaphragm and become pelvic abscesses in case of severe abscesses.

12.1.4 Scrotum and Spermatic Cord

A. Scrotum

1. Location and Function of the Scrotum

   The scrotum is a pouch that harbors the testis, epididymis, and the lower part of the spermatic cord and hangs below the pubic symphysis. The wall of the scrotum consists of skin and the dartos coat. The skin is thin and soft, with folds and pigmentation and little pubic hair. The dartos coat (a superficial fascia) lacks fat tissue and contains dense connective tissue, elastic fibers, and smooth muscle, and it extends along the midline to the deeper part, forming the scrotal septum that divides the scrotum into the left and right parts.
2. Relationships of the scrotum, coverings of spermatic cord and tunica vaginalis of testis with the layers of the abdominal wall

   The deep surface of the scrotum refers to coverings that envelop the testis and spermatic cord (Fig. 12.9), including the following layers (in order from the outside to the inside): the external spermatic fascia, the cremaster, and the internal spermatic fascia. They are continuous with the layers of the

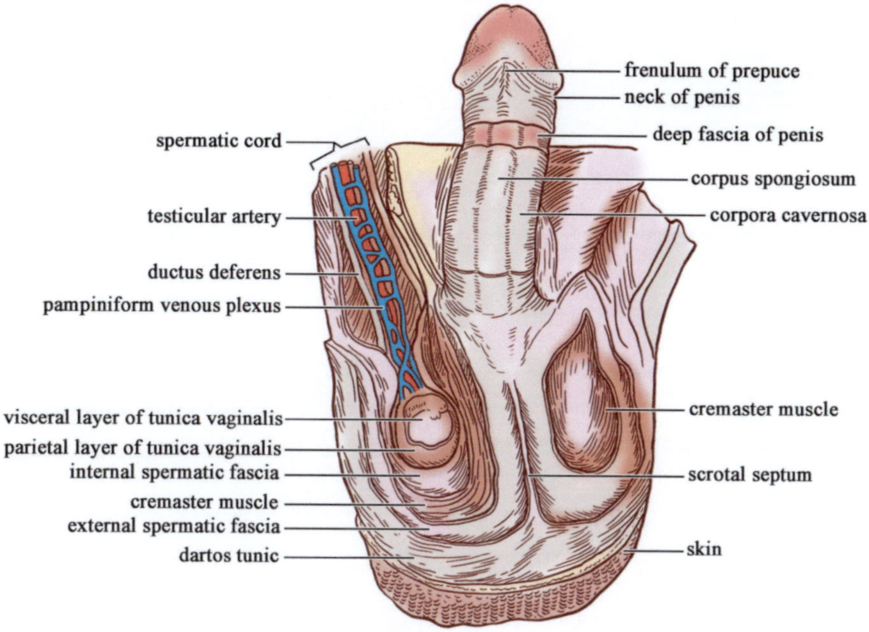

Fig. 12.9 Coverings of testis and spermatic cord

anterolateral abdominal wall (Fig. 12.10). In addition, the testis is surrounded by tunica vaginalis of testis.

The tunica vaginalis of the testis is divided into a visceral layer and a parietal layer. The visceral layer covers the testis and epididymis, while the parietal layer is attached to the inner surface of the spermatic cord fascia. The space between the two layers is the tunica vaginalis cavity, which contains a small amount of serous fluid. Excessive accumulation of fluid in the tunica vaginalis cavity is called testicular syringomyelia. To open the tunica vaginalis cavity, it is necessary to cut through the skin, the dartos coat, the external fascia of the spermatic cord, the cremaster muscle, the internal fascia of the spermatic cord, and the parietal layer of the tunica vaginalis of testis from outside to inside.

B. Spermatic Cord

The spermatic cords are a pair of soft, round, cord-like structures that originate from the deep ring of the inguinal canal and end at the upper posterior end of the testis.

1. Contents of the spermatic cords

The main contents of the spermatic cord include the vas deferens, testicular artery, pampiniform plexus, nerves, lymphatic vessels, and vaginal ligament. The vas deferens, which is located in the posteromedial aspect of the other structures within the spermatic cord, has a thick wall and narrow lumen and is easily palpable in vivo with a hard cord-like sensation. The testicular artery is thin and nourishes the testis and epididymis. The pampiniform

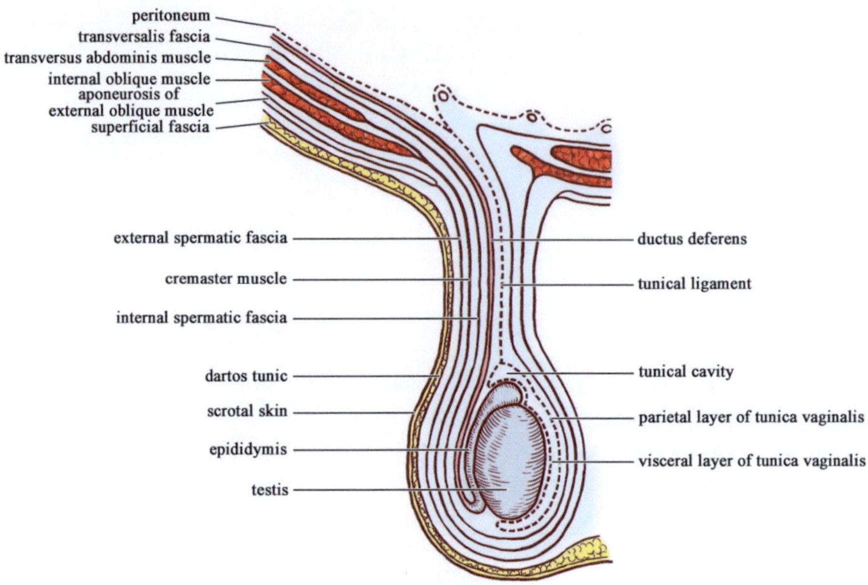

Fig. 12.10 Layers of abdominal wall and scrotum

plexus, which originates from the testis and epididymis, consists of 8–12 small veins that encircle the testicular artery and vas deferens and goes upward to form the testicular vein at the deep ring of the inguinal canal. The left testicular vein drains into the left renal vein, while the right testicular vein drains directly into the inferior vena cava. When the testicular venous return is impaired, the pampiniform plexus bends and expands, a condition called varicocele that is more common on the left side.

2. Coverings of the spermatic cord

   The coverings of the spermatic cord are continuous with those of the testis, but the tunica vaginalis of testis does not enclose the spermatic cord (because the vaginal process has been occluded into the ligament), so the layers of the coverings of the spermatic cord include, from the outside to the inside, the extraspermatic fascia, the cremaster muscle, and the internal spermatic fascia (Fig. 12.10).

12.1.5 Dissection of the Perineum

12.1.5.1 Objectives

To characterize the boundary, divisions, layers, and structures of the perineum. To master the location, composition, and contents of the superficial perineal space, deep perineal space, and ischioanal fossa. To master the layers of the scrotum and spermatic cord and the contents of the spermatic cord

12.1.5.2 Procedures of Operation and Observation

Step 1: Place the body and check for bony landmarks.

Place the body on the back with the hips flexed and the knees bent, and divide the two lower limbs to the sides and immobilize them. Slightly anterior on either side of the anus, press firmly on the skin and touch the ischial tuberosity. Touch the ramus of ischium, the inferior ramus of pubis, and the inferior border of the pubic symphysis anteriorly and medially along the ischial tuberosity. On the midline behind the anus, touch the tip of the coccyx.

Step 2: Dissect the urogenital triangle

1. Make incisions in the skin of perineum: (1) a transverse incision medially from the ischial tuberosity and (2) a curved incision around the anus (and in women also around the pudendal cleft). Turn up the skin from the medial side to the anterior and posterior sides to reveal the superficial fascia.
2. Remove the fat from the superficial fascia and expose the deeper layer of the superficial fascia (the superficial perineal fascia).
3. Lift up the superficial perineal fascia with forceps, make a longitudinal incision along the median line or the pudendal cleft, and use the handle of the knife to reach it into the superficial perineal space on its deep side to explore its extent, connection, and continuation of fascial attachments.
4. Slightly anterior to the posterior border of the superficial perineal fascia, incise the superficial perineal fascia laterally from the midline, turn it to the anterior and lateral sides, and observe the structures within the superficial perineal space: In the posterior and lateral sides of the superficial perineal space, perineal arteries, veins, and nerves of the perineum can be seen; remove the connective tissues within the space, and the superficial transverse perineal muscle, bulbospongiosus, and ischiocavernosus are seen; gently peel off the ischiocavernosus and bulbospongiosus muscles, and the crus of penis (clitoris) and bulb of urethra (vestibular bulb) can be seen on the deeper side.
5. Push the bulb of urethra anteriorly. Cut off the crus of penis attachment and turn it upward anteriorly to reveal the inferior fascia of urogenital diaphragm.
6. Remove the urogenital diaphragm and observe the structures within the deep perineal space. Find the dorsal penile artery and the dorsal penile nerve along the ramus of ischium; the deep transverse perineal muscle and the urethral sphincter (urethrovaginal sphincter in female) are visible.

Step 3: Dissect the anal triangle

1. Locate the pudendal canal in the lateral wall of the ischioanal fossa and incise it. Clean the pudendal nerve and its branch, the anal nerve; clean the internal pudendal artery and its branch, the anal artery.
2. Preserve the anal artery and anal nerve, remove the perianal fat, expose the external anal sphincter, and identify its subcutaneous, superficial, and deep parts.

3. Remove the fat from the anal triangle, expose the ischioanal fossa, and observe the fossa tip and the composition of each wall.

Step 4: Dissect the scrotum and spermatic cord

1. Incise the skin longitudinally from the superficial ring of the inguinal canal down to the lower edge of the scrotum and turn it to the sides.
2. The dartos is visible on the deep side of the skin. Incise the dartos and turn it to sides, and explore the scrotal septum in the deep side of the dartos toward the midline.
3. Isolate the spermatic cord with forceps from the superficial ring down to the upper end of the testis. Incise and isolate the external spermatic fascia, the cremaster, and the internal spermatic fascia layer by layer, from outside to inside. Inside the spermatic cord, separate and observe the vas deferens, testicular artery, and pampiniform plexus.
4. Incise longitudinally the parietal layer of tunica vaginalis, open the tunica vaginalis cavity, and explore the extent of the cavity with the knife handle.

12.2 Clinical Application of Key Anatomical Structures of the Perineum

The anatomy of the perineum, as the outlet of the pelvis and the supporting structure for the pelvic organs, varies much between men and women. This anatomical difference also gives rise to different clinical significance, and surgeries involving the perineum need to be performed according to the requirements set by different clinical departments. Therefore, this section is divided into two parts to introduce the female perineum and male perineum, respectively.

12.2.1 Clinical Application of Key Anatomical Structures of Female Perineum

During human evolution, the upright posture allows the human pelvis to change, distinguishing humans from the quadrupedal walking animals. These changes assist in the balance between the intra-abdominal pressure and the support of visceral structures. The downward pressure acts on the remodeled perineum and pelvic muscles. The pelvic floor is composed primarily of muscles and fascial structures that serve to close the abdominal-pelvic cavity, urethra, vagina, and rectum. Normal pelvic support comes from the interaction between the pelvic floor muscles and fascia. In most cases, the pelvic floor muscles and fascia provide a firm and elastic base for these organs. Adequate support of the perineum and pelvic floor is necessary to maintain the pelvic organs in their normal anatomical positions.

In females, the endopelvic fascia becomes the primary support structure when the pelvic floor muscles are damaged or decline in function due to pregnancy, childbirth, old age, or other injuries. Over time, the pressure of the pelvic organs counteracts the force of the endopelvic fascial attachments and eventually causes the pelvic organs to lose their normal anatomical position by fracturing, stretching, or weakening the support of the endopelvic fascia, thereby resulting in some common female clinical conditions, such as pelvic floor dysfunction and pelvic organ prolapse. The principle and purpose of pelvic floor repair surgery is to restore these organs to their proper position and repair the damaged supporting structures through surgery. The following is an example of surgical treatment of pelvic floor organ prolapse (anterior pelvis), a common pelvic floor disorder in women, to describe the clinical application of the key anatomical structures of the female perineum.

12.2.1.1 Determine the Perineal Skin Puncture Points

The first is the crosspoint at the level of the urethral orifice that intersects with the outer edges of the bilateral inferior ramus of pubis (thigh skin folds), that is, the internal edges of the medial margins of the obturator triangle on both sides; the second point is at 1 cm outer from both sides of the first puncture point and then 2 cm below the first puncture point (i.e., the internal edge of the obturator triangle) (Fig. 12.11).

12.2.1.2 Establish a Surgical Path

The procedure is performed through the transvaginal route, with the patient in the lithotomy position. Retract the cervix and pull it out of the external vaginal opening. Inject saline into the space between the anterior vaginal wall and the bladder for hemostasis and separation. Make a longitudinal incision 3 cm below the external orifice of urethra in the anterior vaginal wall at the top of the vagina, cut open the anterior vaginal wall, and preserve the pubocervical fascia. Separate along the vaginal and bladder space toward the pubic branch of the ischial spine on both sides, till reaching the ramus of ischium of the pubic bone and posteriorly close to the margin of the obturator foramen, and then continue to separate along the white line up to the level of the ischial spine, where the obturator foramen internus is palpable, and the pelvic fascial tendon arch is palpable between the pubic symphysis and the ischial spine. At this point, completely separate the bulging bladder from the vaginal wall.

12.2.1.3 Puncture and Place the Mesh

Insert the puncture needle vertically from the first puncture point; pass it through the obturator foramen at the pubic end of the pelvic fascia tendon arch from the retropubic bone, sequentially through the external obturator muscle, the obturator membrane, the obturator internus, and the pelvic endopelvic fascia around the bladder and the urethra; and finally go out at the vaginal incision. Connect the needle to the long arm of the upper edge of the mesh and carry the mesh out of the first puncture

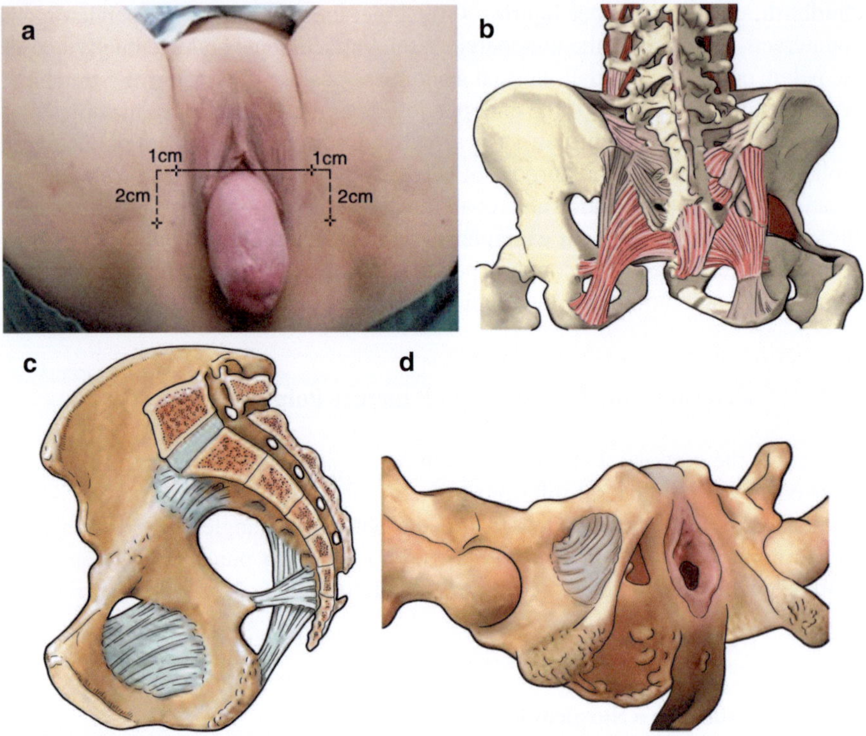

Fig. 12.11 Key anatomical structures of female perineum. (**a**) Location of perineal skin puncture point. (**b**) Schematic of ischial spine and sacrospinous ligament (posterior view). Intraoperative palpation of the ischial spine can help to determine the position of the sacrospinous ligament. (**c**) Schematic of obturator foramen. The puncture needle should be close to the sciatic end of the pubic bone as it passes through the obturator foramen to avoid the obturator canal (because the obturator vessels and nerves pass through here). (**d**) Schematic of obturator membrane. The puncture through the obturator membrane should be made close to the medial margin of the inferior ramus of pubis

point. Insert the needle vertically from the second puncture point and palpate the pelvic fascia tendon arch at the medial aspect of the ischial spine. Guide the needle through the pelvic fascia tendon arch, to the paravaginal space, and then finally out through the vaginal incision, where the needle is attached to the long arm of the lower edge of the mesh and brings the mesh out to the second puncture point. Place the mesh tension-free in the vesicovaginal space, underneath the bladder, to support the bulging bladder and urethra.

12.2.2 Clinical Application of Key Anatomical Structures of Male Perineum

Male urethral injury is the most common injury of the urinary system. Male urethra is divided into anterior and posterior parts by urogenital diaphragm, and the injury of posterior urethra (urethro-prostatic and urethral membrane parts) is mostly complicated by pelvic fracture, which is more serious and difficult to deal with, together with various sequelae. Anterior urethral injuries mainly manifest as bulbar urethral injuries caused by perineal straddle injuries, which are mild and easier to handle. Such injuries may contain contusion, laceration, or complete rupture. Urethral contusion may be only shown as edema and bleeding and can heal by itself. Urethral lacerations can cause periurethral hematomas and urinary extravasation, and after healing, scarring urethral strictures may arise. Complete urethral rupture causes regression and separation of the severed ends, with a large hematoma and urinary retention, which can lead to extravasation of urine during forced urination.

In bulbar urethral injuries, blood and urine leak into the superficial perineal pouch surrounded by the superficial perineal fascia, causing swelling of the perineum, scrotum, and penis, which sometimes extends upward to the abdominal wall. Urine does not extravasate into the femur on either side. When patients develop bulbar urethral scarring stricture secondary to perineal straddle injuries after conservative treatment, if urethrography confirms that the stenosis is within 2 cm in length, resection of scarring stenosis segment and end-to-end anastomosis should be performed; if the stenosis is more than 2 cm, it can be replaced by mucosal tissues (the most widely used mucosal tissues are lingual mucous membranes and buccal mucous membrane tissues). The following case is a 1.5 cm bulbar urethral stricture with proposed scar resection and end-to-end anastomosis, which illustrates the clinical application of the male perineum and anterior urethral anatomical structures.

12.2.2.1 Expose the Anterior Urethra

Make an inverted Y incision at the perineum to cut open the skin and subcutaneous tissues, expose the bulbospongiosus muscle, and isolate the urethral segment initially palpated scarred and stenotic in this plane (Fig. 12.12a).

12.2.2.2 Establish a Surgical Approach

Incise the bulbospongiosus muscle longitudinally, and separate the urethra bluntly from the bulbospongiosus muscle along the surface of the urethral corpus cavernosum to the sides and up and down. Free the scarred and stenotic segment of the urethra completely from the penile corpus cavernosum to the normal urethra

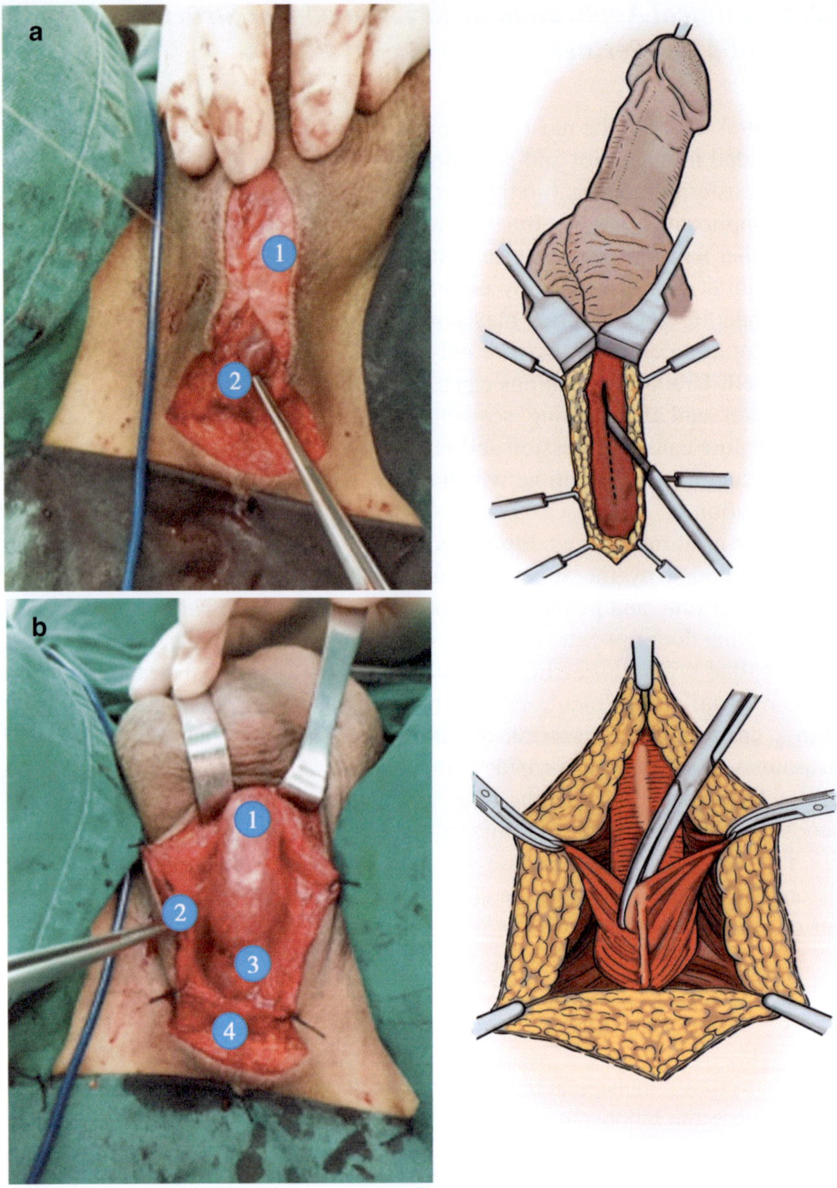

Fig. 12.12 Schematic of establishing surgical approach. (**a**) Superficial perineal fascia layer: bulbospongiosus muscle (1. superficial perineal fascia, i.e., Colles' fascia; 2. bulbospongiosus muscle). (**b**) Bulbospongiosus muscle is dissected to reveal urethral corpus cavernosum (1. urethral corpus cavernosum; 2. bulbospongiosus muscle; 3. bulbous urethra; 4. central tendon of the perineum). (**c**) Posterior aspect of penile corpus cavernosum is revealed, and the crus can be reached

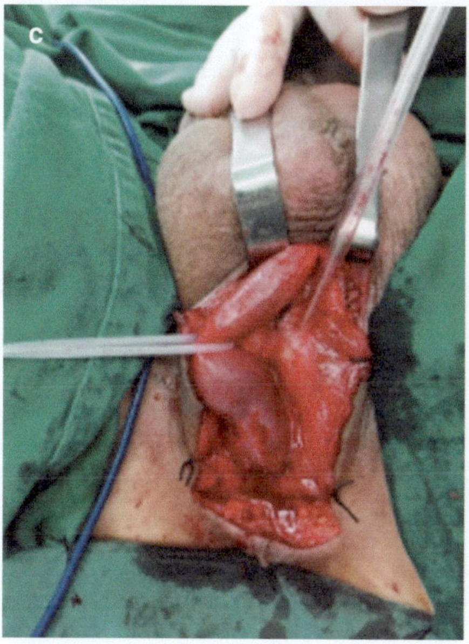

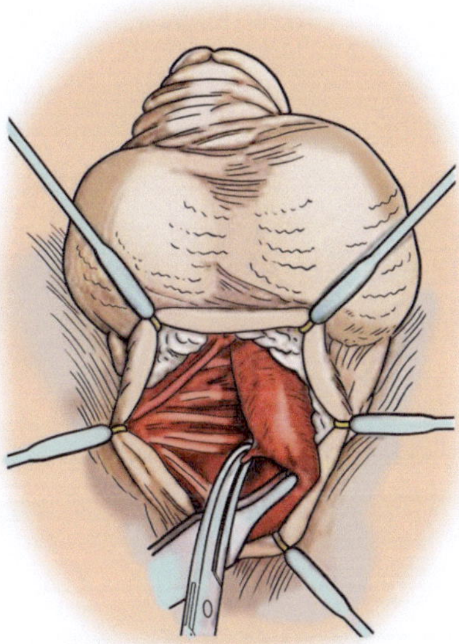

Fig. 12.12 (continued)

(Fig. 12.12b), and the crus of penis located on both sides of the corpus cavernosum are visible after freeing the ventral side of the urethral corpus cavernosum (Fig. 12.12c). Insert the metal urethral probe from the external urethral orifice to the distal end of the stricture, and transversely cut off the normal urethra, clamp the distal broken end of the urethra with tissue forceps to stop the hemorrhage, then cut off the proximal normal urethra, and finally completely resect the scarred and stenotic segment of the urethra. Use absorbable materials to anastomose the broken ends of the urethra with interrupted external sutures. Suture the bulbospongiosus muscle, superficial perineal fascia, and skin.